Primary Care DERMATOLOGY

Primary Care DERMATOLOGY

KENNETH A. ARNDT, M.D.
Dermatologist-in-Chief
Beth Israel Deaconess Medical Center
Professor of Dermatology
Harvard Medical School
Boston, Massachusetts

BRUCE U. WINTROUB, M.D.
Executive Vice Dean
Professor of Dermatology
Department of Dermatology
University of California, San Francisco,
School of Medicine
San Francisco, California

JUNE K. ROBINSON, M.D.
Professor of Dermatology and Surgery
Departments of Dermatology and Surgery
Northwestern University Medical School
Chicago, Illinois

PHILIP E. LEBOIT, M.D.
Associate Professor of Pathology and Dermatology
University of California, San Francisco,
School of Medicine
San Francisco, California

W.B. SAUNDERS COMPANY
A Division of Harcourt Brace & Company
Philadelphia London Toronto Montreal Sydney Tokyo

W.B. SAUNDERS COMPANY
A Division of Harcourt Brace & Company

The Curtis Center
Independence Square West
Philadelphia, Pennsylvania 19106

Library of Congress Cataloging-in-Publication Data

Primary care dermatology/[edited by] Kenneth A. Arndt . . . [et al.].—1st ed.

p. cm.

ISBN 0–7216–6096–7

1. Skin—Diseases. 2. Primary care (Medicine). 3. Dermatology.
I. Arndt, Kenneth A. [DNLM: 1. Skin Diseases—therapy. 2. Skin Diseases—diagnosis. WR 140 D435134 1997]

RL71.D458 1997 616.5—dc20

DNLM/DLC 96–44227

PRIMARY CARE DERMATOLOGY ISBN 0–7216–6096–7

Printed in the United States of America.

Last digit is the print number: 9 8 7 6 5 4 3 2 1

To Our Families

CONTRIBUTORS

Samar Alaiti, M.D.
Resident, Department of Dermatology, University of Illinois at Chicago, Chicago, Illinois
Alopecia Areata

Philip C. Anderson, M.D., A.B.
Professor, Dermatology and Medicine; Chairman, Dermatology Department, University of Missouri Medical Center and Medical School, Columbia, Missouri
Toxic Spider Bites

Richard J. Antaya, M.D.
Resident in Dermatology, Duke University School of Medicine, Durham, North Carolina
Viral Rashes (Those With Consequences and Those Without)

Jack L. Arbiser, M.D., Ph.D.
Instructor in Dermatology, Harvard Medical School; Howard Hughes Medical Institute, Children's Hospital, Boston, Massachusetts
Lichen Simplex Chronicus (Neurodermatitis)

Kenneth A. Arndt, M.D.
Dermatologist-in-Chief, Beth Israel Deaconess Medical Center; Professor of Dermatology, Harvard Medical School, Boston, Massachusetts
Important Considerations for Topical Corticosteroid Therapy

Timothy G. Berger, M.D.
Associate Clinical Professor, Department of Dermatology, University of California, San Francisco, School of Medicine, San Francisco, California
Varicella; Herpes Simplex; Zoster

Jeffrey D. Bernhard, M.D.
Professor of Medicine and Director, Division of Dermatology, University of Massachusetts Medical School, Worcester, Massachusetts
Itch

Patricia F. Bilden, M.D.
Resident in Dermatology, University of Massachusetts Medical Center, Worcester, Massachusetts
Itch

John Q. Binhlam, M.D.
Senior Resident, Division of Dermatology, Department of Medicine, Vanderbilt University School of Medicine, Nashville, Tennessee
Erythroderma

Kathryn E. Bowers, M.D.
Instructor in Dermatology, Harvard Medical School; Associate Dermatologist, Beth Israel Deaconess Medical Center, Boston, Massachusetts
Anogenital Pruritus

K. Robin Carder, M.D.
Clinical Research Fellow in Dermatology, Massachusetts General Hospital, Harvard Medical School, Boston, Massachusetts
Tinea (Pityriasis) Versicolor

Geetinder Kaus Chattha, M.D.
Clinical Instructor, Department of Dermatology, University of California, San Francisco, School of Medicine, San Francisco, California
Abscess; Cellulitis

Lisa M. Cohen, M.D.
Department of Dermatology, Children's Hospital; Department of Pathology, Beth Israel Deaconess Medical Center; Instructor in Dermatology and Pathology, Harvard Medical School, Boston; Associate Pathologist, Pathology Services, Inc., Cambridge, Massachusetts
Pregnancy Rashes

Thomas G. Cropley, M.D.
Assistant Professor, Division of Dermatology, Department of Medicine, University of Massachusetts Medical School, Worcester, Massachusetts
Seborrheic Dermatitis

Ponciano D. Cruz, Jr., M.D.
Associate Professor and Director of Residency Training Program, University of Texas Southwestern Medical Center, Dallas, Texas
Contact Dermatitis

Zoe Diana Draelos, M.D.
Clinical Assistant Professor, Department of Dermatology, Bowman Gray School of Medicine of Wake Forest University, Winston-Salem; Central Carolina Dermatology Clinic, High Point, North Carolina
Skin Care Maintenance

Daniel B. Dubin, M.D.
Instructor in Dermatology, Harvard Medical School; Associate Physician, Brigham and Women's Hospital, Boston, Massachusetts
Important Considerations for Topical Corticosteroid Therapy; Inflamed Epidermal Cysts

Daniella Duke, M.D., M.P.H.
Laser Fellow, Massachusetts General Hospital, Harvard Medical School, Boston, Massachusetts
Pityriasis Rosea

Lawrence F. Eichenfield, M.D.
Assistant Professor of Pediatrics and Medicine (Dermatology) and Chief, Division of Pediatric Dermatology, University of California, San Diego, School of Medicine; Chief, Pediatric Dermatology and Laser Surgery, Children's Hospital and Health Center, San Diego, California
Impetigo

Virginia C. Fiedler, M.D.
Professor and Interim Head, Department of Dermatology, University of Illinois College of Medicine, Chicago, Illinois
Alopecia Areata

Ilona J. Frieden, M.D.
Associate Clinical Professor, Dermatology and Pediatrics, University of California, San Francisco, School of Medicine, San Francisco, California
Diaper Dermatitis

Sheila Fallon Friedlander, M.D.
Assistant Clinical Professor, University of California, San Diego, School of Medicine; Staff, Children's Hospital and Health Center, San Diego, California
Impetigo

Michelle M. Goller, M.D.
Resident, Department of Dermatology, University of Texas Medical School at Houston, Houston, Texas
Molluscum Contagiosum

Jane M. Grant-Kels, M.D.
Professor and Chief, Division of Dermatology, Director of Dermatopathology, University of Connecticut School of Medicine, Farmington, Connecticut
Atopic Dermatitis

Suzanne Grevelink, M.D.
Clinical Assistant in Medicine, Children's Hospital Medical Center; Instructor, Department of Dermatology, Harvard Medical School, Boston, Massachusetts
Hidradenitis Suppurativa; Warts

Pearl E. Grimes, M.D.
Clinical Associate Professor, Division of Dermatology, University of California at Los Angeles School of Medicine; Director, Vitiligo and Pigmentation Center of Southern California, Los Angeles, California
Melasma; Vitiligo

Arnold W. Gurevitch, M.D.
Professor and Chief, Division of Dermatology, University of Southern California School of Medicine, Los Angeles, California
Nummular Dermatitis

Adelaide A. Hebert, M.D.
Associate Professor of Dermatology, Pediatrics, Pediatric Dentistry, University of Texas Medical School at Houston, Houston, Texas
Molluscum Contagiosum

Maria K. Hordinsky, M.D.
Associate Professor, Department of Dermatology, University of Minnesota Medical School—Minneapolis, Minneapolis, Minnesota
Balding and Hair Loss

Larisa C. Kelley, M.D.
Department of Dermatology, Beth Israel Deaconess Medical Center; Instructor, Harvard Medical School, Boston, Massachusetts
Stasis Dermatitis

A. Paul Kelly, M.D.
Professor of Medicine (Dermatology), Charles R. Drew University of Medicine and Science; Clinical Professor of Medicine (Dermatology), University of California, Los Angeles, School of Medicine; Chief, Division of Dermatology, Department of Internal Medicine, King-Drew Medical Center, Los Angeles, California
Folliculitis; Pseudofolliculitis

Lloyd E. King, Jr., M.D.
Chief, Division of Dermatology, Department of Medicine, Vanderbilt University School of Medicine, Nashville, Tennessee
Erythroderma

Neil J. Korman, Ph.D., M.D.
Assistant Professor, Department of Dermatology, Case Western Reserve University School of Medicine, Cleveland, Ohio
Bullous Pemphigoid and Other Immunologically Mediated Blistering Diseases

Andrew Paul Lazar, M.D., M.P.H.
Associate Professor of Clinical Dermatology, Northwestern University Medical School, Chicago, Illinois
Hand and Foot Dermatitis

Agnes M. Lynch, B.S.
Study Coordinator, Dermatology Clinical Investigations Unit, Massachusetts General Hospital, Harvard Medical School, Boston, Massachusetts
Candidiasis

Steven M. Manders, M.D.
Assistant Professor of Clinical Medicine, Division of Dermatology, Department of Medicine, University of Medicine and Dentistry of New Jersey, Robert Wood Johnson Medical School at Camden, Camden, New Jersey; Clinical Associate, Department of Dermatology, University of Pennsylvania, Philadelphia, Pennsylvania
Perioral Dermatitis

Toby A. Maurer, M.D.
Assistant Clinical Professor, Department of Dermatology, University of California, San Francisco, School of Medicine, San Francisco, California
Varicella; Herpes Simplex; Zoster

Theodora Mauro, M.D.
Assistant Professor in Residence, Department of Dermatology, University of California, San Francisco, School of Medicine; Assistant Service Chief, Dermatology Service, San Francisco Veterans Hospital, San Francisco, California
Leg Ulcers

S. Teri McGillis, M.D.
Staff Physician, Department of Dermatology, Section of Mohs Micrographic Surgery and Cutaneous Surgery, Cleveland Clinic Foundation, Cleveland, Ohio
Common Skin Cancers (Basal Cell and Squamous Cell)

John W. Melski, M.D.
Clinical Associate Professor of Dermatology, University of Wisconsin School of Medicine, Madison; Dermatologist, Department of Medical and Surgical Dermatology, Marshfield Clinic, Marshfield, Wisconsin
Lyme Borreliosis

Clark C. Otley, M.D.
Assistant Professor of Dermatology, Mayo Medical School; Senior Associate Consultant, Mayo Clinic, Rochester, Minnesota
Actinic Keratosis; Seborrheic Keratosis

Julie S. Prendiville, M.B., M.R.C.P.I., F.R.C.P.(C.)
Clinical Associate Professor in Pediatrics, University of British Columbia; Head, Division of Pediatric Dermatology, British Columbia's Children's Hospital, Vancouver, British Columbia, Canada
Erysipelas

Neil S. Prose, M.D.
Associate Professor of Medicine (Dermatology), and Pediatrics, Duke University School of Medicine, Durham, North Carolina
Viral Rashes (Those With Consequences and Those Without)

James E. Rasmussen, M.D.
Professor of Dermatology, Department of Dermatology, University of Michigan Medical School; Professor of Dermatology, Ann Arbor Veterans Administration Medical Center, Ann Arbor, Michigan
Lice; Scabies

Jason K. Rivers, B.Sc., M.D., F.R.C.P.(C.)
Associate Professor, University of British Columbia; Active Staff, British Columbia Cancer Agency, Vancouver, British Columbia, Canada
Moles and Melanoma

June K. Robinson, M.D.
Professor of Dermatology and Surgery, Departments of Dermatology and Surgery, Northwestern University Medical School, Chicago, Illinois
Biopsy (Punch, Shave, Saucerization, and Elliptical); Destructive Methods

Marti Jill Rothe, M.D.
Associate Professor of Medicine, Division of Dermatology, University of Connecticut School of Medicine, Farmington, Connecticut
Atopic Dermatitis

Neil S. Sadick, M.D., F.A.C.P.
Clinical Associate Professor, Cornell University Medical College; Assistant Attending Physician, The New York Hospital, New York, New York
Human Immunodeficiency Virus–Related Cutaneous Disease

Christopher R. Shea, M.D.
Associate Professor of Pathology and Medicine, Duke University School of Medicine; Attending Pathologist and Director of Dermatopathology, Duke University Medical Center, Durham, North Carolina
How Do You Care for Normal Skin?

Debra Karp Skopicki, M.D.
Harvard Medical School, Boston; Pathology Services, Inc., Cambridge, Massachusetts
Rocky Mountain Spotted Fever

Shondra L. Smith, B.A., M.P.H., M.D.
Dermatology Resident, Dermatology Division, Department of Internal Medicine, University of Kansas Medical Center, Kansas City, Kansas
Fungal Infections

Nicholas A. Soter, M.D.
Professor of Dermatology, New York University School of Medicine; Medical Director, Charles C. Harris Skin and Cancer Pavilion; Attending Physician, Tisch Hospital—The University Hospital of New York University, New York, New York
Vasculitis

Robert S. Stern, M.D.
Associate Professor of Dermatology, Harvard Medical School; Dermatologist, Beth Israel Deaconess Medical Center, Boston, Massachusetts
Cutaneous Drug Reactions; Psoriasis; Toxic Epidermal Necrolysis and Stevens-Johnson Syndrome

Matthew J. Stiller, M.D.
Assistant Professor of Dermatology, Harvard Medical School; Chief, Dermatology Clinical Investigations Unit, Massachusetts General Hospital, Boston, Massachusetts
Candidiasis; Fungal Infections; Tinea (Pityriasis) Versicolor

Charles R. Taylor, M.D.
Instructor in Dermatology, Harvard Medical School; Assistant Dermatologist, Director of Phototherapy, Massachusetts General Hospital, Boston, Massachusetts
Sunburn

Michael D. Tharp, M.D.
Professor and Chairman, Department of Dermatology, Rush-Presbyterian–St. Luke's Medical Center, Chicago, Illinois
Urticaria

Diane M. Thiboutot, M.D.
Assistant Professor of Medicine, Division of Dermatology, Pennsylvania State University College of Medicine, Hershey, Pennsylvania
Acne; Rosacea

Marcia G. Tonnesen, M.D.
Associate Professor of Dermatology and Medicine, State University of New York at Stony Brook School of Medicine, Stony Brook; Chief, Dermatology, Veterans Affairs Medical Center, Northport, New York
Erythema Multiforme

Hensin Tsao, M.D., Ph.D.
Resident in Dermatology, Harvard Medical School, Boston, Massachusetts
Hand and Foot Dermatitis; Raynaud's Disease/Phenomenon

Bruce U. Wintroub, M.D.
Executive Vice Dean and Professor of Dermatology, Department of Dermatology, University of California, San Francisco, School of Medicine, San Francisco, California
Seborrheic Dermatitis

PREFACE

PRIMARY CARE DERMATOLOGY is written to assist primary care physicians and other health care providers as they care for patients with skin disorders and other common cutaneous problems. Care delivered to patients with skin disease has long rested to a large extent in the hands of internists, general practitioners, family physicians, and other primary care providers. As the landscape of medicine has changed, even more of the care of patients with cutaneous disease will rest initially, if not entirely, with primary care physicians and nurse practitioners. This book will help these clinicians diagnose and understand skin disease, explain how it comes about, and give their patients practical, straightforward, and detailed instructions on how to care for skin problems.

PRIMARY CARE DERMATOLOGY is organized in a fashion that should be of great use to clinicians. Major subjects include: (1) What are the important considerations for treatment of the skin? (2) What are the common dermatologic disorders and how they are treated? (3) Dermatologic emergencies and critical problems. (4) Procedures. The most common skin diseases and those disorders that are most important to patients seen by primary care physicians are included in this book. More esoteric topics seen primarily by specialists are not discussed. Each chapter begins with a definition and description of clinical findings followed by a description of the disease, detailed discussion of treatment, and a unique feature entitled "Pitfalls and Problems" that points out difficulties primary care clinicians may encounter. "Referral/Consultation Guidelines" are provided to guide primary care clinicians as the value of referral for specialty care is considered. Each chapter contains a few selected references and high-quality color pictures illustrating each disorder in order to allow greater accuracy in diagnosing skin conditions. The last section of the book describes common procedures that most primary care physicians may carry out in the office. These include biopsies, cryosurgery, electrosurgery, and other simple surgical procedures. Each procedure is illustrated with line drawings clearly showing the best techniques available.

This is the first dermatology text that has been written for primary care health care providers. Other dermatology books and atlases have been written for medical students and residents, but none has been conceptualized from inception to be especially useful to primary care physicians. We hope that PRIMARY CARE DERMATOLOGY's clear and practical information will be of value to clinicians as they care for the skin and its disorders and to patients as they receive care in our changing health care system.

KENNETH A. ARNDT
BRUCE U. WINTROUB
JUNE K. ROBINSON
PHILIP E. LEBOIT

CONTENTS

SECTION III

Dermatologic Emergencies and Critical Problems

SECTION IV

Procedures

NOTICE

Dermatology is an ever-changing field. Standard safety precautions must be followed, but as new research and clinical experience broaden our knowledge, changes in treatment and drug therapy become necessary or appropriate. Readers are advised to check the product information currently provided by the manufacturer of each drug to be administered to verify the recommended dose, the method and duration of administration, and contraindications. It is the responsibility of the treating physician relying on experience and knowledge of the patient to determine dosages and the best treatment for the patient. Neither the publisher nor the editor assumes any responsibility for any injury and/or damage to persons or property.

THE PUBLISHER

PLATE 1

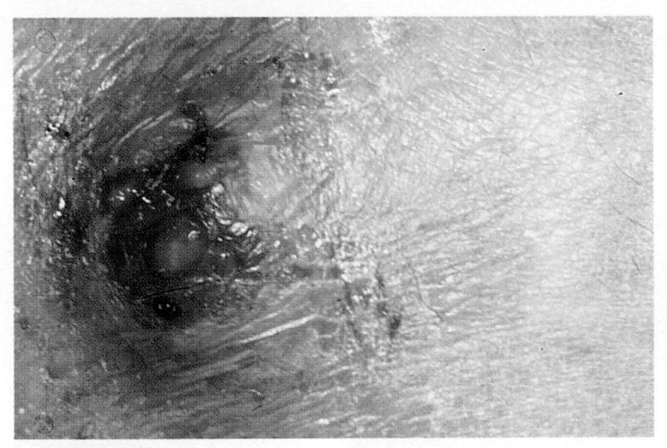

FIGURE 5–1

Carbuncle with multiple draining sites on the surface.

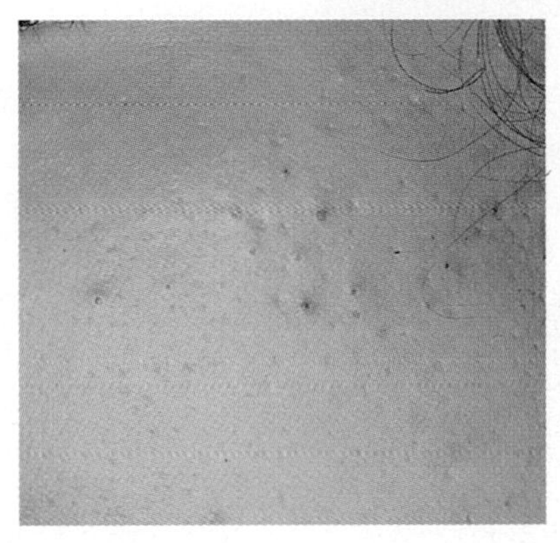

FIGURE 6–1

Open and closed comedones. The noninflammatory lesions are the first manifestation of acne vulgaris.

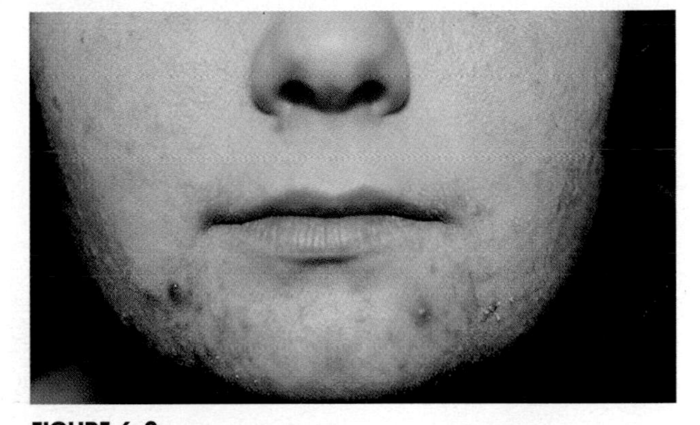

FIGURE 6–2

Inflammatory lesions such as papules and pustules are often found on the chin of adult females with acne.

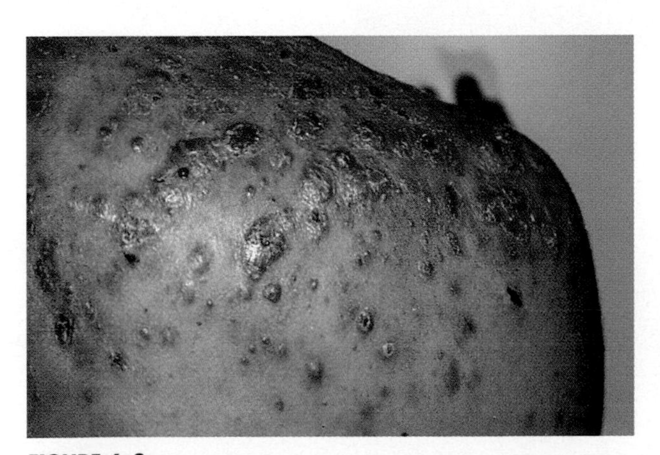

FIGURE 6–3

Cystic acne affects the face, chest, and back. Lesions on the back are most resistant to treatment and can result in extensive scarring.

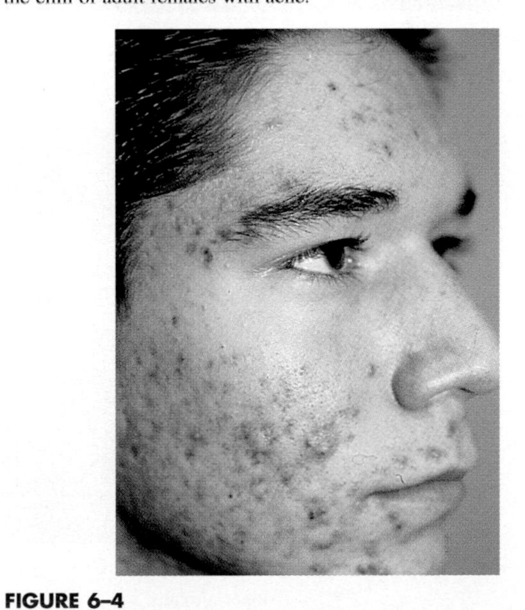

FIGURE 6–4

Hyperpigmented macules (postinflammatory lesions) can appear red to brown. It may take 6 to 12 months for these to resolve. Acne scarring is characterized by pits or depressions in the surface of the skin following resolution of cystic or inflammatory lesions.

PLATE 2

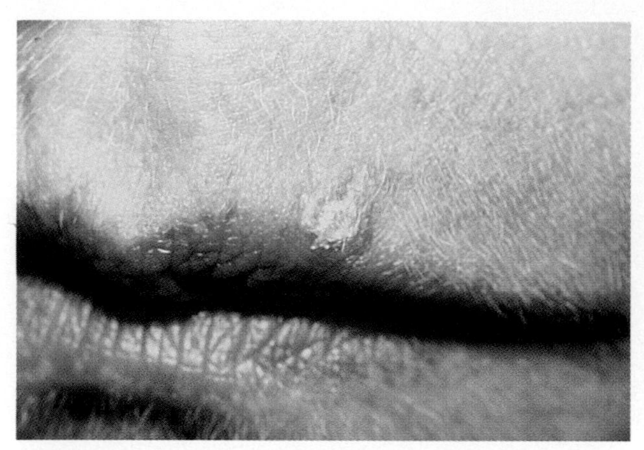

FIGURE 7–1

Typical isolated actinic keratosis with white adherent scale. (Courtesy of Richard A. Johnson, M.D.)

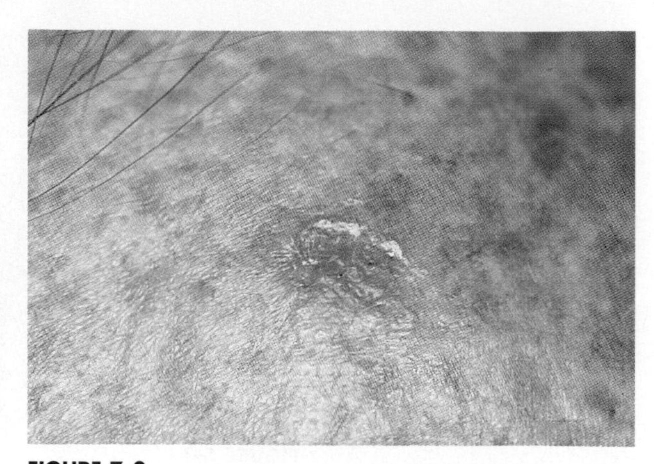

FIGURE 7–2

Erythematous, macular actinic keratosis. (Courtesy of Richard A. Johnson, M.D.)

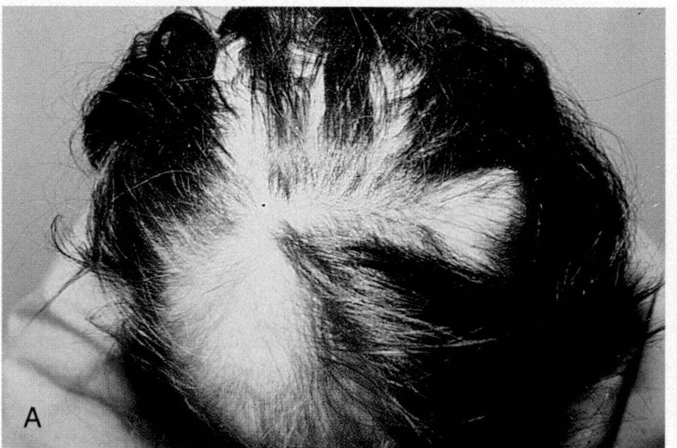

B

FIGURE 8–1

A and *B,* Patchy alopecia areata.

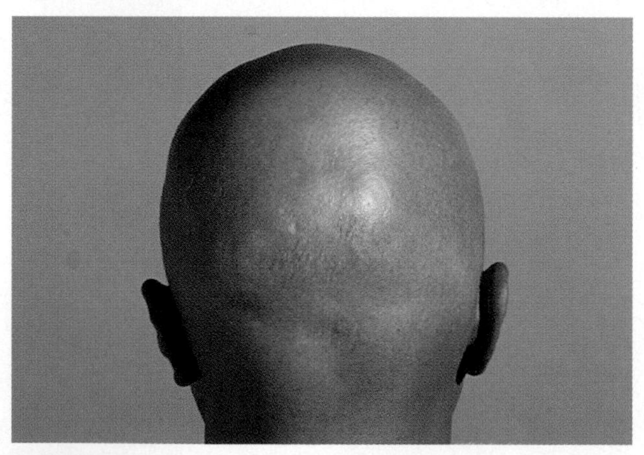

FIGURE 8–2

Alopecia totalis.

PLATE 3

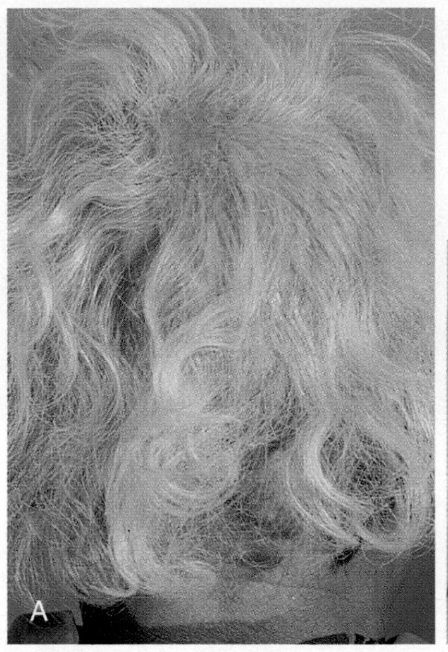

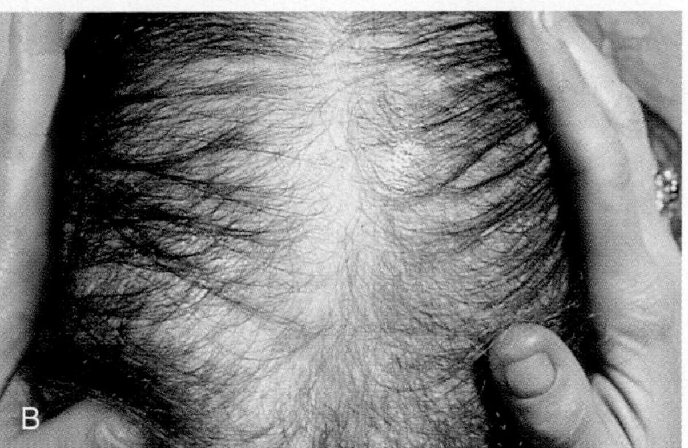

FIGURE 8–3
A and *B,* Diffuse alopecia areata.

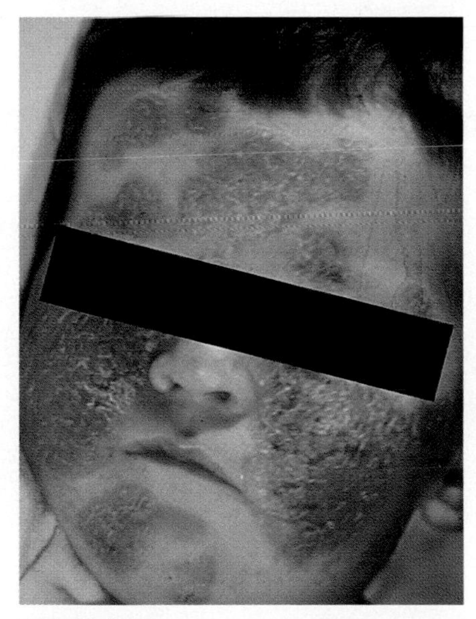

FIGURE 10–1
Facial plaques of acute infantile atopic dermatitis.

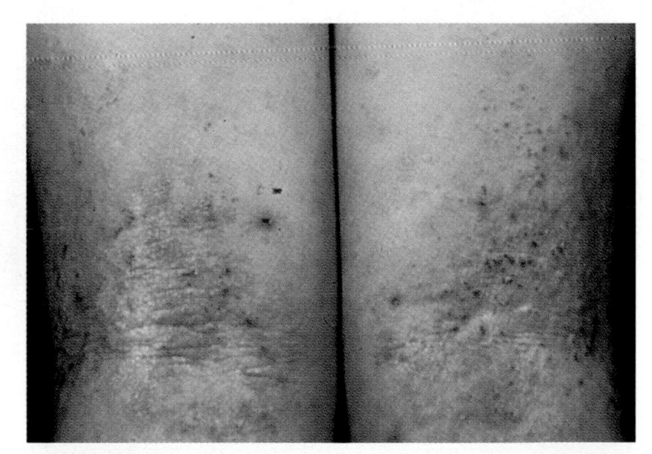

FIGURE 10–2
Excoriated flexural plaques of chronic adult atopic dermatitis.

PLATE 4

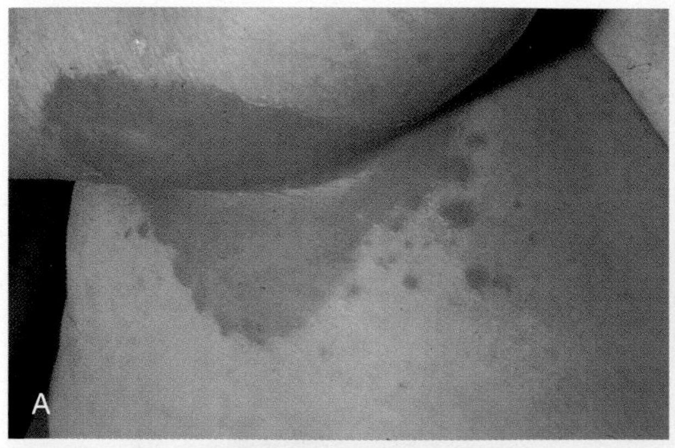

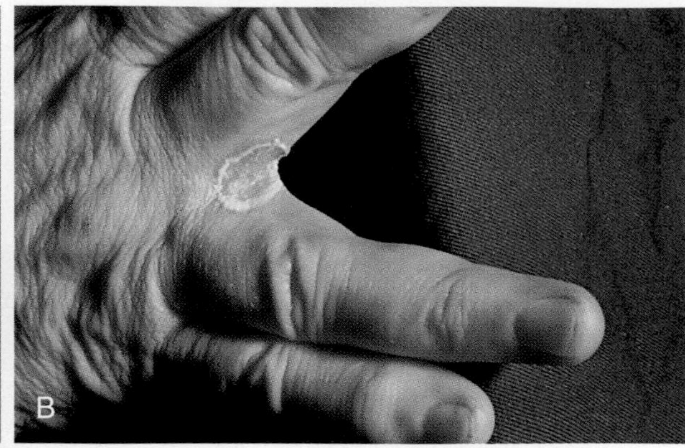

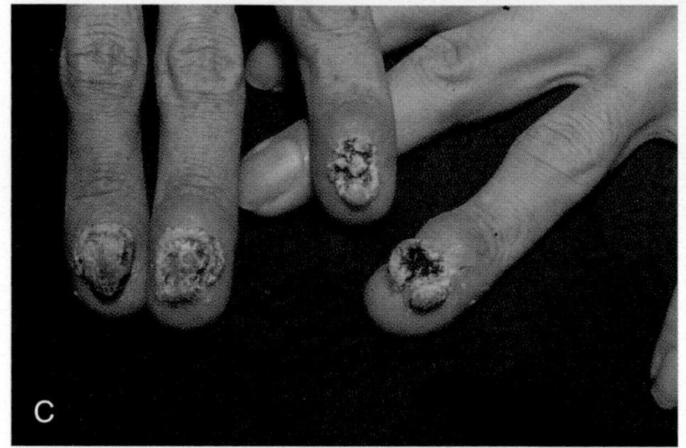

FIGURE 12–1

A, Submammary *Candida* intertrigo. The well-demarcated annular border and satellite lesions are important clinical features. *B,* Interdigital candidiasis (erosio interdigitalis blastomycetica) most commonly occurs between the middle digit and the ring finger in individuals whose hands are chronically exposed to water, e.g., bartenders, waiters, and dishwashers. *C,* Severely dystrophic fingernails in a patient with chronic mucocutaneous candidiasis.

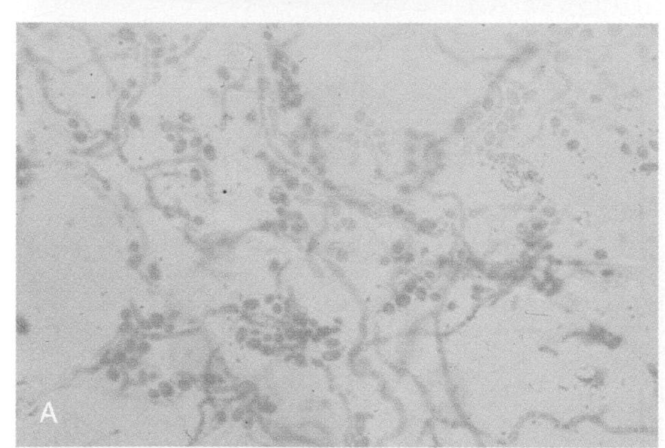

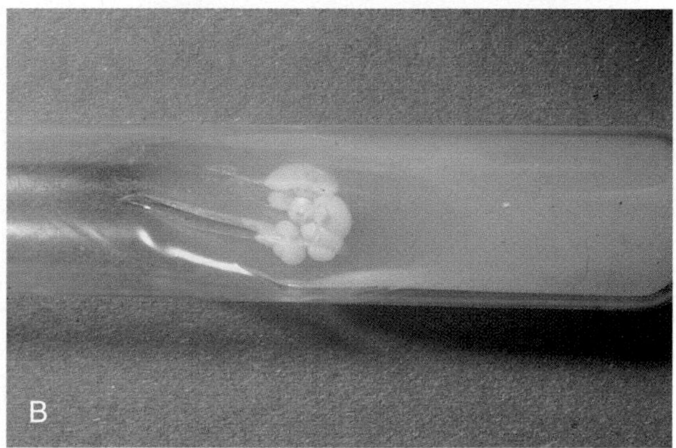

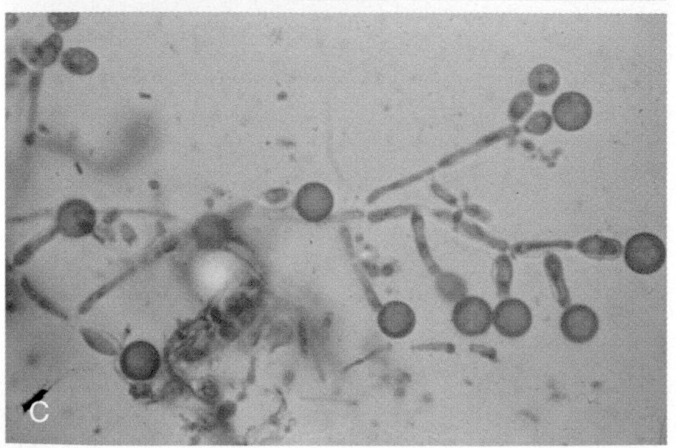

FIGURE 12–2

A, A potassium hydroxide wet mount preparation from the nail fold of a patient with paronychia, showing a characteristic combination of yeast and mycelial-phase organisms. *B,* A culture tube showing *Candida albicans* growing on Sabouraud dextrose agar. *C,* Of all species of *Candida, C. albicans* is the most pathogenic in humans. Formation of chlamydoconida, as seen here after inoculation on corn meal agar with Tween 80, is one of the most useful laboratory tests for speciation of *C. albicans.*

PLATE 5

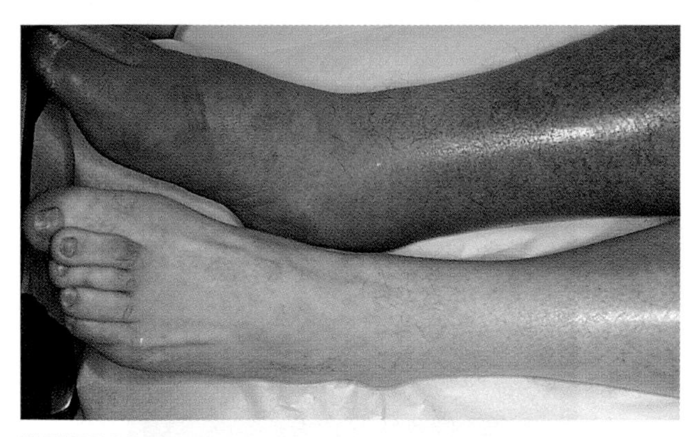

FIGURE 13–1

Lower leg cellulitis. (Courtesy of Raza Aly, M.D.)

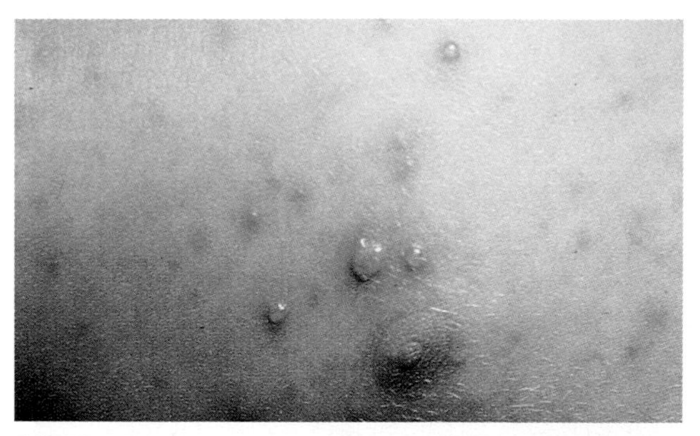

FIGURE 14–1

Varicella.

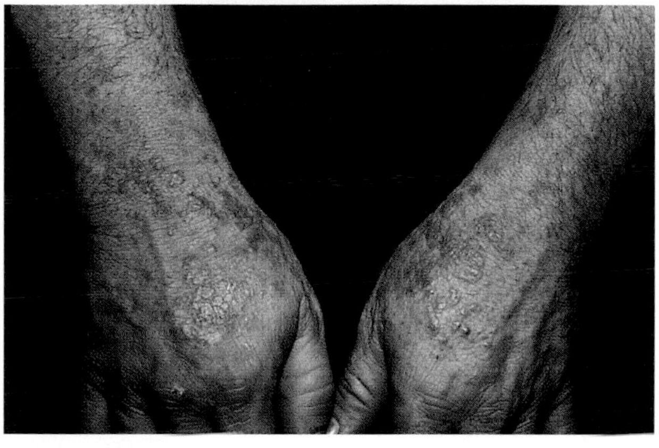

FIGURE 16–1

Contact dermatitis can begin as small red papules and plaques. This patient's condition was due to epoxy resin hypersensitivity. (From Callen JP, Greer KE, Hood AF, et al: Color Atlas of Dermatology. Philadelphia: WB Saunders, 1993, p 74.)

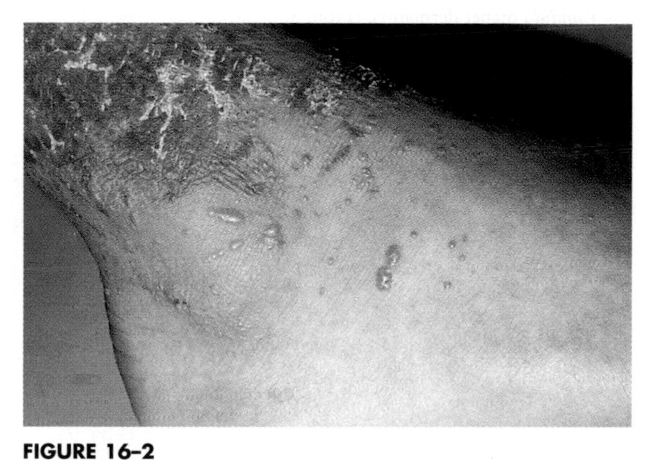

FIGURE 16–2

Contact dermatitis. (From Callen JP, Greer KE, Hood AF, et al: Color Atlas of Dermatology. Philadelphia: WB Saunders, 1993, p 273.)

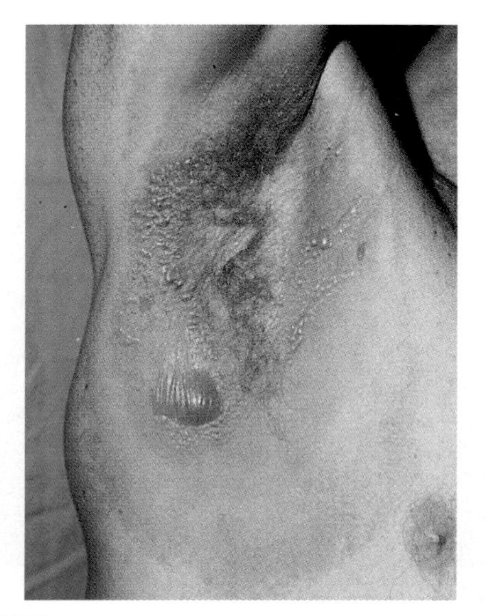

FIGURE 16–3

Contact dermatitis. (From Callen JP, Greer KE, Hood AF, et al: Color Atlas of Dermatology. Philadelphia: WB Saunders, 1993, p 322.)

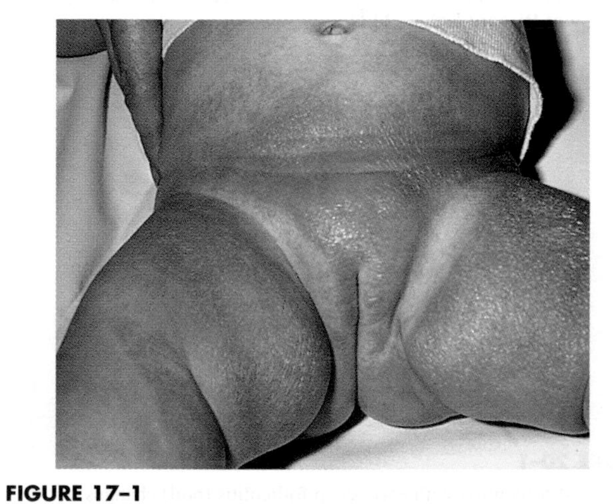

FIGURE 17–1

Severe irritant diaper dermatitis. Note the sparing of the inguinal folds.

PLATE 8

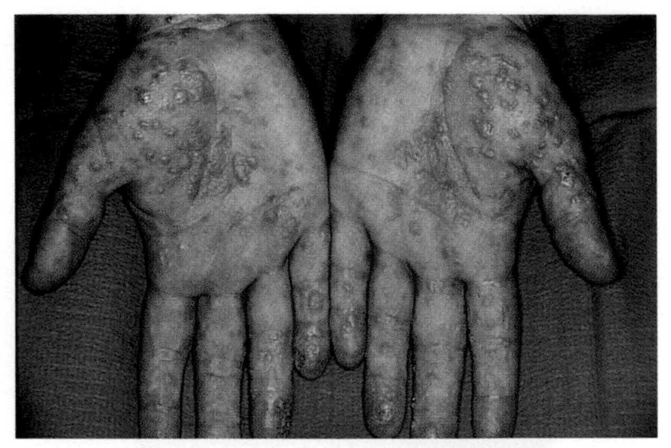

FIGURE 23–1
Dyshidrotic eczema. (Courtesy of Fernando Botero, M.D.)

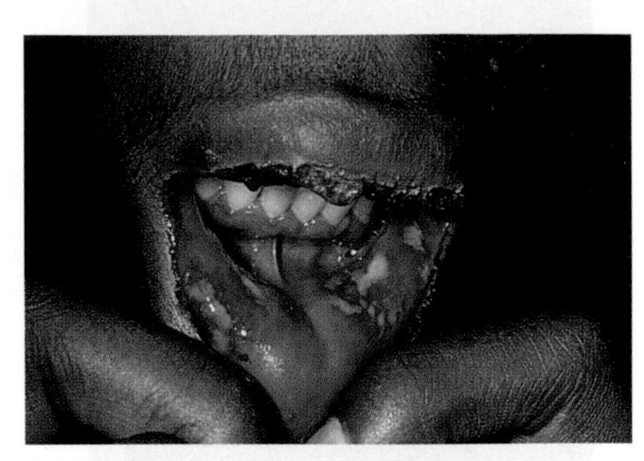

FIGURE 24–1
Orolabial herpes simplex.

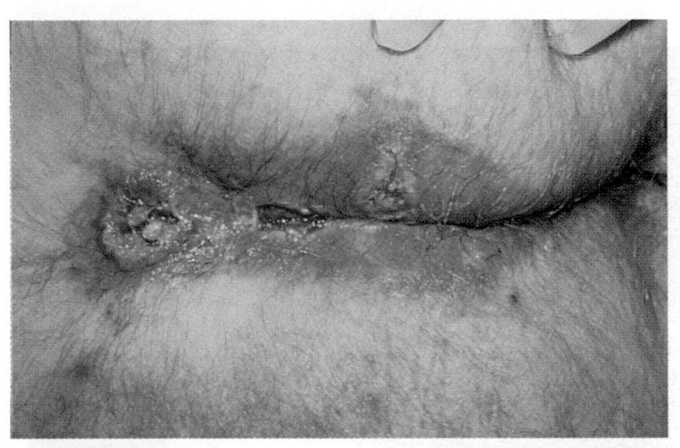

FIGURE 24–2
Perirectal herpes simplex.

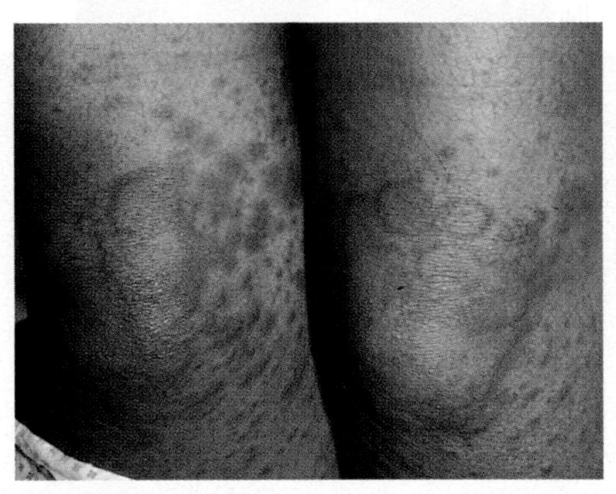

FIGURE 24–3
Erythema multiforme secondary to herpes simplex.

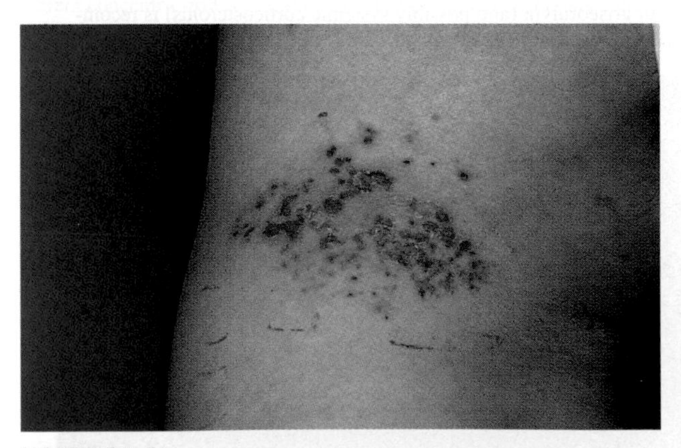

FIGURE 25–1
Grouped blisters on an erythematous base, consistent with herpes zoster.

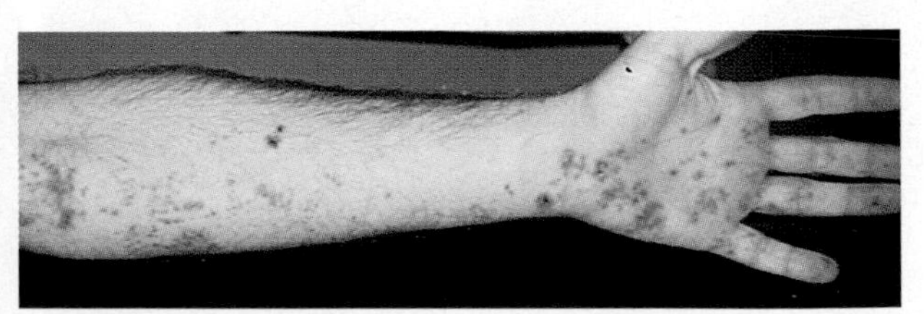

FIGURE 25–2
Grouped blisters—dermatomal distribution consistent with herpes zoster.

PLATE 9

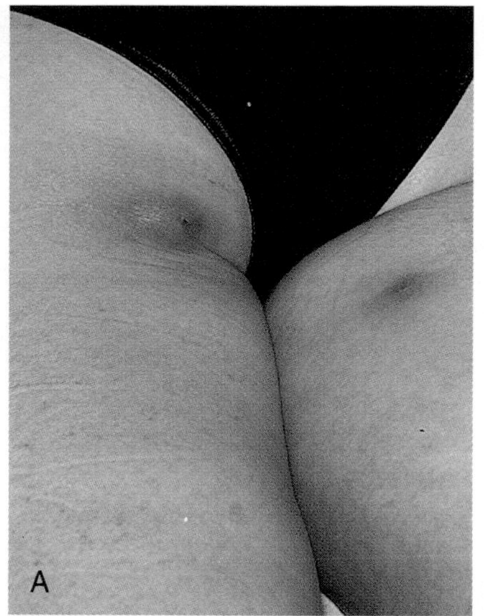

FIGURE 26–1
A and *B,* Hidradenitis of the buttock.

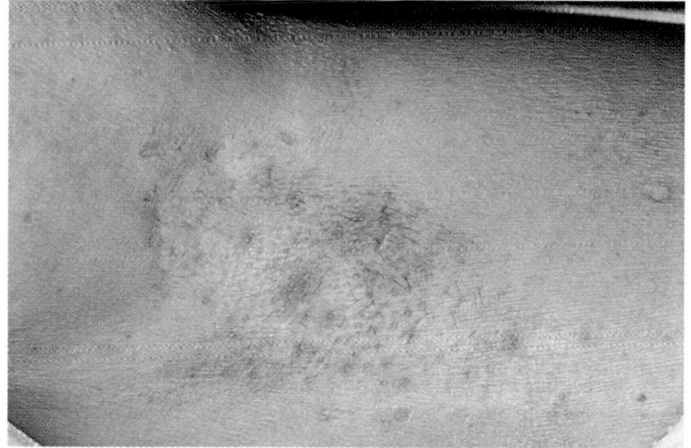

FIGURE 26–2
Hidradenitis of the axilla.

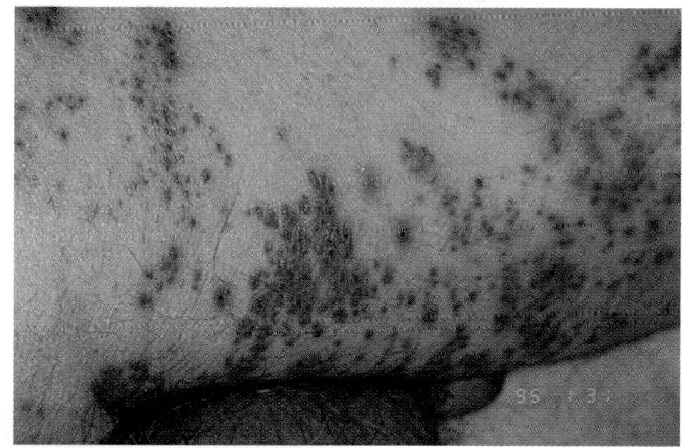

FIGURE 27–1
Herpes zoster. Crusted dermatomal lesions.

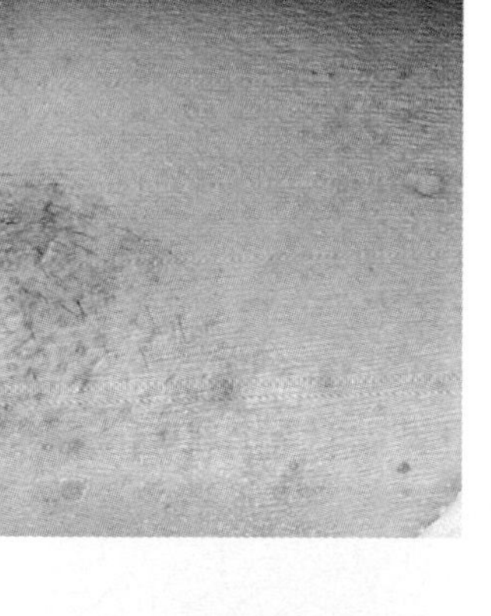

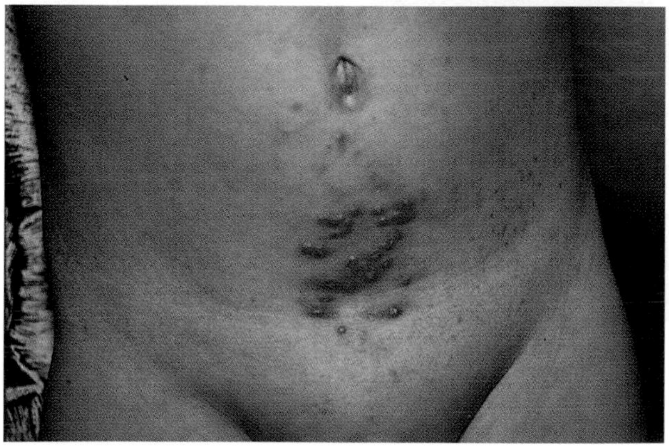

FIGURE 27–2
Molluscum contagiosum. Erythematous umbilicated papules.

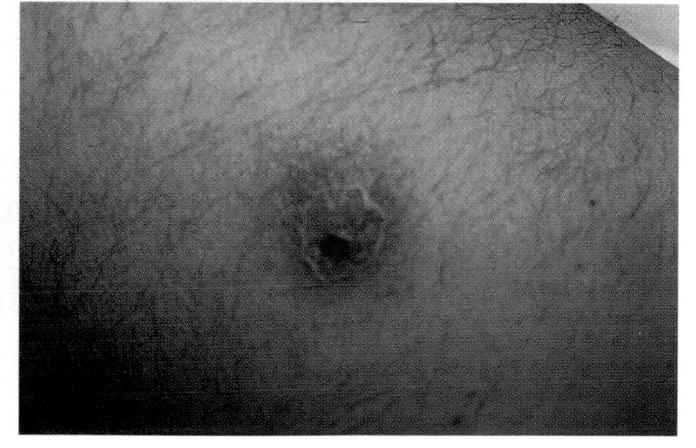

FIGURE 27–3
Mycobacterium avium-intracellulare. Necrotic ulcer.

PLATE 14

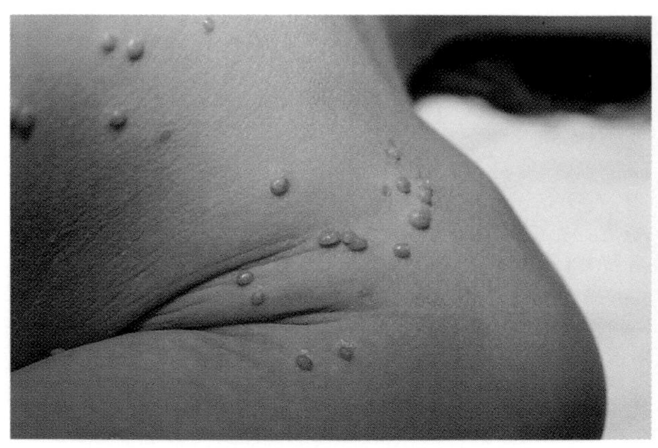

FIGURE 35–1
Multiple molluscum on the upper trunk of a child.

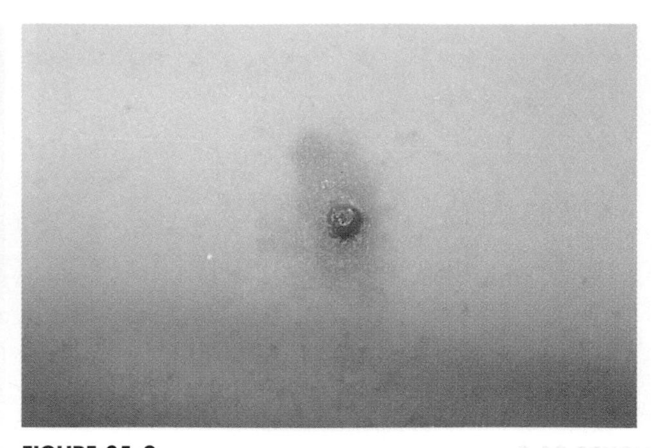

FIGURE 35–2
A single molluscum lesion that is inflamed owing to trauma.

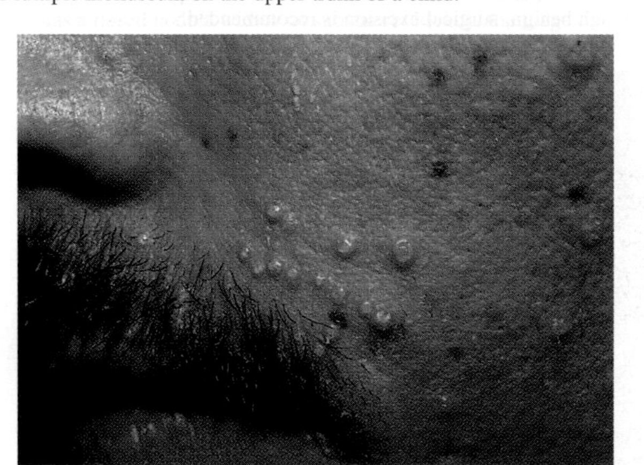

FIGURE 35–3
Large molluscum contagiosum on the face of patient who is positive for the human immunodeficiency virus.

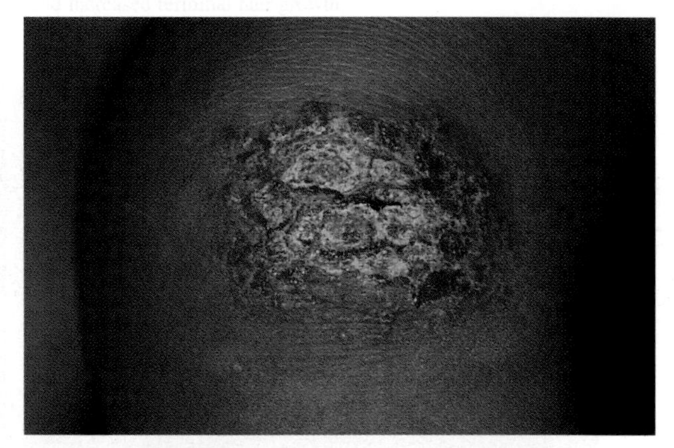

FIGURE 36–1
Exudative and crusted eruption of nummular dermatitis.

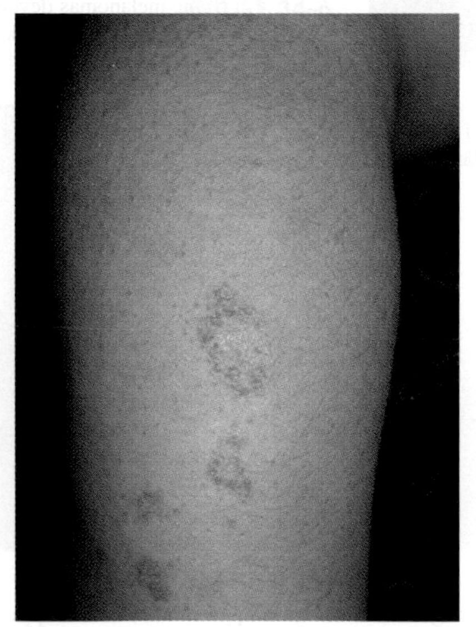

FIGURE 36–2
Dry, scaling patches of nummular dermatitis.

PLATE 15

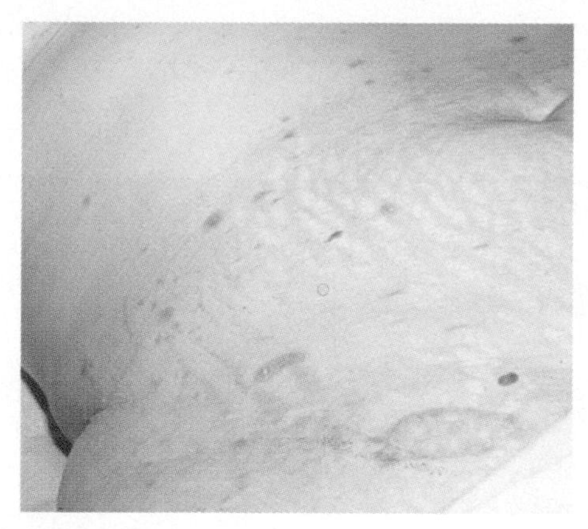

FIGURE 38–1

Herald patch and secondary lesions of pityriasis rosea.

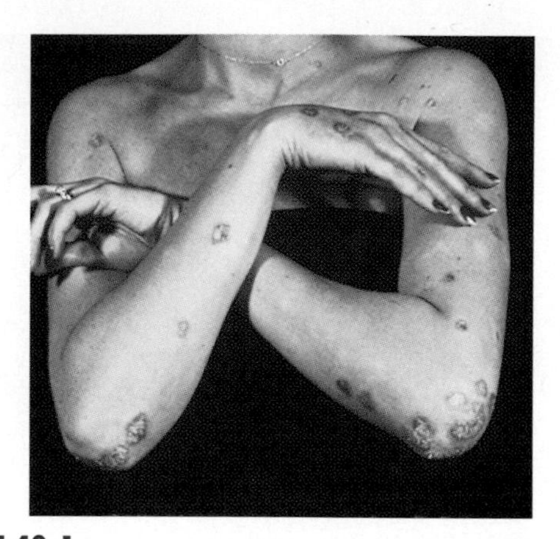

FIGURE 40–1

Small-plaque psoriasis. These sharply demarcated lesions are erythematous and only moderately scaly. Note the accentuation over the elbows.

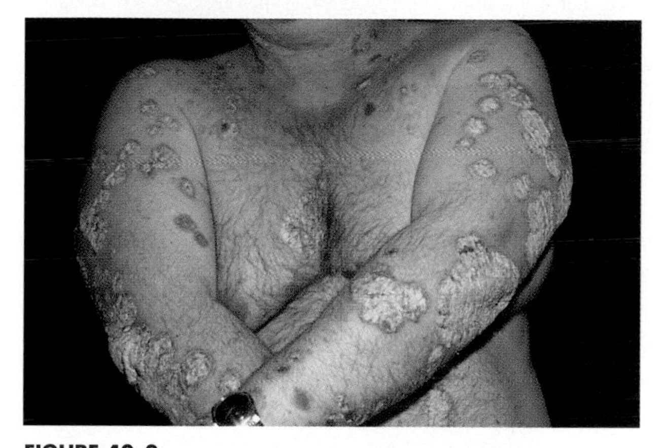

FIGURE 40–2

Large-plaque psoriasis. These well-demarcated erythematous lesions are covered by a thick, mica-like scale. Note the variability in the size and degree of scale.

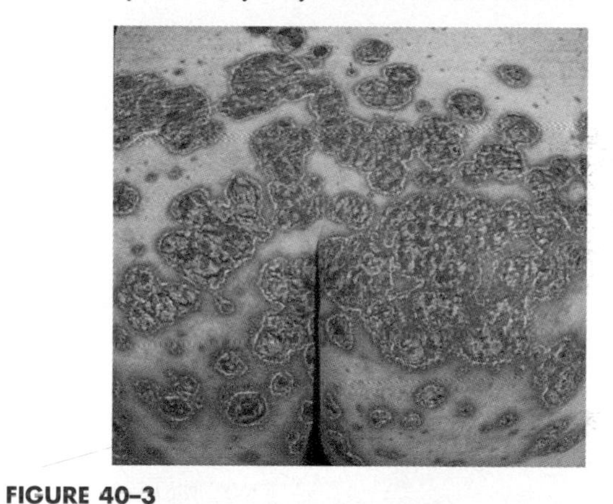

FIGURE 40–3

Well-demarcated erythematous plaques of the buttocks. Scale is limited. Lesions are typical of those on the buttocks and lower back.

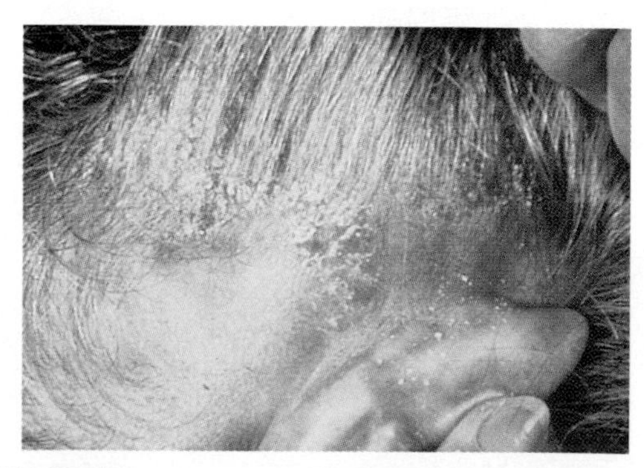

FIGURE 40–4

Scaling plaques on the scalp and behind the ears are typical of psoriasis. These plaques are thicker and more sharply demarcated than the scalp changes typically seen in seborrheic dermatitis.

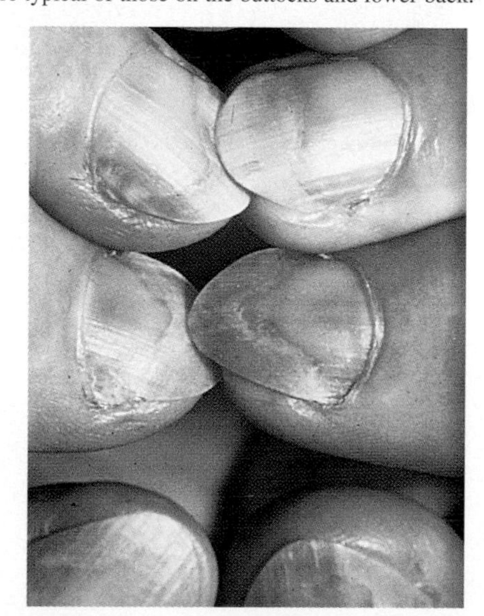

FIGURE 40–5

Nail changes of psoriasis include onycholysis, oil streaks (at the proximal edge of onycholysis), and nail dystrophy.

PLATE 16

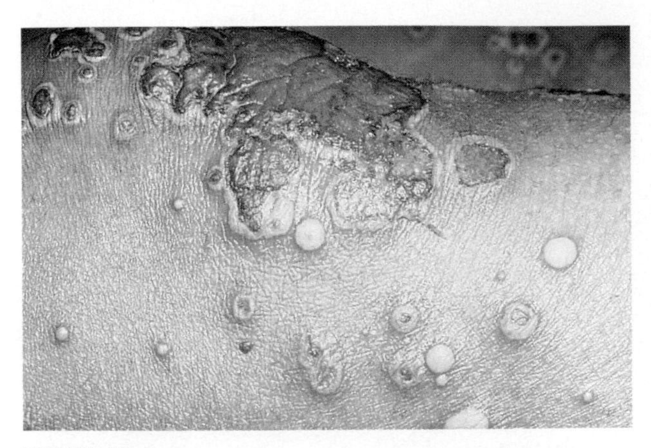

FIGURE 40–6

Localized pustular psoriasis in conjunction with plaque psoriasis of the knee. These pustules are sterile.

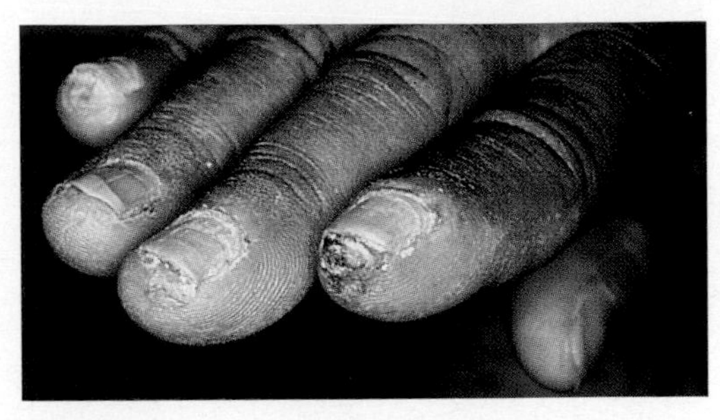

FIGURE 41–1

Scleroderma. This patient has severe Raynaud's phenomenon with ulceration of the distal fingertip. (From Callen JP, Greer KE, Hood AF, et al: Color Atlas of Dermatology. Philadelphia: WB Saunders, 1993, p 340.)

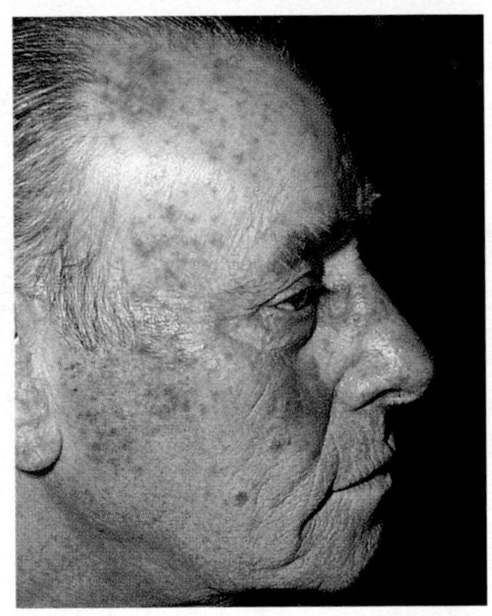

FIGURE 42–1

Extensive inflammatory papules and pustules of rosacea involving the central and lateral face.

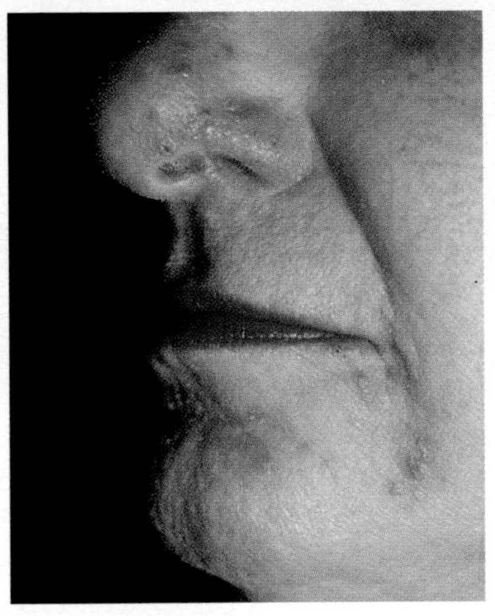

FIGURE 42–2

Erythematous papules, pustules, and telangiectasia in a woman with rosacea. Note the prominent nasal involvement.

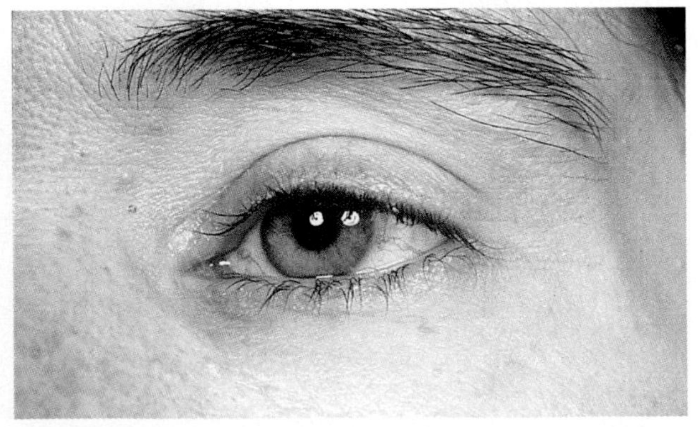

FIGURE 42–3

Ocular findings of rosacea include conjunctivitis, erythema, and telangiectasia of the eyelid margins.

PLATE 17

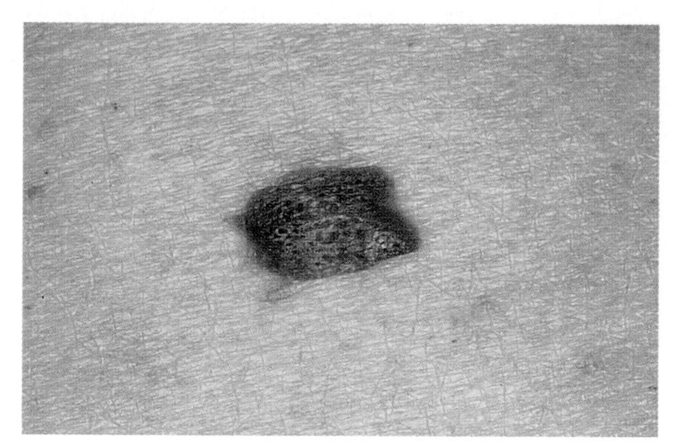

FIGURE 45–1

Typical seborrheic keratosis with horn cysts. (Courtesy of Richard A. Johnson, M.D.)

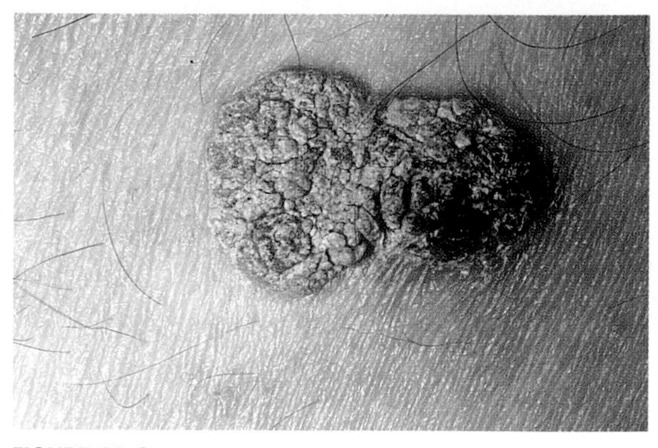

FIGURE 45–2

Irritated seborrheic keratosis with crusting and peripheral erythema. (Courtesy of Richard A. Johnson, M.D.)

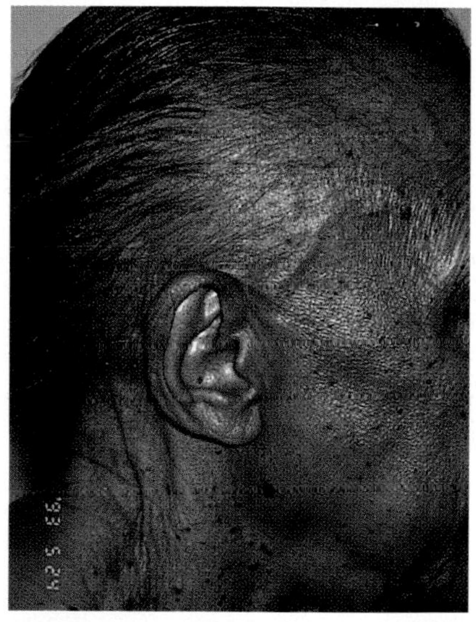

FIGURE 45–3

Numerous small, dark seborrheic keratoses, typical of dermatosis papulosa nigra. (Courtesy of Richard A. Johnson, M.D.)

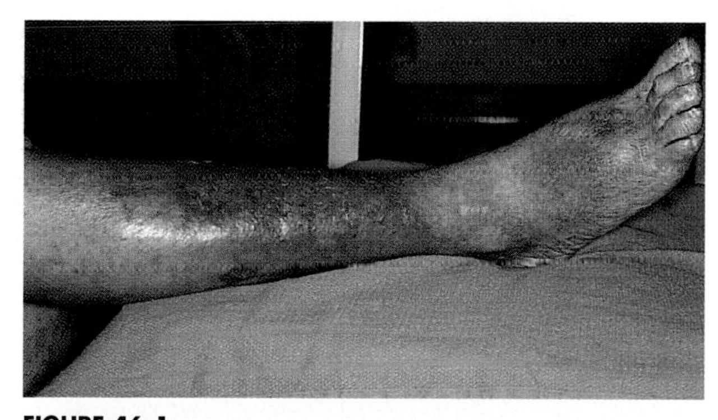

FIGURE 46–1

An eczematous plaque of acute stasis dermatitis. Note the edema, erythema, and crusting.

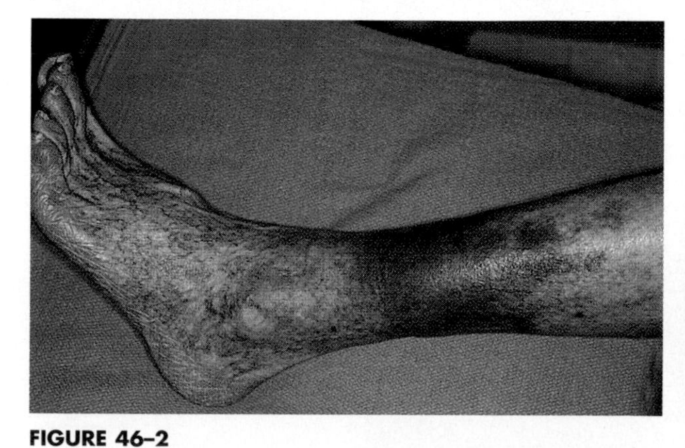

FIGURE 46–2

Chronic stasis dermatitis with hyperpigmentation, atrophy, and dilated reticular veins.

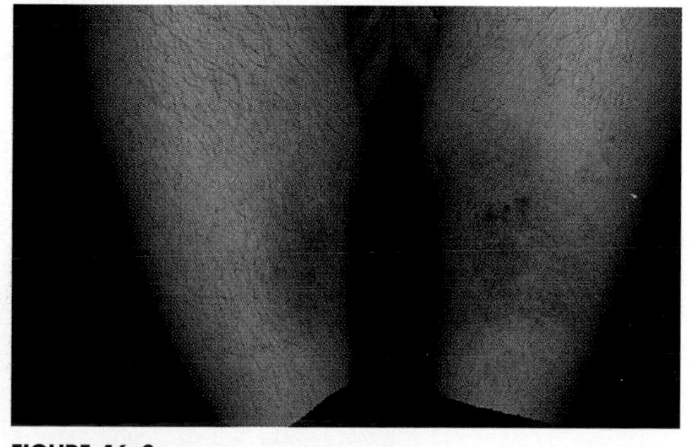

FIGURE 46–3

Early lipodermatosclerosis. These indurated plaques produce loss of the subcutaneous tissue that, without treatment, will increase over time. (Courtesy of Susan B. Mallory.)

PLATE 18

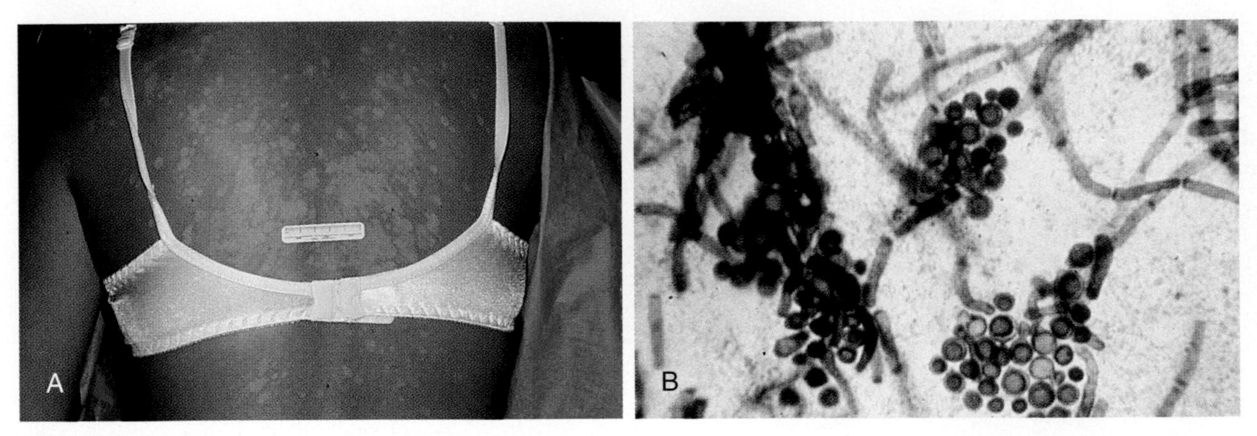

FIGURE 48–1

Tinea versicolor. *A,* Typical hypopigmented, sharply marginated, coalescing macules with fine scale, prominent on the upper back of this patient. *B,* Characteristic "spaghetti and meatballs" appearance of the blastospores and hyphae of *Malassezia furfur* seen on potassium hydroxide examination. (Polychrome blue stain, ×400.) (*A* and *B,* Courtesy of Stanley A. Rosenthal, Ph.D.)

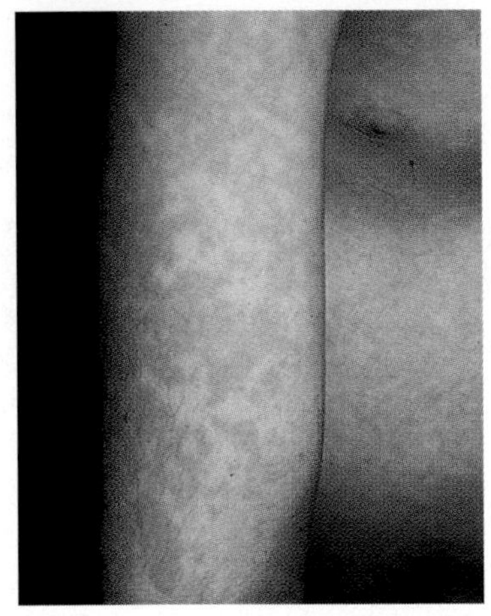

FIGURE 50–1

Reticulated or marbled erythema on the extremities characteristic of erythema infectiosum (fifth disease).

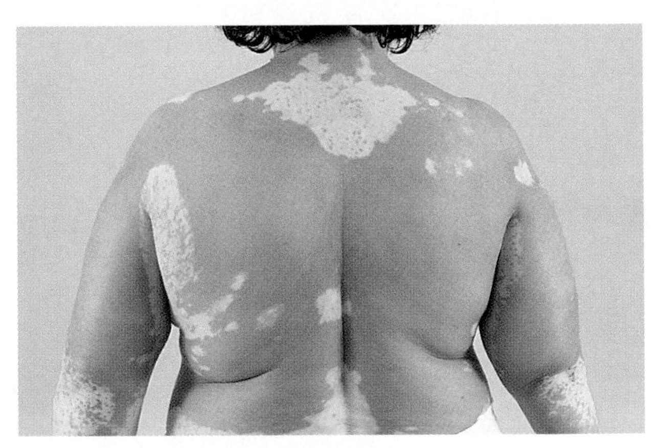

FIGURE 51–1

Extensive depigmentation caused by vitiligo.

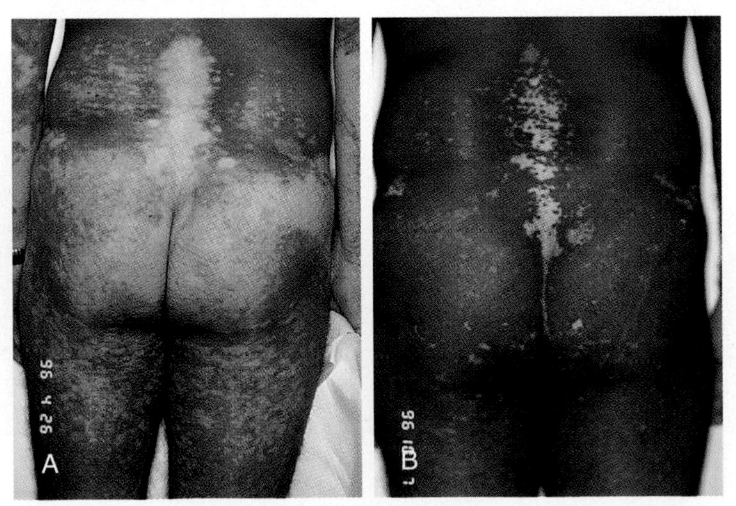

FIGURE 51–2

Extensive psoralen plus ultraviolet A (PUVA)–induced repigmentation.

PLATE 19

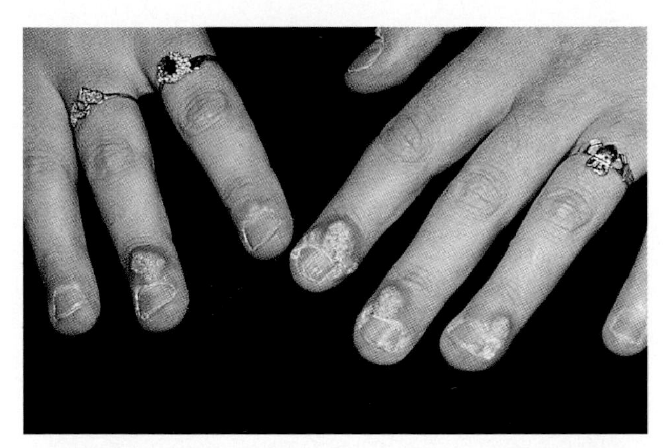

FIGURE 52–1
Common warts.

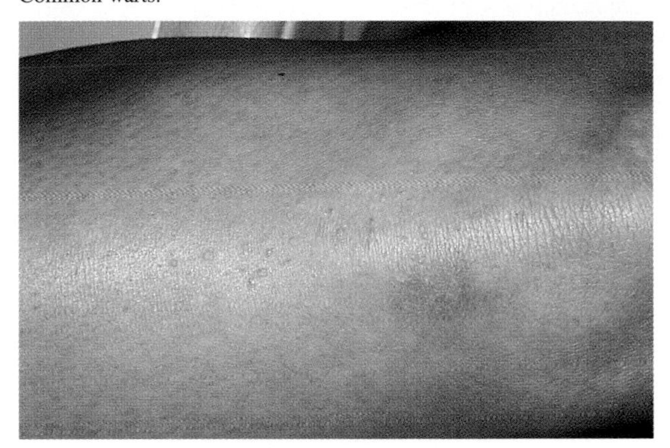

FIGURE 52–2
Flat warts.

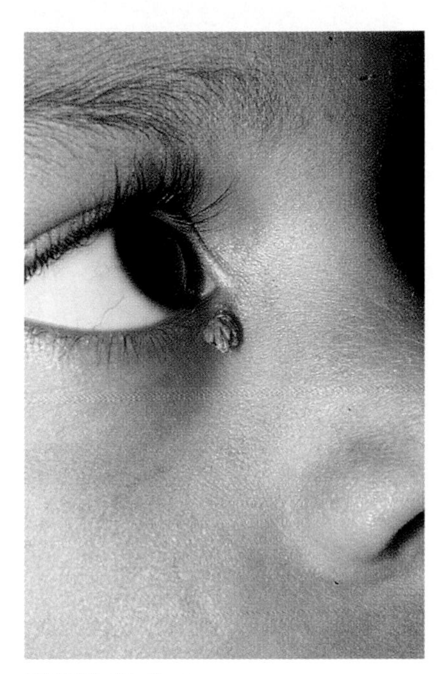

FIGURE 52–3
Filiform wart.

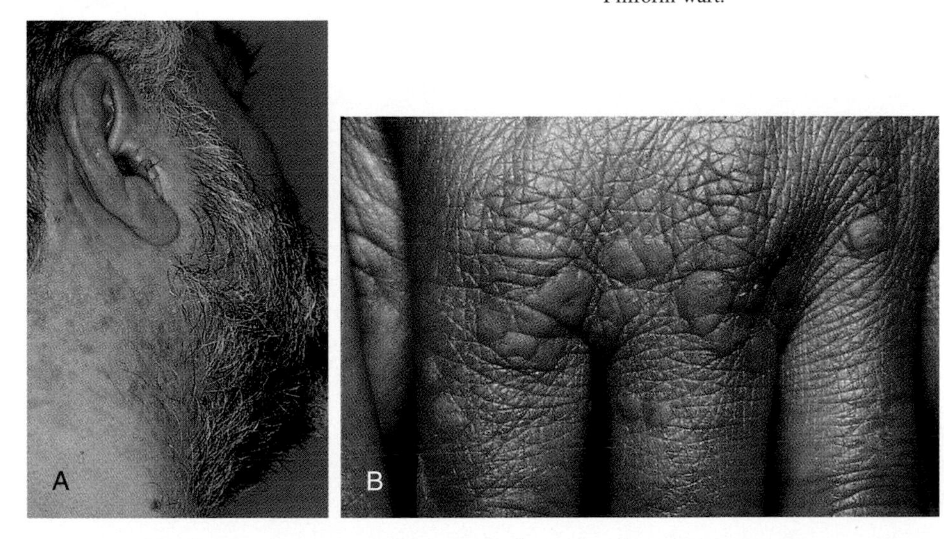

FIGURE 52–4
A and *B*, Epidermodysplasia verruciformis. (*B*, From Callen JP, Greer KE, Hood AF, et al. Color Atlas of Dermatology. Philadelphia: WB Saunders, 1993, p 285.)

PLATE 20

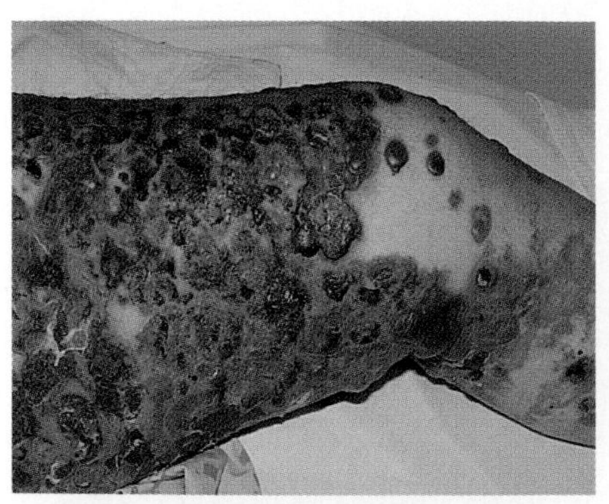

FIGURE 53–1

Extremity of a patient with severe bullous pemphigoid showing confluent tense blisters of underlying erythematous urticarial skin.

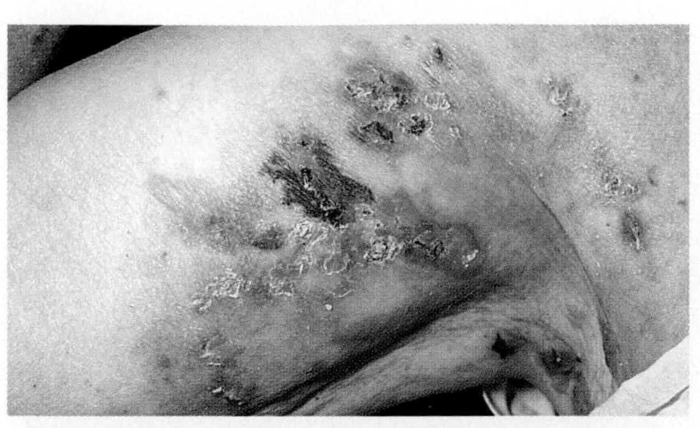

FIGURE 53–2

Extremity of a patient with inflammatory epidermolysis bullosa acquisita showing underlying erythema with blisters and erosions.

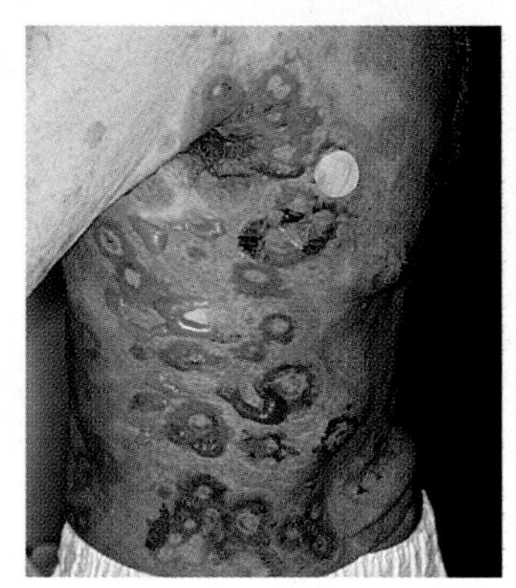

FIGURE 53–3

Trunk of a patient with linear immunoglobulin A bullous dermatosis showing numerous tense arcuate blisters.

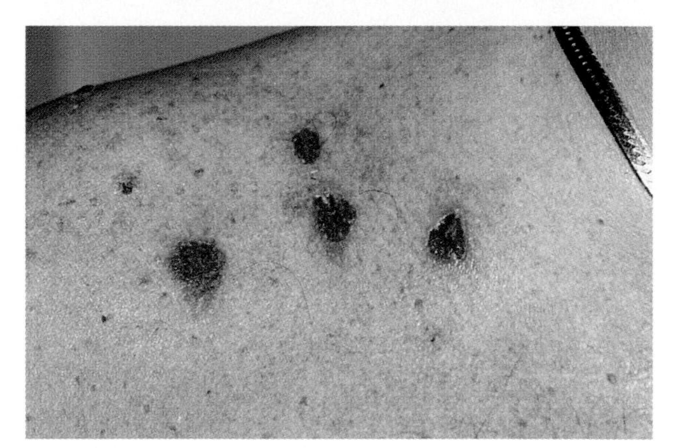

FIGURE 53–4

Upper trunk of a patient with pemphigus vulgaris showing eroded lesions at sites of previous flaccid blisters.

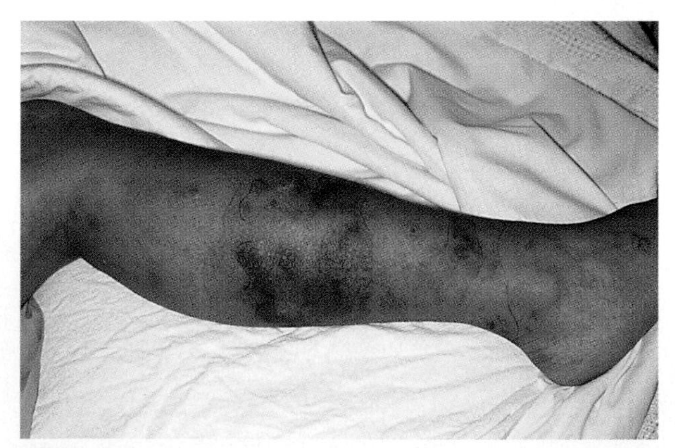

FIGURE 54–1

Typical lesions of erysipelas.

PLATE 21

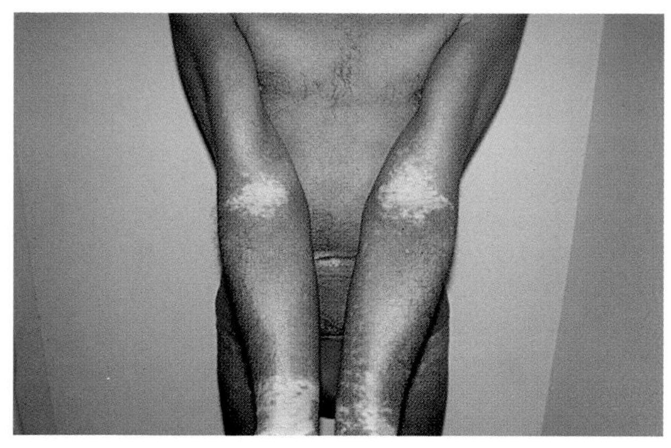

FIGURE 55–1

Drug-induced erythroderma in a middle-aged man. Only the wrists and antecubital fossae are spared.

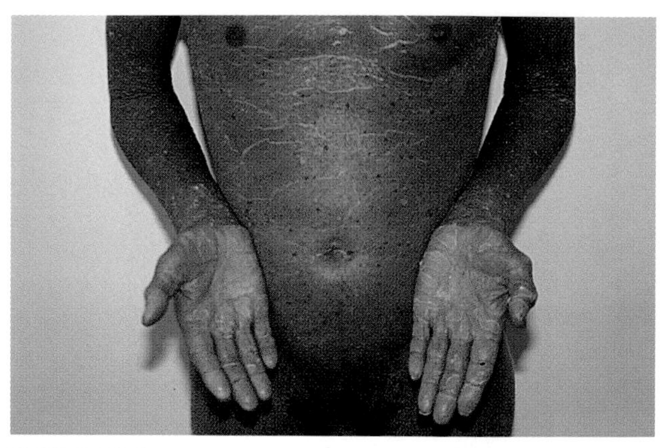

FIGURE 55–2

Chronic erythroderma.

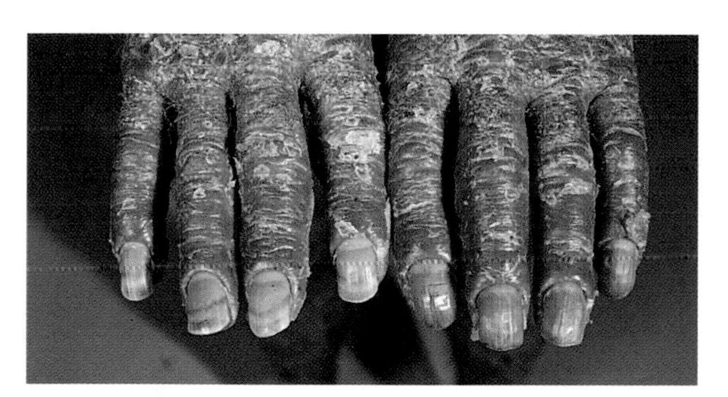

FIGURE 55–3

Hand and nail changes in exfoliative dermatitis.

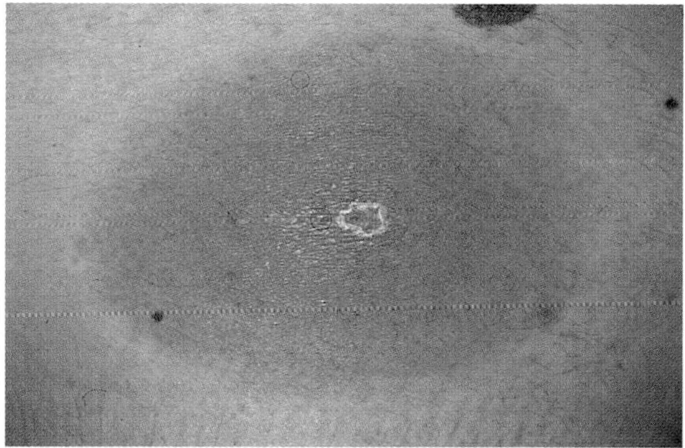

FIGURE 56–1

Primary erythema migrans (EM). Solid erythema with an early collarette of scale. (From Melski JW: Lyme borreliosis in Wisconsin. Fitzpatrick's J Clin Dermatol 1994; May/June, pp 14–25.)

PLATE 24

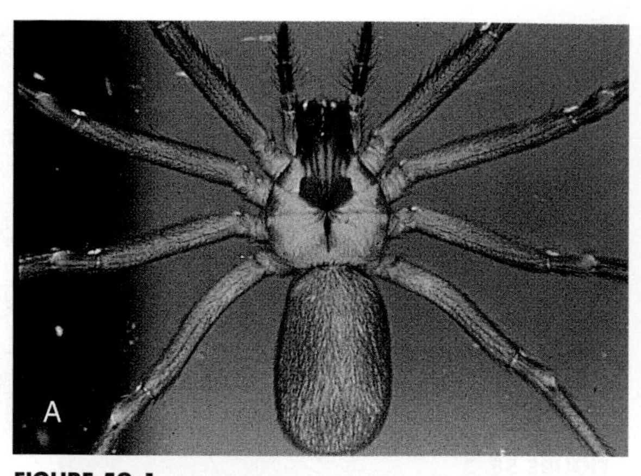

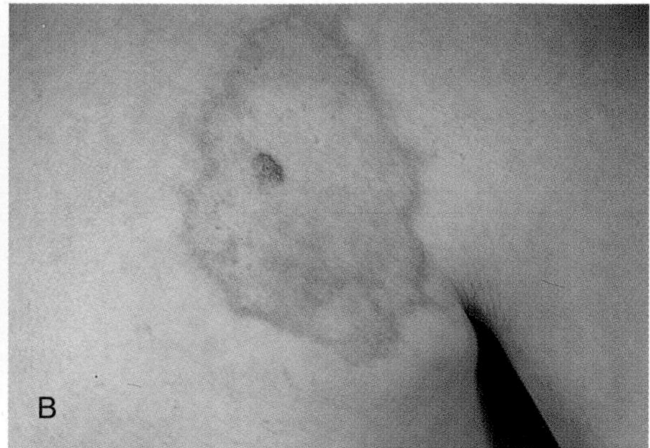

FIGURE 59–1

A, Brown recluse spider. *B,* Typical bite of the brown recluse spider.

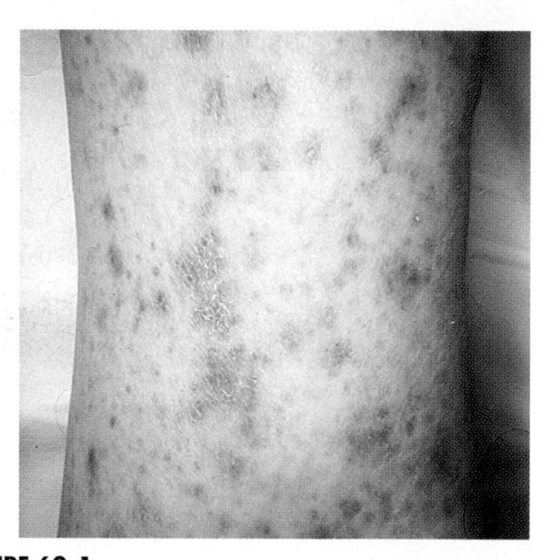

FIGURE 60–1

Palpable purpura as a manifestation of cutaneous necrotizing venulitis in a patient with coexistent Sjögren's syndrome.

SECTION

I

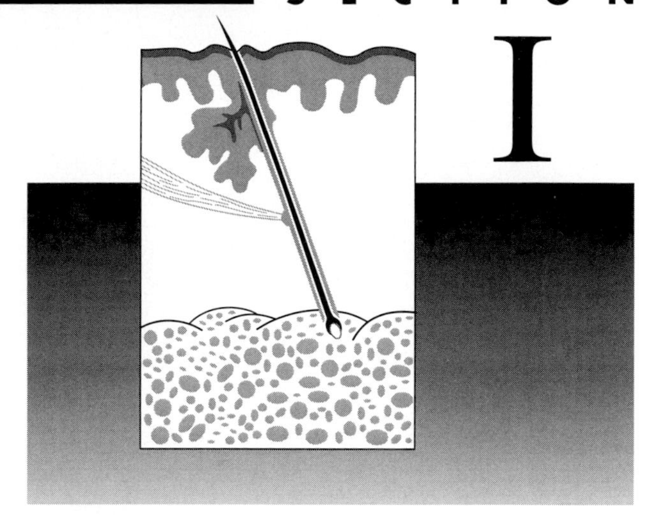

What Are the Important Considerations for Treatment of the Skin?

CHAPTER 1

How Do You Care for Normal Skin?

Christopher R. Shea

Production and sale of goods related to the care and embellishment of normal skin is a multibillion-dollar industry in the United States. Much of this total is in strictly cosmetic products such as makeup and scent, which are discussed in other texts.[1] This chapter addresses the related needs to keep the skin and hair clean, odor-free, appropriately hydrated, and protected from environmental hazards.

SOAP

Soap was discovered by the ancient Phoenicians, who first hydrolyzed the triglycerides of animal fat with lye to yield sodium salts of fatty acids by the saponification reaction still used today. Soap forms spherical micelles with hydrophobic lipids in the center and hydrophilic, anionic regions outside. This amphophilic structure permits grease and dirt to be dissolved in water and rinsed away. Additives include fragrances and antibacterial agents, such as triclorsan, that reduce body odor resulting from bacterial action on axillary sweat.

Soap can be a primary irritant, especially when used in excess.[2] Irritancy is assessed experimentally using prolonged contact at high concentration, which exaggerates the irritation and thus discriminates among different products for their irritating potential. Allergic sensitization can occur to fragrances, dyes, antibacterial agents, or other additives.

True soaps are alkaline. Synthetic detergents share many properties of soap but can be formulated at a pH approximating that of normal skin (pH 5 to 6). In the past, alkaline soaps were considered likely to disrupt the natural acid mantle of the skin. However, it now appears more likely that, under conditions of daily use on normal skin, the pH of skin cleansers has relatively little effect on their irritancy, which probably results mainly from the extraction of lipids from the stratum corneum.[3] Persons with oily skin or acne benefit from relatively harsh, defatting soaps (e.g., Dial or Lever 2000), whereas those with dry, sensitive skin do better with milder products (e.g., Dove or Cetaphil).

SHAMPOO

Sebum, the product of the oil gland associated with the hair follicle, is a chemical trap for environmental dirt, smoke, and odor. Its removal is the central function of a shampoo. The cleansing ingredients in shampoos are anionic, cationic, amphoteric, or nonionic detergents (surfactants) that have different abilities to cleanse, lather, and mix with other ingredients.[4] Nonprescription shampoos include Neutrogena, Prell, and Free & Clear. In addition, shampoos contain numerous other ingredients such as foam stabilizers, preservatives, fragrances, thickeners, and opacifiers. Baby shampoos (e.g., Johnson's Ultra Sensitive Baby Shampoo) have very low detergency and irritancy, so that the eyes are not harmed by contact.

Simply removing sebum can result in dull, dry hair that is easily tangled. Conditioning shampoos (e.g., Clinique Daily Wash or Extra Benefits Shampoo) contain additional ingredients to coat damaged hair and impart desired properties such as body and luster. The particular product needed depends on the character of the hair and scalp, the type of styling to be done, and the frequency of shampooing. Because the addition of conditioner to a shampoo formulation can compromise its cleansing function, it is more efficient if less convenient to use a separate conditioner after shampooing, if required (e.g., BioComplex 5000 Revitalizing Conditioner and Clinique Extra Benefits Conditioner).

DEODORANT AND ANTIPERSPIRANT

Human sweat is of two kinds. Eccrine sweat serves primarily to cool the skin by evaporation. It is produced by intradermal glands that are anatomically and embryologically distinct from the hair follicles, and these glands are most numerous on the palms and soles. Apocrine sweat is the holocrine secretion of glands associated with the hair follicles of the axilla, groin, perineum, and breast. Axillary sweat is an originally odorless secretion of both the eccrine and the apocrine glands. Bacterial metabolism produces a variety of odorific compounds, including androgens and other steroids. It is believed that apocrine sweat evolved as a chemical signal for mating behavior (pheromone). In our modern world, however, the effect is the contrary.

Antiperspirants block secretion from both the eccrine and the apocrine glands, reducing moisture and staining as well as the possible subsequent development of odor. Most antiperspirants are aluminum salts that work by forming a plug in the sweat duct. Pure deodorants inhibit bacterial growth and thus block the metabolism of apocrine sweat; they have no antiperspirant effects. Fragrance-free deodorants are made by Almay and Clinique.

MOISTURIZER

Dry skin (xerosis) may occur in otherwise normal skin or reflect an underlying dermatosis such as atopic dermatitis or ichthyosis. It is a common cause of itching. Xerotic skin has a fine scale and is dry and rough to the touch; when xerosis is severe, it creates a pattern likened to the cracked texture of old porcelain (eczema craquelé). Xerotic skin has a thickened stratum corneum with fine fissures and a tendency to desquamate as groups of cells rather than singly. In more severe cases, intercellular edema of the epidermis and a dermal lymphocytic infiltrate (asteatotic dermatitis) occur. Xerosis is exacerbated by environmental factors such as low humidity and exposure to wind. It is usually worse in winter, when forced-air heating causes the level of humidity inside many dwellings to plummet. It may not be necessary or advisable to shower and scrub as often or as vigorously in winter as in the sticky summer months. Use of an air humidifier can also benefit xerotic skin in winter.

Water can both cause and cure xerosis. Overvigorous washing, especially with harsh soaps, strips the stratum corneum of its natural lipids and thereby exacerbates xerosis; frequent hand washing, for instance, can lead to a frank irritant contact dermatitis. On the other hand, the essential treatment of xerosis is to rehydrate the stratum corneum, and this requires water. Moisturizing products supply water directly to the skin or prevent its loss. Humectants such as urea (e.g., Ultra Mide 25) and lactate (e.g., Lac-Hydrin, Lac-Hydrin Five, and Eucerin Plus) are hygroscopic compounds that increase the water-holding capacity of the stratum corneum. Occlusives such as petrolatum and mineral oil restore the lipid barrier between cells of the stratum corneum and thus reduce transepidermal water loss.

Moisturizers are formulated with a broad range of lipid-water ratios. The heavier, more lipidized products (e.g., Aquaphor) are excellent occlusives but may be objectionably greasy. Experimentation may be necessary to find the right balance between effectiveness and cosmetic elegance. Water-repellent pure hydrocarbon ointments such as petrolatum are mainly used for treatment of severe xerosis or other dermatoses. Hydrophilic petrolatum is a somewhat less greasy, absorbent ointment consisting of petrolatum and emusifier. Water-in-oil emulsions such as lanolin and traditional cold cream are acceptable to many users but are not water-soluble and therefore are difficult to wash off. Oil-in-water creams are more washable and feel and look less greasy. Finally, emollient lotions (e.g., Lubriderm, LactiCare, and Complex 15) are dilute dispersions of emulsified lipids in water. These provide the smoothest application and the most rapid hydration if applied to dry skin, but the least protective effect on the lipid barrier.

Careless overbathing ultimately dries the skin, but a regimen of soaking can help prevent or treat xerosis. Soaking is intended to saturate, not clean the skin; if necessary for hygiene, a brief, cleansing shower with mild soap and a thorough rinse can precede soaking.

Soaking should be done for about 15 minutes in soap-free water that is comfortably warm but not hot. Many patients enjoy adding an oil to the bath water, but this probably does not add much to the objective benefit. On emerging, the body should be toweled gently to avoid mechanical irritation and leave a thin film of water on the surface—a good method is to wrap the torso in an absorbent, cotton terry-cloth robe rather than to rub down. Most important, soaking should be promptly followed by application of an appropriate moisturizer to all affected areas.

HAIR REMOVAL

Shaving is a common cause of skin irritation, which can be lessened by application of a moisturizer after shaving. Razor blades should be changed frequently to reduce drag on the beard. Shaving creams (e.g., Clinique Shave Cream) and gels (e.g., Edge) hydrate and soften the beard and make the skin surface slippery. Paradoxically, the opposite effect is the purported benefit of dry shaving aids that contain alcohol or other astringents, to be applied before use of an electric razor. In black men especially, shaving too close permits the resultant sharpened, tightly coiled hairs to retract beneath the skin surface and penetrate the follicular wall from within or else to reenter the epidermis from without, causing painful, unattractive "razor bumps" (pseudofolliculitis barbae). The best treatment is simply to grow a beard, but this may not be acceptable to the patient, employer, or family. Less-close shaving (e.g., Bump Fighter razor) or use of a mild depilatory is an alternative. Chemical depilatories remove hair by reducing the disulfide bonds of cysteine residues. They contain thioglycollates as the reducing agents, in conjunction with an alkali such as CaOH. Sulfides are also effective depilatories but these produce hydrogen sulfide, which has an obnoxious smell. *Epilation,* in contrast to depilation, refers to the physical removal of hair, generally with a wax that extracts hair when it is pulled off the skin surface. New techniques using the neodymium:yttrium-aluminum-garnet (Nd:YAG) and ruby lasers for permanent hair removal are becoming available in spas and physician's offices.

PHOTOPROTECTION

Photoprotection from the sun's ultraviolet radiation (UVR) is increasingly important. Atmospheric pollution from chlorinated fluorocarbons in recent decades has reduced the stratospheric ozone layer, which blocks ultraviolet C (UVC) (wavelengths < 290 nm) and reduces the penetration of ultraviolet B (UVB) (wavelengths 290 to 320 nm) to the earth's surface. This environmental hazard is increasing at a time when outdoor leisure activities and travel to tropical locales are becoming more popular. The talismanic allure of the suntan as a mark of sophistication and apparent health remains a formidable obstacle to the use of sensible photoprotection.

Erythema (sunburn) is a familiar acute result of UVB overexposure, typically beginning 2 to 8 hours after irradiation and peaking at 24 to 36 hours. The lighter the complexion, the more severe the risk of sunburn. Threshold values (minimal erythema dose [MED]) of UVB for fair-skinned white people are about 20 to 70 joules of incident radiant energy per square centimeter of skin surface. Erythema is followed in about 1 week by hyperpigmentation (suntan) as a result of increased epidermal biosynthesis of melanin. After severe overexposure, desquamation (peeling) occurs, reflecting transient changes in keratinocyte proliferation.

Chronic effects of UVR exposure are more insidious and important. A wealth of data from studies in cells and animals proves that UVR is mutagenic and carcinogenic, and this conclusion is confirmed epidemiologically by the clear relationship in humans between the incidence of skin cancer and such variables as skin color, geographic latitude, and history of occupational and leisure-time exposure to sunlight. Chronic, excessive sun exposure has many other unattractive effects, collectively designated *photoaging*—the leathery, wrinkled, unevenly pigmented skin that reflects not chronologic age per se but rather the accumulation of years of actinic abuse. The chronic effects of UVR may result from a long accumulation of relatively low-level exposures, each below the threshold for acute erythema.

Sunscreens (e.g., Sundown, Bullfrog, Neutrogena, Bain de Soleil, Oil of Olay, and PreSun) are key ingredients in a photoprotection program.[5] They prevent erythema and reduce the incidence of actinic keratoses, a marker of chronic photodamage associated with development of squamous cell carcinoma.[6] Chemical blockers that absorb UVB, and thereby prevent its transmission into the skin, include para-aminobenzoic acid and its esters, salicylates, and cinnamates. Benzophenones and dibenzoylmethanes absorb ultraviolet A (UVA) (wavelengths 320 to 400 nm), a portion of the spectrum that is much less effective at causing erythema than UVB but that contributes to acute and chronic photodamage.

UVA is also important in photosensitivity diseases and in photoallergic and phototoxic reactions to medications. Opaque pastes such as zinc oxide and micronized reflecting powders such as titanium dioxide scatter and reflect UVR and thereby act as physical rather than chemical UVR blockers. Sunscreens should be applied ½ hour before exposure. Reapplication may be advisable after swimming or sweating, but this does not reset the clock—any accumulated UVR dose will still have its effects.

The U.S. Food and Drug Administration defines the sun protection factor (SPF) as the ratio of the MED in treated versus untreated skin, under controlled conditions involving careful, copious application and calibrated exposure to a solar-simulator xenon arc lamp. The actual protection provided by a sunscreen in everyday use is often less. The SPF predominantly assesses protection against UVB; UVA contributes about 15% of the erythemogenic radiation from sun exposure. Commercial sunscreens have SPFs ranging from as low as 2 to greater than 30. The need for strong sunscreens (SPF 15 and above) can be addressed by considering the exposure anticipated in daily activities. At noon during the summer in California, a fair-skinned person receives 1 MED in only 20 minutes; thus the unprotected skin might receive up to 12 MED if exposed for the 4 peak hours around high noon, a UVR dose that would cause severe erythema, edema, and probably blistering. Liberal use of a sunscreen with an SPF of only 10 in such a case would result in $^{12}/_{10}$ of a sunburn, that is, an effective UVR exposure greater than 1 MED. Note that even a sunscreen with SPF 15 would still permit accumulation of about $^{12}/_{15}$ MED, an effective dose that would cause mild acute inflammation and contribute to chronic photodamage.

Many people consider sunscreens messy, inconvenient, and expensive and fail to use them. Therefore, behavioral aspects of photoprevention also need to be learned. UVR irradiance is most intense at midday; planning to do outdoor activities early in the morning or late in the afternoon is perhaps the simplest form of photoprotection. Seeking shade from an umbrella, awning, or building is also effective. Cloud cover may reduce brightness and heat, but it is an unreliable shield against solar UVR. On the other hand, ordinary window glass blocks UVB but transmits visible light and UVA. When outdoors, it is important to protect oneself not only against direct exposure from the solar disk but also from diffuse UVR scattered by the atmosphere and reflected by sand or snow on the ground. Sunburn is usually considered a summertime malady, but in fact, the terrestrial UVB flux reaches up to 80% of its peak intensity by midspring, and so photoprotection measures should be initiated in spring and continued into fall. Persons traveling to a different climate may encounter unaccustomed UVR exposures. UVR irradiance increases in proportion to altitude above sea level; this explains why sunburn is a hazard on winter ski slopes. More importantly, UVR intensity increases progressively with proximity to the equator.

Clothing is another important tool for photoprotection. A broad-brimmed hat efficiently shields the face, neck, and ears from UVR. Ordinary woven cloth garments vary markedly in their ability to reflect and absorb UVR and typically have an SPF of about 6. Special clothing that provides an SPF of 30 or greater (e.g., Sun Precautions, Frogskin) is more reliable for prevention of erythema in humans and also protects against photocarcinogenesis in mice.[7]

PROTECTION FROM CONTACT DERMATITIS

Many patients need protection from *Toxicodendron* spp. (poison ivy, oak, and sumac) or other environmental allergens.[8] Barrier creams and gels (e.g., Stokes Gard Outdoor Cream), consisting of hydrocarbons, silicone, or chelating agents such as ethylenediaminetetraacetate, are intended to block penetration of allergens through the stratum corneum. Barriers must be thoroughly washed off after exposure, lest any allergen be transferred to unprotected skin. The clinical efficacy of current barriers is unimpressive.[9] Unfortunately, it will probably prove very difficult to develop barriers as effective as sunscreens. The inherent amplifying action of the activated immune system magnifies reactions to even a small number of molecules, and an almost-total blockade of contact with the allergen may be needed for complete protection.

As with photoprotection, basic knowledge and preventive behaviors can reduce the hazard of exposure to environmental allergens. The offending resin of poison ivy is present throughout the year in stalks and stems as well as leaves. Severe reactions can occur from exposure to smoke from burning plants in the fall. Thick-weave or impermeable clothing is an effective protection against exposure, but the resin may persist on it and lead to rechallenge if not removed by cleaning. Washing of exposed skin in the first hours after exposure reduces the antigenic load and the intensity of subsequent inflammation and also helps to prevent spread to other areas of the body. Exposed pets carry the allergen on their coats and should also be washed to prevent further spread.

PROTECTION FROM ARTHROPODS

Protection from arthropod assaults is important not only to prevent painful, itchy local reactions but also to guard against serious arthropod-borne infectious diseases. The most commonly used repellent (in preparations such as Off! and Ultrathon) is diethyltoluamide (DEET); it is effective against mosquitoes, flies, midges, fleas, ticks, and mites. Other repellents include ethyl hexanediol and benzyl benzoate. Unfortunately, effective repellents against bees, wasps, fire ants, and spiders are not yet available. Mosquitos respond to the convection currents of warm, moist air surrounding their prey as well as to the trail of carbon dioxide vapor they exhale. DEET does not act as a negative attractant but rather blocks the ability of mosquitos to perceive and respond appropriately to these stimuli.[10] DEET must be applied liberally over the entire exposed surface and reapplied every hour or so. Application to clothes can prevent bites through them. Up to 17% of the applied dose may be percutaneously absorbed into the systemic circulation, with an elimination half-life of 5 days.[11] DEET is generally safe, but there have been rare reports of acute manic psychosis, toxic encephalopathy, and bullous reactions following its topical use, and ingestion can be lethal.

REFERRAL GUIDELINES

Care of truly normal skin requires no referral. However, the primary care practitioner should be aware of potential complications of normal skin care products. If a patient develops erythema, itching, or other signs of inflammation, an allergic hypersensitivity reaction to fragrance, preservative, lanolin, sunscreen, and the like should be suspected. Persistence after discontinuation of the product is grounds for referral to a dermatologist. Counseling about cross-reaction to other products and the performance and interpretation of patch-testing are best done by an experienced specialist. Remember also that what the patient may consider normal may in fact represent a disease. For instance, dandruff may be a clue to psoriasis, dry skin may indicate ichthyosis, and easy sunburning may be a sign of lupus erythematosus, porphyria, or a phototoxic drug reaction. Any strong deviation from normal deserves investigation and possible referral.

REFERENCES

1. Draelos ZD: Cosmetics in Dermatology. 2nd ed. New York: Churchill Livingstone, 1995.
2. Wolf R: Has mildness replaced cleanliness next to godliness? Dermatology 1994; 189:217–221.
3. Ostreicher MI: Detergents, bath preparations, and other skin cleansers. Clin Dermatol 1988; 6:29–36.
4. Bouillon C: Shampoos and hair conditioners. Clin Dermatol 1988; 6:83–92.
5. Lowe NJ, Friedlander J: Prevention of photodamage with sun protection and sunscreens. *In* Gilchrest BA (ed): Photodamage. Cambridge, MA: Blackwell Science, 1995; pp 201–220.
6. Thompson SC, Jolley D, Marks R: Reduction of solar keratoses by regular sunscreen use. N Engl J Med 1993; 329:1147–1151.
7. Menter JM, Hollins TD, Sayre RM, et al: Protection against UV photocarcinogenesis by fabric materials. J Am Acad Dermatol 1994; 31:711–716.
8. Mathias CG: Prevention of occupational contact dermatitis. J Am Acad Dermatol 1990; 23:742–748.
9. Pigatto PD, Bigardi AS, Legori A, et al: Are barrier creams of any use in contact dermatitis? Contact Dermatitis 1992; 26:197–198.
10. Wright RH: Why mosquito repellents repel. Sci Am 1975; 233(1):104–111.
11. Robbins PJ, Cherniak MG: Review of the biodistribution and toxicity of the insect repellent *N,N*-diethyl-*m*-toluamide (DEET). J Toxicol Environ Health 1986; 18:503–525.

CHAPTER 2

Skin Care Maintenance

Zoe Diana Draelos

SCOPE OF SKIN CARE PRODUCTS

Skin care maintenance embodies all topically applied products for general hygiene, enhanced skin function, and environmental protection. Basic product categories include cleansers, astringents, moisturizers, and sunscreens. Variations in formulation allow product development for different skin-type needs, resulting in a plethora of consumer choices.

PRODUCT DESCRIPTIONS

Cleansers

Cleansing of the skin is the most important aspect of skin care maintenance to prevent infection and remove both excess sebum and environmental dirt while minimizing damage to the stratum corneum protective barrier. This is a challenge for any cleanser, since a balance between adequate and excessive removal of sebum in different consumer hands is impossible to achieve.[1]

Basically, skin cleansers can be divided into deodorant soaps, true soaps, and synthetic detergent soaps. These soaps can be manufactured in the form of opaque bars, translucent bars, transparent bars, lotions, creams, and gels, but the three levels of cleansing remain.[2] Deodorant soaps (e.g., Dial, Lever 2000, Safeguard) contain triclosan or triclocarban as topical antibacterial agents and are useful in decreasing body odor, preventing bacterial spread, and assisting in the treatment of cutaneous infections. True soaps (e.g., Ivory) mechanically remove bacteria and are effective at removing all sebum and environmental dirt. Synthetic detergent bars (e.g., Dove, Oil of Olay), also known as syndet bars, are generally milder on the skin and compose the group of products known as beauty bars.[3] These soaps are milder on the skin, in that sebum is less thoroughly removed, and generally based on sodium cocoate isethionate.[4]

One last formulation of cleanser deserves mention: lipid-free cleansers (e.g., Cetaphil, Aquanil). These products are the mildest of all cleansers and can be applied to dry skin and wiped away or used with water as a liquid cleanser.[5]

Astringents

Astringents, also known as toners, skin fresheners, and balancing lotions, among others, are alcohol solutions originally designed to remove soap scum residue from the face.[6] With the development of improved detergents and public water treatment facilities, soap scum following facial cleansing is minimal. Astringents remain popular, however, to remove any sebum or cosmetics left behind following cleansing, to deliver topical acne preparations to the skin (e.g., salicylic acid), and to provide the aesthetic values of skin tightness or freshness.

Moisturizers

Moisturizers are intended to mimic the function of sebum on the skin, either supplementing decreased sebum production or replacing overly aggressive sebum removal through cleansing.[7] Moisturizers function based on two mechanisms: occlusion and humectancy.[8] Occlusion employs an oily substance (e.g., petrolatum, lanolin, cocoa butter, mineral oil) to prevent evaporation of water from the skin, a phenomenon known as *transepidermal water loss.*[9] Humectancy applies substances that attract moisture to the skin (e.g., glycerin, sorbitol, propylene glycol, some proteins) either from the atmosphere, when ambient humidity exceeds 70%, or more commonly from the upper dermis. Humectants can also allow water within the moisturizer formulations to remain on the skin longer. The best moisturizer products combine both occlusive and humectant properties.[10]

Modern moisturizer formulations must not only enhance cutaneous water content but also provide emollient and protective qualities.[11] Emollients (e.g., silicone oils, propylene glycol, isopropyl palmitate, octyl stearate) function to increase skin smoothness by filling gaps in the stratum corneum created by dry, contracted skin cells. Some emollients can also function as skin protectants (e.g., diisopropyl dilinoleate, isopropyl isostearate) if they soothe the symptoms of pruritus due to exposed, traumatized nerve endings.

Sunscreens

Sunscreens are of paramount importance in protecting the skin from premature aging (dermatoheliosis) and, more importantly, from carcinogenesis. Two methods of sun protection exist: chemical sunscreens and physical sunscreens (Table 2–1). Chemical sunscreens function to transform light energy to heat energy primarily in the ultraviolet B (UVB) or sunburn spectrum. Physical sunscreens provide broad-spectrum protection by reflecting energy in both the UVB and the ultraviolet A (UVA) wavelengths, thus protecting against both UVB-induced sunburn and UVA-induced tanning and premature aging. Better sunscreen formulations combine both chemical and physical agents.[12]

TABLE 2–1

Examples of Sunscreening Agents

Common Chemical Sunscreening Agents	Common Physical Sunscreening Agents
Anthranilates	Titanium dioxide
Benzophenones	Iron oxide
Methoxycinnamates	Zinc oxide
Aminobenzoates	Magnesium silicate
Salicylates	Magnesium oxide
	Kaolin

SKIN CARE MAINTENANCE ROUTINES

A basic formulation of cleanser, astringent, moisturizer, or sunscreen can be altered and adapted to a variety of patient needs (infants, adolescents, and mature patients) with dry, normal/combination, oily, and sensitive skin types.

Infancy

The skin of an infant is unique in that it produces minimal sebum, but it is subject to the cutaneous insult of possibly prolonged contact with urine and feces. This creates the need for more frequent bathing. Cleansers selected for the infant should be of the synthetic detergent or lipid-free type, and astringents should be avoided. Moisturizers are important in the diaper area to minimize skin-excrement contact and should be of the occlusive ointment type, with petrolatum as the primary ingredient. Ointment moisturizers (e.g., petroleum jelly, Aquaphor) are generally too occlusive for the body, however, resulting in follicular irritation and sweat duct occlusion, a condition known as *miliaria,* commonly called *prickly heat.* Cream formulations (e.g., dimethicone [Moisturel] cream, Eucerin cream) with water as the first ingredient, combining both occlusive and humectant agents, are preferred. Baby oil, composed primarily of mineral oil, is a thin occlusive agent but has no humectant properties. Sunscreen, recommended for use only on infants older than 6 months, should be a cream formulation with microsized titanium dioxide as the primary physical screening agent (e.g., Neutrogena Sensitive Skin Sunscreen SPF 17).

Adolescent/Oily Skin

With the onset of puberty, sebaceous gland secretions become more abundant, resulting in oilier skin. Antibacterial soaps (e.g., Dial) are preferred to decrease body odor, remove sebum, and aid in the treatment of early acne. Antibacterial astringents (e.g., Clean & Clear), if desired, can be used by the patient for the same reasons outlined previously. Some treatment astringents, such as those containing salicylic acid as a keratolytic, may be useful in comedonal acne (blackheads, whiteheads). Moisturizers, if necessary to smooth skin scale induced by drying topical acne treatment products (benzoyl peroxide, tretinoin), should be oil-free and based on silicone derivatives (dimethicone, cyclomethicone). Oil-free sunscreens are also available in gel (e.g., Solbar,

Coppertone) or spray (e.g., Presun, Clinique) formulations.

Normal/Combination Skin

Most patients who classify their skin as normal in actuality possess combination skin. Normal anatomic distribution of the sebaceous glands places larger, more numerous glands on the central face (central forehead, nose, medial cheeks, central chin) with fewer, smaller glands on the lateral face. Thus, the central face is oily and the lateral face is dry. True soaps or synthetic detergent soaps may be used, depending on personal preference, with an astringent applied only to the central face and a lotion moisturizer to the lateral face. A sunscreen-containing moisturizer (e.g., Purpose Moisturizer SPF 15, Neutrogena Moisture SPF 15, Eucerin for Face SPF 25) applied each morning is valuable in preventing sun damage.

Mature/Dry Skin

Sebum production gradually decreases 23% or more over the lifetime of an individual, beginning at age 20 years. The ability of the stratum corneum to slough also decreases, accounting for much of the increased scaling and roughness observed in elderly individuals.[13, 14] Thus, achieving smooth skin requires minimizing sebum removal, enhancing moisture retention, and encouraging corneocyte desquamation. Synthetic detergent cleansers should be used at least once weekly to mechanically remove bacteria from the skin, possibly in combination with a lipid-free cleanser in patients with extreme xerosis. Sometimes water-only cleansing is appropriate if environmental dirt is minimal. Astringents are generally not indicated, but moisturizers and sunscreens assume greater importance. Daytime moisturizers should combine occlusive, humectant, and sunscreen agents (DML Facial Moisturizer SPF 15), whereas nighttime creams can be heavier formulations (e.g., Eucerin Creme, Moisturel Cream, Cetaphil Cream).

Some mature individuals may wish to use some of the newer therapeutic moisturizer formulations, attempting to correct physiologic changes associated with aging. For example, decreased corneocyte desquamation can be enhanced by disrupting ionic bonding through the use of alpha-hydroxy acids, such as glycolic acid (e.g., Neutrogena Healthy Skin) or lactic acid (e.g., Lac-Hydrin), or beta-hydroxy acids, such as salicylic acid.[15] The water-holding capacity of the skin can be improved through the application of urea in combination with lactic acid (e.g., Eucerin Plus cream and lotion). Further formulations attempt to speed skin barrier repair through the addition of raw materials required to reduce water loss, such as essential fatty acids (e.g., Dermasil).

A further important area of concern in the mature patient is sun protection. The damage induced by solar radiation results from the production of highly energetic oxygen radicals that damage collagen and elastin fibers in the skin. This has led to an interest in topical antioxidants, such as vitamins C, E, and A.[16] Some therapeutic moisturizers combine antioxidants, as well as chemical and physical sunscreens, to maximize sun protection. Mature patients should use broad-spectrum, creamy, moisturizing sunscreen products (Solbar, Presun) on a daily basis. In women, these sunscreening agents can be incorporated into facial foundations or daytime moisturizers. Waterproof, rubproof, and sweatproof products (Neutrogena Sunblock SPF 30) should be selected under conditions of water contact, high humidity, or heavy perspiration.

Sensitive Skin

An amazing 50% of consumers, when surveyed, claim to have sensitive skin.[17] However, there are no clearly defined manufacturing specifications to which sensitive skin products must adhere. Thus, sensitive skin products are labeled as such primarily for marketing purposes. Nevertheless, patients frequently present who supply long lists of products to which they are allergic or claim irritation. From a cutaneous standpoint, patients with sensitive skin possess one or more of the following: deficient barrier function, heightened immune system, or altered neurosensory input. These patients require skin care products that are fragrance-free, contain a paucity of ingredients, and do not contain volatile substances and cutaneous irritants (e.g., lactic acid, glycolic acid, urea, salicylic acid, witch hazel, strong detergents).

It can be difficult to select usable products for these patients, since their needs vary greatly. Sometimes use-testing is the best method to allow patients to self-select products that can be tolerated.[18] This technique can aid in the selection of moisturizers and sunscreens, but not astringents or cleansers. Use-testing of leave-on facial products involves applying a small amount of the substance to the area lateral to the eye at the temple for 5 days. If no erythema, desquamation, or vesiculation is present, generally the product can be safely used by the patient. It should be recognized, however, that products are frequently reformulated with or without packaging changes, resulting in problems for the patient.

SUMMARY

Skin care maintenance principles and practice are an important aspect of dermatologic care to prevent or decrease disease recurrence.

REFERENCES

1. Willcox MJ, Crichton WP: The soap market. Cosmet Toilet 1989; 104:61–63.
2. Wortzman MS: Evaluation of mild skin cleansers. Dermatol Clin 1991; 9:35–44.
3. Prottey C, Ferguson T: Factors which determine the skin irritation potential of soap and detergents. J Soc Cosmet Chem 1975; 26:29.
4. Jackson EM: Soap: A complex category of products. Am J Contact Dermatitis 1994; 5:173–175.
5. Mills OH, Berger RS, Baker MD: A controlled comparison of skin cleansers in photoaged skin. J Geriatr Dermatol 1993; 1:173–179.
6. Wilkinson JB, Moore RJ: Astringents and skin toners. *In* Harry's Cosmeticology. 7th ed. New York: Chemical Publishing, 1982; pp 74–81.
7. Goldner R: Moisturizers: A dermatologist's perspective. J Toxicol Cutan Ocul Toxicol 1992; 11(3):193–197.
8. Boisits EK: The evaluation of moisturizing products. Cosmet Toilet 1986; 101:31–39.
9. Wu MS, Yee DJ, Sullivan ME: Effect of a skin moisturizer on the water distribution in human stratum corneum. J Invest Dermatol 1983; 81:446–448.
10. Reiger MM: Skin, water and moisturization. Cosmet Toilet 1989; 104:41–51.
11. Brand HM, Brand-Garnys EE: Practical application of quantitative emolliency. Cosmet Toilet 1992; 107:93–99.
12. Shaath NA: The chemistry of sunscreens. *In* Lowe NJ, Shaath NA (eds): Sunscreens: Development, Evaluation and Regulatory Aspects. New York: Marcel Dekker, 1990; pp 223–225.
13. Wepierre J, Marty JP: Percutaneous absorption and lipids in elderly skin. J Appl Cosmetol 1988; 6:79.
14. Potts RO, Buras EM, Chrisman DA: Changes with age in the moisture content of human skin. J Invest Dermatol 1984; 82:97.
15. Van Scott JE, Yu RJ: Hyperkeratinization, corneocyte cohesion and alpha hydroxy acids. J Am Acad Dermatol 1984; 11:867–879.
16. Rieger MM: Oxidative reactions in and on skin: Mechanism and prevention. Cosmet Toilet 1993; 108:43.
17. Johnstone A: Sensitive skin and the consumer. Presentation at the First International Symposium on Irritant Contact Dermatitis, Gröningen, Neth: October 1991.
18. Draelos ZD: Contact dermatitis. *In* Draelos ZD (ed): Cosmetics in Dermatology. New York: Churchill Livingstone, 1996; pp 261–266.

CHAPTER 3

Itch

Patricia F. Bilden and Jeffrey D. Bernhard

CLINICAL APPEARANCE

Itch is defined as an unpleasant sensation that provokes the desire to scratch. It is a *symptom* of a multitude of dermatologic and internal disorders and, as such, has no characteristic rash (Fig. 3–1). It is one of the more frustrating sensations, as scratching the itch often gives initial relief, only to further intensify the itch. In addition, scratching can lead to changes in the skin and nerve receptors that make the skin more pruritic. The sensation of pruritus is occasionally severe enough to cause depression and even suicidal ideation. Pruritus can affect all ages, all ethnic groups, and all socioeconomic groups. It affects males and females and all ages, save for small infants who lack the motor skills to scratch and the verbal skills to express their sensation of itch.

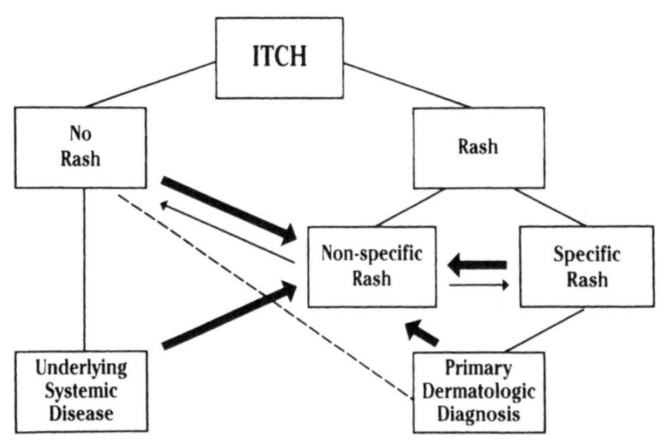

FIGURE 3–1

Connections and pathways between the causes and the manifestations of itching. The *broad arrows* represent transitions created by rubbing and scratching. The *narrow arrows* represent transitions that may occur after spontaneous or therapeutic improvement. The most important implication of this figure is that both underlying systemic and specific dermatologic diseases may present with nonspecific cutaneous changes or with no detectable cutaneous changes at all. Furthermore, a rash that is not diagnostic at one point in time may have diagnostic features at a later date. Reexamination over time is, therefore, a critical aspect of the approach to the patient with generalized pruritus or an undiagnosed pruritic eruption. (From Bernhard JD: Pruritus in skin diseases. *In* Bernhard JD [ed]: Itch: Mechanisms and Management of Pruritus. New York: McGraw-Hill, 1994; p 40. Reprinted by permission of The McGraw-Hill Companies.)

Although pruritus is frequently a sign of a dermatologic disease, many significant and sometimes fatal systemic diseases (such as Hodgkin's disease) lead to itching. Scratching may lead to a secondary, nonspecific rash that confounds the diagnostic problem. Some important diseases with pruritus as a major component include Hodgkin's lymphoma, cutaneous T-cell lymphoma, polycythemia vera, and malignancies of the gastrointestinal tract, lung, and central nervous system.[1]

This chapter considers itching in clinical situations in which a primary disease process cannot be identified or treated. Table 3–1 lists the clinical states in which pruritus is a major symptomatic problem.

Xerosis, or dry skin, is more common in the winter owing to decreased lipid production and to the fact that low humidity and heated, forced air are common living conditions. Xerosis is also a particular problem among elderly people because aged skin does not retain water as well as young skin. This can lead to extreme generalized pruritus, frequently accompanied by fine scaling and fissuring and erythema of the skin, known as *eczema*

TABLE 3-1

Causes of Pruritus

Malignancy: Hodgkin's lymphoma; non-Hodgkin's lymphoma; cutaneous T-cell lymphoma; polycythemia vera; malignancies of the gastrointestinal tract, lung, and central nervous system
Atopic dermatitis
Folliculitis: bacterial, yeast, and dermatophyte
Infestations: scabies, lice, and other mites
Pruritus of chronic renal failure
Cholestatic pruritus
Iron deficiency
Pruritus of pregnancy: pemphigoid gestationis, pruritic urticarial papules and plaques of pregnancy, prurigo of pregnancy, cholestasis of pregnancy
Psychiatric disease: neurotic excoriations, delusions of parasitosis
Allergic contact dermatitis, irritant contact dermatitis
Aging
Prurigo nodularis, lichen simplex chronicus
Lichen planus
Human immunodeficiency virus: infection, infestation, seborrheic dermatitis, psoriasis, atopic dermatitis, drug exanthem, urticaria, eosinophilic pustular folliculitis, iron deficiency, folliculitis
Exanthematous eruptions
Urticaria
Endocrine disease: thyroid disease, diabetes, mastocytosis
Aquagenic pruritus
Psoriasis

craquelé. It is often worsened by bathing but responds to hydration therapy.

TREATMENT OF PRURITUS AND XEROSIS[2]

Pruritus

Because pruritus has such a multitude of causes, the treatment needs to be tailored to the specific cause. In the absence of a diagnosis, repeated efforts must be made to establish one. General principles include the use of topical corticosteroids to decrease inflammation, systemic H_1 antihistamines to decrease pruritus when it is histamine-related or to cause drowsiness when it is not, topical or systemic antibiotics to counter diagnosed infection, topical antihistamines to deal locally with pruritus, and hydration in the form of bland emollients and hydrating baths (oilated colloidal oatmeal baths). Topical corticosteroids are divided into ultrapotent (e.g., clobetasol propionate [Temovate], diflorasone diacetate [Psorcon]), high potency (e.g., halcinonide [Halog], fluocinonide [Lidex]), medium potency (e.g., hydrocortisone valerate [Westcort], alclometasone dipropionate [Aclovate]), and low potency (1 to 2.5% hydrocortisone). Systemic H_1 antihistamines include sedating (hydroxyzine, diphenhydramine, chlorpheniramine) and nonsedating (terfenadine, astemizole, loratadine) types. Topical anesthetics include pramoxine and pramoxine plus hydrocortisone. Doxepin (Zonalon) is a topical antihistamine. Colloidal oatmeal is antipruritic, and if the oilated version is used, additional hydration is achieved through the bath.

Xerosis

Older skin has less natural lubrication and is subjected to low-humidity heated air through most of the winter. It can become quite eczematous. Hydration by bathing daily followed by emollient application is the mainstay of therapy. Treatment also includes increasing the humidity in the air with a humidifier, avoiding harsh detergents, avoiding hot water (which is quite drying), and liberally applying emollients, preferably ointment-based. These should be applied immediately after bathing and at one other time of the day. Examples of good bland emollients include Moisturel cream, DML Forte or lotion, Curel, Eucerin, and petroleum jelly. Excellent humectants, which actually draw moisture into the skin, include Lac-Hydrin 12% lotion (ammonium lactate) and the numerous alpha-hydroxy preparations available over-the-counter, such as Penecare cream or Lubriderm Moisture Recovery Lotion. One caveat with the use of these creams and lotions is that they will cause stinging if applied to broken or fissured skin. Occasionally, severely xerotic and inflamed skin will require a low- to midpotency topical steroid applied twice a day for a short period of time.

PITFALLS AND PROBLEMS

Both acute and chronic pruritus are incredibly frustrating to patients. Many want and expect instantaneous relief, so expectations must be managed. Many are also disheartened that the cause of their condition is not clear and it is not curable, only treatable.

Long-term use of topical corticosteroids, even low-potency ones, can lead to atrophy, striae formation, telangiectasia, or even a rebound effect of the condition if the steroid is stopped abruptly. Patients must be cautioned about these side effects.

Most importantly in generalized pruritus, with or

without a rash, is the possibility of underlying systemic disease. The physician must remain vigilant to this and physically reexamine the patient and repeat laboratory work periodically.

REFERRAL GUIDELINES

Referral to a dermatologist should be considered (1) when the diagnosis is in question, (2) if there is a lack of response, or (3) if refractory chronic disease such as psoriasis or eczema is present. Ultraviolet B or psoralen plus ultraviolet A phototherapy treatment requires referral to an appropriate physician or facility.

REFERENCES

1. Goldman BD, Koh HK: Pruritus and malignancy. *In* Bernhard JD (ed): Itch: Mechanisms and Management of Pruritus. New York: McGraw-Hill, 1994; pp 299–319.
2. Bernhard JD: General principles, overview, and miscellaneous treatments of itching. *In* Bernhard JD (ed): Itch: Mechanisms and Management of Pruritus. New York: McGraw-Hill, 1994; pp 367–381.

BIBLIOGRAPHY

Bernhard JD (ed): Itch: Mechanisms and Management of Pruritus. New York: McGraw-Hill, 1994.

Greaves MW: Pathophysiology and clinical aspects of pruritus. *In* Fitzpatrick TB, Eisen AZ, Wolff K, et al (eds): Dermatology in General Medicine. 4th ed. New York: McGraw-Hill, 1993; pp 413–421.

CHAPTER 4

Important Considerations for Topical Corticosteroid Therapy

Daniel B. Dubin and Kenneth A. Arndt

Topical corticosteroids constitute mainstay therapy for superficial inflammatory dermatoses. The key to the successful use of topical corticosteroids is to closely match drug potency and delivery to severity of disease. The chemical structure of the steroid, the delivery vehicle, the epidermal thickness and hydration of the affected site, and the concomitant use of dressings all influence the potency of topical corticosteroids. Less-potent corticosteroids will barely budge nonfacial acute allergic contact dermatitis; on the other hand, indiscriminate use of potent corticosteroids for mild to moderate dermatoses, especially over the face, can rapidly induce atrophy and telangiectasia. Specific guidelines for designing topical corticoid therapy are detailed in this chapter.

MECHANISM OF ACTION

On the molecular level, corticosteroids penetrate cutaneous cell membranes and bind to cytosolic steroid receptors. These receptor–steroid ligand complexes translocate to the nucleus, where they bind to specific gene regulatory elements and either enhance or inhibit the transcription of certain genes. As a consequence of these molecular events, topical corticosteroids exert a broad spectrum of anti-inflammatory effects including decreasing neutrophil emigration into sites of cutaneous inflammation, suppressing helper T-cell proliferation, and inhibiting the production of inflammatory mediators, such as interleukins 1, 2, and 6, prostaglandins, leukotrienes, interferon-gamma, tumor necrosis factor, and colony-stimulating factors.

POTENCY

Modification of both the ring structure and the side chains of cortisone has resulted in the development of a vast array of topical corticosteroids of varying activities (Fig. 4–1*A*). Within a finite range, increases in concentration of a particular corticosteroid in a defined vehicle will increase potency. However, once the concentration is optimized, permeability, stability, and steroid receptor affinity of a topical steroid preparation limit potency. Application of topical corticosteroids beyond local receptor saturation will not increase local efficacy and may result in increased systemic absorption. Epidermal integrity and thickness, delivery vehicle, hydrophilicity of the corticosteroid, chemical stability, and occlusive dressings all influence epidermal penetration.

Psoriatic and eczematous lesions are significantly

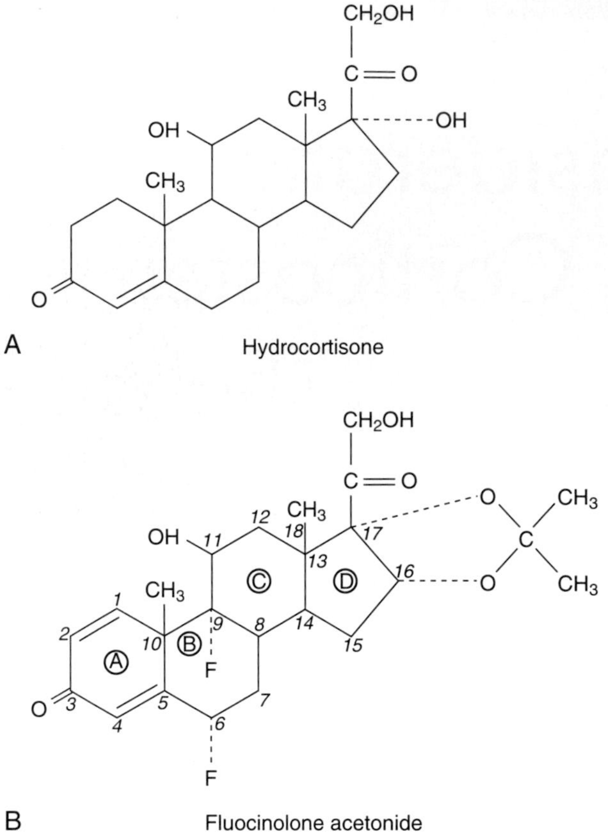

A Hydrocortisone

B Fluocinolone acetonide

FIGURE 4-1

Corticosteroid structures. *A*, Hydrocortisone. *B*, Fluocinolone acetonide (with basic corticosteroid labeling shown).

more permeable to topical corticosteroids than undiseased skin. Anatomic regions with thin epidermis are significantly more permeable to topical steroids than thick-skinned areas; for example, scrotal skin absorbs topical steroids 42 times more avidly than forearm skin. As a rule of thumb, ointment preparations of a particular topical corticosteroid allow better percutaneous drug absorption and are, therefore, more potent than corresponding cream formulations. One exception to this rule—beware that superpotent topical corticosteroids, for example, betamethasone dipropionate (Diprolene AF) cream, may be packaged in ''optimized'' cream vehicles.

Hydrophilic corticosteroids most readily penetrate the stratum corneum. However, lipophilic compounds are more efficient at entering viable cells and binding to cytosolic corticoid receptors, thus resulting in physiologically more potent corticoid compounds. Esterification at the 16 and 17 positions enhances potency by increasing lipophilicity. Introduction of a C1-2 double bond into the A ring structure renders the corticosteroid resistant to metabolic inactivation, thus increasing longevity and potency. Fluorination at the 6 or 9 position, or both, enhances steroid receptor binding and potency (Fig. 4–1*B*).

Occlusive dressings promote cutaneous hydration and significantly increase absorption and potency. Among several local physiologic effects, topical corticosteroids induce cutaneous vasoconstriction commensurate with their potency. The standard vasoconstriction bioassay provides potency measurements that correlate well with clinical anti-inflammatory efficacy. For practical purposes, topical steroids can be subdivided into four groups: superpotent (Class I), potent (Classes II to III), intermediate (Classes IV–V), and mild (Classes VI to VII) (Table 4–1). A Class I topical steroid, such as clobetasol propionate (Temovate) ointment, is about 1000 times more potent than 1% hydrocortisone. It is helpful for clinicians to be well acquainted with one or two ointments, creams, and lotions from each of these groups in order to provide a solid framework from which to initiate therapy of inflammatory dermatoses. Table 4–2 details the indications and precautions for the use of each class of topical corticosteroid.

ANATOMIC CONSIDERATIONS IN ADULTS (Fig. 4–2)

Superpotent corticosteroids, generally, are reserved for severe dermatoses over nonfacial/nonintertriginous areas. They are especially useful over the palms and soles, which maintain a thick stratum corneum and thus resist topical corticosteroid penetration. Potent to intermediate-strength topical corticosteroids are appropriate for moderate to mild nonfacial/nonintertriginous dermatoses as well as for severe to moderate facial/intertriginous dermatoses, respectively. Eyelid and genital dermatoses should be initially managed with 1 to 2.5% hydrocortisone. Treat facial, intertriginous, and genital dermatoses for short 1- to 2-week intervals, as these areas are most susceptible to corticosteroid-induced atrophy, telangiectasia, and acneiform eruption. Extra care is required when treating the eyelids, since posterior cataracts and glaucoma may complicate long-term application of topical corticosteroids.

PEDIATRIC CONSIDERATIONS

As a general rule, children under 12 years old should not use topical corticosteroids of greater than intermediate

TABLE 4-1

Topical Corticosteroid Potency

Class	Examples
I (Most potent)	Betamethasone dipropionate cream, ointment 0.05% (optimized vehicle) (Diprolene) Clobetasol propionate cream, ointment 0.05% (optimized vehicle) (Temovate) Diflorasone diacetate ointment 0.05% (optimized vehicle) (Psorcon) Halobetasol propionate cream, ointment 0.05% (Ultravate)
II	Amcinonide ointment 0.1% (Cyclocort) Augmented betamethasone dipropionate cream 0.05% (Diprolene AF) Betamethasone dipropionate ointment 0.05% (Diprosone) Desoximetasone cream, ointment 0.25% (Topicort) Desoximetasone gel 0.05% (Topicort) Diflorasone diacetate ointment 0.05% (Florone, Maxiflor) Fluocinonide cream, gel, ointment (0.05%) (Lidex) Halcinonide 0.1% cream (Halog) Mometasone furoate ointment 0.1% (Elocon) Triamcinolone acetonide ointment 0.5% (Kenalog)
III	Amcinonide cream, lotion 0.1% (Cyclocort) Betamethasone benzoate gel 0.025% (Benisone, Uticort) Betamethasone dipropionate cream 0.05% (Diprosone) Betamethasone valerate ointment 0.1% (Valisone) Desoximetasone emollient cream 0.05% (Topicort LP) Diflorasone diacetate cream 0.05% (Florone, Maxiflor) Fluticasone propionate ointment 0.005% (Cutivate) Fluocinonide cream 0.05% (Lidex E) Halcinonide ointment 0.1% (Halog) Triamcinolone acetonide ointment 0.1% (Aristocort A), cream 0.5% (Aristocort-HP)
IV	Betamethasone benzoate ointment 0.025% (Benisone, Uticort) Betamethasone valerate lotion 0.1% (Valisone) Desoximetasone cream 0.05% (Topicort LP) Fluocinolone acetonide cream 0.2% (Synalar-HP) Fluocinolone acetonide ointment 0.025% (Synalar) Flurandrenolide ointment 0.05% (Cordran) Halcinonide cream 0.025% (Halog) Hydrocortisone valerate ointment 0.2% (Westcort) Mometasone furoate cream 0.1% (Elocon) Triamcinolone acetonide ointment 0.1% (Aristocort, Kenalog)
V	Betamethasone benzoate cream 0.025% (Benisone, Uticort) Betamethasone dipropionate lotion 0.02% (Diprosone) Betamethasone valerate cream 0.1% (Betatrex, Valisone) Clocortolone cream 0.1% (Cloderm) Fluocinolone acetonide cream 0.025% (Fluonid, Synalar) Fluocinolone acetonide oil 0.01% (Derma-Smoothe/FS) Flurandrenolide cream 0.05% (Cordran SP) Fluticasone propionate cream 0.05% (Cutivate) Hydrocortisone butyrate cream 0.1% (Locoid) Hydrocortisone valerate cream 0.2% (Westcort) Predincarbate 0.1% cream (Dermatop) Triamcinolone acetonide cream 0.025% (Artistocort)
VI	Aclometasone dipropionate cream, ointment 0.05% (Aclovate) Betamethasone valerate lotion 0.1% (Valisone) Desonide cream 0.05% (DesOwen, Tridesilon) Fluocinolone acetonide cream, solution 0.01% (Synalar) Triamcinolone acetonide cream, lotion 0.1% (Kenalog)
VII (Least potent)	Dexamethasone sodium phosphate cream 0.1% (Decadron Phosphate) Hydrocortisone 0.5%, 1.0%, 2.5% (generic, Hytone, others)

From Arndt KA: Manual of Dermatologic Therapeutics. 5th ed. Boston: Little, Brown, 1994; adapted from Cornell RC, Stoughton RB: Use of topical steroids in psoriasis. Dermatol Clin 1984; 2:399; and Stoughton RB, Cornell RC: Review of super-potent topical corticosteroids. Semin Dermatol 1987; 6:73.

TABLE 4-2

Indications and Precautions for Selecting Topical Corticosteroid Potency

Class	Indications and Precautions
Class I	Severe inflammatory dermatoses in adults
	Acute allergic contact dermatitis
	Palm/sole inflammatory dermatoses
	Avoid usage in children under 12 years old
	Do not use on face, groin, axillae, under breasts
Classes II–III	Severe inflammatory dermatoses in children or on adult facial (noneyelid) or intertriginous skin; use for no longer than 5–7 days
	Moderate inflammatory dermatoses in adults
Classes IV–V	Mild inflammatory dermatoses in adults
	Moderate inflammatory dermatoses in children or on adult facial (noneyelid) or intertriginous skin
Classes VI–VII	Eyelid and genital skin inflammatory dermatoses
	Very mild inflammatory dermatoses or maintenance therapy in adults
	Mild inflammatory dermatoses in children or on adult facial (noneyelid) or intertriginous skin
	Start with 1–2.5% hydrocortisone

strength; however, very severe inflammatory dermatoses may merit 5- to 14-day courses of potent corticosteroids. Superpotent topical corticosteroids should be avoided in young children. Application of mild- or intermediate-potency corticosteroids to large areas or focally under occlusion may result in systemic absorption sufficient to suppress the hypothalamic-pituitary-adrenal (HPA) axis in children.

VEHICLE CHOICE

Although ointments often provide optimal cutaneous penetration of a corticosteroid moiety, they are cosmetically displeasing owing to their greasy texture and potential for staining apparel. Overnight application of ointments often alleviates these cosmetic concerns. Ointments rarely sting or burn when applied to injured epidermis. Creams can be rubbed entirely into the skin and are often more cosmetically appealing than ointments, but creams sometimes sting dermatitic skin and diminish patient compliance with therapy. Lotions, solutions, and gels are most suitable for hair-bearing areas. However, since many of these vehicles contain alcohol, they tend to sting the most. Newer water-based gels tend not to sting and are particularly useful in weepy acute contact dermatitis. Benzocaine (Orabase) is a resilient base that is useful for delivering topical steroids to the oral mucosa. Oral suspensions and aerosolized steroids are alternative vehicles for mucous membrane therapy. Keratolytic preparations, such as salicylic acid, or alpha-hydroxy acids, such as lactic acid (e.g., Lac-Hydrin 12% lotion) or glycolic acid, may benefit the treatment of hyperkeratotic inflammatory dermatoses by enhancing cutaneous penetration of topical corticosteroids.

FREQUENCY OF APPLICATION

Dosing of topical corticosteroids more frequently than two to three times daily is neither indicated nor of proven benefit for nonmucosal, superficial inflammatory dermatoses. Once- to twice-daily application is sufficient. In fact, recent studies suggest that once-daily application of superpotent topical corticosteroids is just as effective as twice-daily dosing and may result in less systemic absorption and fewer local side effects. Oral mucosal inflammatory disorders, however, require three- to five-times-daily application in order to ensure delivery of an effective dose.

Self-limited dermatoses such as acute contact dermatitis can be relatively safely managed with twice-daily application of a superpotent topical steroid for 2 to 3 weeks. However, chronic disorders such as atopic dermatitis and psoriasis require management of acute flares with potent therapy, followed by careful tapering to an acceptable maintenance regimen. After achieving control of the disease flare, usually within 1 to 2 weeks, reduction of dosing from twice daily to once daily to every other day to twice weekly should be encouraged. Application of lubricants between doses often allows patients to smoothly taper the frequency of application. Successful reduction of dosing frequency should be followed by a substitution of potent topical corticosteroids with lubricants and judicious application of mild- to intermediate-strength preparations to quell signs of reflares. To achieve optimal penetration and efficacy, topical steroids should be applied to moist skin after bathing or soaking in water.

TACHYPHYLAXIS

Repeated application of potent topical steroids may result in diminished efficacy as early as 1 week after institution of therapy. Restoration of efficacy usually returns within 4 days of withholding topical steroids. To avoid tachyphylaxis when managing chronic in-

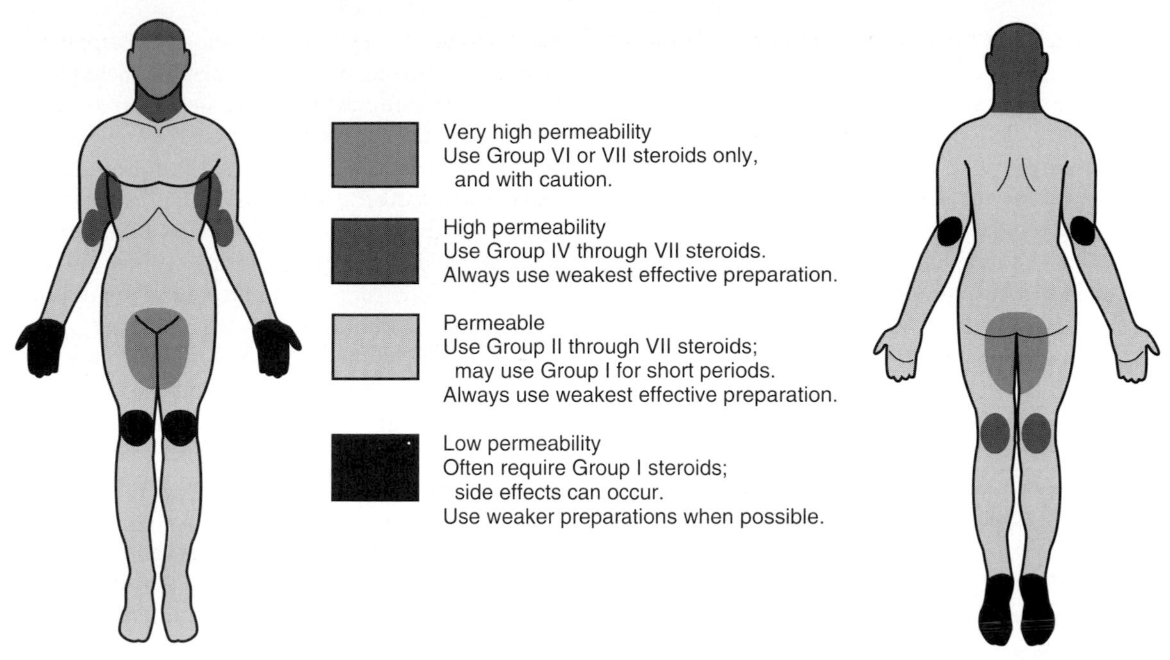

FIGURE 4-2

Regions of skin permeability. (Redrawn by permission of the publisher from Trozak DJ: Topical corticosteroid therapy in psoriasis vulgaris. Cutis 46:341–350. Copyright 1990 by Quadrant Healthcom, Inc.)

flammatory dermatoses, potent topical steroid therapy should be tapered, if possible, within 2 weeks, after which patients should be encouraged to attempt pulse therapy consisting of twice-daily application for 1 or 2 consecutive days each week; bland lubricants should be liberally applied on off days.

OCCLUSIVE DRESSINGS

Occlusive dressings prevent normal transepidermal water loss, thus creating a well-hydrated epidermis that is optimally receptive to penetration of topical corticosteroids. Occlusion can enhance topical corticosteroid potency by as much as 100-fold. Cellophane wraps, for example, Saran Wrap, secured with paper tape, plastic bags for the feet, vinyl gloves, plastic shower caps for the scalp, as well as plastic suits and wraps are available for occlusive topical corticosteroid therapy. Before occlusive therapy, bathe the affected area to remove keratotic debris and moisten the skin.

Erythroderma due to psoriasis or atopic dermatitis is typically initially managed with intermediate- to mild-potency topical corticoids, for example, fluocinolone acetonide (Synalar) 0.025% ointment, under occlusion twice to once daily for 6-hour periods for several days to achieve disease control. Be aware that topical corticosteroid therapy of erythroderma will be accompanied by a pharmacologically significant systemic dose. A recent report suggests that 1 to 2 days of betamethasone dipropionate in optimized vehicle (Diprolene) ointment, a superpotent agent, under occlusion hastens resolution of erythroderma and can shorten hospitalization. Occlusive therapy must not be abruptly halted even though rapid improvement is often noted within 1 to 3 days, as rebound flares will occur; gradual tapering to nonocclusive treatment is necessary. Furthermore, it is essential not to assess patients shortly after removing their wraps, as the vasoconstrictive effects of topical steroids can mask the erythema of an active inflammatory process. Alternatively, the baths that precede occlusive therapy dilate cutaneous vasculature and heighten erythema. Patients are best examined shortly before pretreatment bathing.

Certain localized chronic inflammatory dermatoses, such as atopic dermatitis, lichen simplex chronicus, psoriasis, lichen planus, and prurigo nodularis, are greatly exacerbated by scratching and picking. Therefore, occlusive dressings not only optimize permeability but also protect inflammatory lesions and permit topical steroids to work optimally. Flurandrenolide (Cordran) tape is an occlusive dressing, impregnated with an intermediate-strength corticosteroid, that offers a convenient option for providing potent corticosteroid therapy to localized inflammatory lesions. Hydrocolloid bioocclusive dressings (e.g., DuoDerm extra thin) applied over potent to intermediate-strength steroid ointments and left in place for 3 to 7 days are very helpful in managing thick chronic inflammatory dermatoses. Plastic shower cap occlusion enhances the ability of steroid solutions to ameliorate scalp inflammatory dermatoses, such as refractory seborrheic dermatitis and psoriasis. The potential side effects of occlusive therapy include irritancy from sweat retention, folliculitis, and systemic absorption that may suppress the HPA axis.

SIDE EFFECTS

Cutaneous

Superpotent and potent topical corticosteroids may induce atrophy, telangiectasia, and striae as early as 2 to 3 weeks following daily application. Purpura may be noted in atrophic areas, especially in thin-skinned areas. However, inappropriate chronic use of intermediate- or mild-potency topical corticosteroids can induce similar changes. Intertriginous and thin-skinned highly penetrable areas are particularly susceptible to atrophic changes. Corticosteroid-induced cutaneous atrophy usually recovers within weeks to months if therapy is discontinued as soon as atrophic changes are noted. Use potent topical corticosteroids sparingly when treating conditions such as cutaneous collagen vascular disease, for example, dermatomyositis, and stasis dermatitis, disorders whose natural course predisposes to cutaneous atrophy. Prolonged use of topical steroids may induce an acneiform eruption characterized by monomorphous follicular pustules that resolve with discontinuance of corticosteroid treatment, usually without scarring. Chronic application of topical steroids to the face may induce a dry, scaly eruption with scattered follicular pustules around the mouth, termed *perioral dermatitis*.

Although topical steroids may initially soothe the burning pustular inflammation associated with moderate to severe rosacea, abrupt discontinuance of therapy is frequently followed by a severe rebound vasodilatory flare that prompts patients to use topical corticosteroids chronically. Such chronic application of topical steroids in rosacea often leads to marked atrophy and telangiectasia; however, withdrawal of steroids, although mandatory, must consist of gradual tapering to avoid severe rebound flares. Similar steroid withdrawal syndromes may be encountered in patients using topical corticosteroids chronically to treat anogenital inflammatory dermatoses. Tapering of topical therapy includes gradual reduction of both potency and dosing frequency at 2-week intervals until steroid use is completely discontinued. Topical anesthetics or antipruritics such as pramoxine (PrameGel), lidocaine and prilocaine (EMLA) cream, or doxepin (Zonalon) cream are useful in decreasing patient discomfort during withdrawal.

Topical corticosteroids predispose to the development of cutaneous fungal infections. Signs of fungal or bacterial skin infections or scabetic infestation may be masked by inappropriate use of topical corticosteroids. Ironically, allergic sensitization to topical corticosteroid preparations also occurs. Most often, vehicles or preservatives are the sensitizing agents; however, contact allergy against the steroid moiety itself is possible. Topical corticosteroid–induced contact allergy should be suspected in patients with chronic dermatoses that appear to be exacerbated by topical corticosteroid therapy. If substitution with hypoallergenic steroid ointments devoid of preservatives, for example, fluocinolone acetonide 0.025% ointment, does not improve the condition, referral to a dermatologist experienced in patch-testing should be considered. Chronic periorbital application of topical steroids can precipitate glaucoma and, rarely, induce posterior subcapsular cataracts.

Systemic

Topical corticosteroids may induce HPA axis suppression. High-potency corticosteroids, chronic use, application to highly permeable areas, treatment of large areas, the use of occlusion, poor skin integrity, liver failure, and young age are factors that render HPA axis suppression more likely. Patients with chronic, relapsing, erythrodermic inflammatory dermatoses are particularly susceptible not only to HPA axis suppression but also to the side effects typically associated with chronic oral or parenteral therapy, such as osteoporosis and exogenous Cushing's syndrome. One to 2.5% hydrocortisone should be initially tried in all children with atopic dermatitis, since widespread routine use of even mild corticosteroids in young children frequently induces HPA axis suppression. Topical corticosteroid–induced growth retardation is always a concern in young children with severe atopic dermatitis. The HPA axis returns to normal within days to weeks, depending on the duration, intensity, and extent of topical steroid therapy. Insidious onset of asthenia, weakness, weight loss, hypotension, and gastrointestinal disturbances indicates significant topical corticosteroid–induced adrenal insufficiency. Patients with adrenal insufficiency demonstrate decreased morning blood cortisol or 24-hour urinary free-cortisol levels as well as blunted adrenal cortisol production in response to parenteral adrenocorticotropic hormone.

COST (Table 4–3)

The brand name superpotent and potent topical corticosteroids tend to cost $15 to $25/15 g; brand name intermediate- to mild-potency corticosteroids garner less than $10 to $15/15 g. Prescribing in bulk quantities, that is, 45- to 60-g tubes to ½-pound jars, significantly lowers the cost per gram of topical steroids. Without surprise, generic preparations tend to be considerably less expensive than comparable brand names. However, generic topical corticosteroid preparations may bear potencies 25 to 75% lower than those of comparable brand name products. Brand name preparations provide the most reliable efficacy. Generic preparations of fluocinonide, triamcinolone acetonide, fluocinolone acetonide, and hydrocortisone offer less-expensive alternatives to patients on tight budgets or restricted by health plan formularies.

TREATMENT OF SELECTED DERMATOSES

Table 4–4 provides guidelines for the topical treatment of selected dermatoses.

INTRALESIONAL CORTICOSTEROID THERAPY

Intralesional triamcinolone acetonide injection can rapidly improve localized plaques of hypertrophic inflammatory dermatoses, such as lichenified psoriasis or eczema, that are refractory to topical therapy. Other conditions that are treated with intralesional corticosteroids include bullous pemphigoid, pemphigus vulgaris, inflammatory acne lesions, inflamed epidermal inclusion cysts, alopecia areata, hypertrophic and keloidal scars, and granuloma annulare.

Overdosing of intralesional triamcinolone acetonide will cause cutaneous atrophy that is often reversible but may be unsightly for several months. Therefore, for facial inflammatory acne lesions, triamcinolone should be diluted to 1 to 3 mg/ml, and only 0.1 to 0.2 ml of corticosteroid should be injected per lesion. Dilutions may be made in sterile saline solution or in 1% lidocaine (Xylocaine) with epinephrine. Injections should be delivered through a 30-gauge needle to allow for optimal control of dosing.

The goal of injection therapy is to insert enough material to slightly distend the dermis. Treatment of nonfacial dermatoses should begin at 5 to 10 mg/ml of triamcinolone, depending on lesion severity. Thick hypertrophic scars and keloids may require 20 to 40 mg/ml, but try 10 mg/ml initially. Thick scars provide marked resistance to injection; therefore, the needle should be completely inserted into the scar and the

TABLE 4–3

Cost of Selected Corticosteroids*

Class	Topical Corticosteroid	Brand	Generic†
I	Temovate (clobetasol propionate) ointment	$37.59/30 g	$29.90/30 g
II	Diprolene AF (betamethasone dipropionate) cream	$63.59/45 g	
II	Elocon (mometasone furoate) ointment	$33.79/45 g	
II	Lidex (fluocinonide) ointment	$34.89/30 g	$43.49/60 g
II	Lidex (fluocinonide) cream	$50.99/60 g	$18.49/60 g
III	Lidex E (fluocinonide) cream	$55.59/60 g	$25.99/60 g
III	Aristocort A (triamcinolone acetonide) 0.1% ointment	$ 9.17/15 g	$ 4.76/15 g
IV	Westcort (hydrocortisone valerate) ointment	$36.59/45 g	
IV	Synalar (fluocinolone acetonide) 0.025% ointment	$73.99/60 g	$32.19/60 g
V	Diprosone (betamethasone dipropionate) 0.02% lotion	$16.91/20 ml	$ 9.89/20 ml
V	Synalar (fluocinolone acetonide) 0.025% cream	$23.75/30 g	$ 8.99/30 g
VI	Synalar (fluocinolone acetonide) 0.1% solution	$22.30/20 ml	$ 7.28/20 ml
VI	Synalar (fluocinolone acetonide) 0.1% cream	$14.12/15 g	$ 3.77/15 g
VI	DesOwen (desonide) cream	$16.82/15 g	$11.96/15 g
VII	Hytone (hydrocortisone) 2.5% ointment	$27.79/30 g	$13.79/30 g
VII	Hytone (hydrocortisone) 2.5% cream	$23.49/30 g	$ 8.69/30 g

*From CVS Pharmacy, Boston.

†The potencies of generic preparations of topical corticosteroids may be significantly less than those of comparable brand name products.

TABLE 4-4

Treatment Guidelines for Selected Dermatoses

Disease	Potency	Vehicle	Comments
Psoriasis			
Intertriginous/face	Mild	Ointment	Treat as sparingly as possible to avoid atrophy and fungal infection
Scalp	Mild to intermediate	Solution	Apply at bedtime under shower cap
Localized, other areas	Intermediate to superpotent	Ointment or optimized cream	Start with intermediate strength and advance potency if necessary May require occlusion Once control is achieved, pulse therapy 1–3 times per week can prevent tachyphylaxis
Erythrodermic	Intermediate to superpotent	Ointment	Under occlusive wraps until control is achieved Systemic absorption a concern
Seborrheic dermatitis	Mild to intermediate	Cream, lotion, solution, ointment	Use mild agents on face and intertriginous areas Solutions and lotions are useful in hair-bearing areas
Atopic dermatitis	Mild to potent depending on extent, age, severity	Ointment, emollient creams	Taper to steroid-free emollients as soon as possible
Irritant dermatitis	Intermediate to superpotent	Ointment	Apply under cotton or vinyl gloves at bedtime for hand dermatitis
Acute allergic contact dermatitis	Superpotent to potent	Gel or cream	Apply after soaking affected area
Chronic allergic contact dermatitis	Intermediate to potent	Ointment, emollient cream, impregnated tape	Eliminate sensitizing agent from environment if possible
Lichen simplex chronicus, prurigo nodularis	Superpotent to potent	Ointment, impregnated tape, hydrocolloid dressing	Lesions may require occlusion or intralesional corticosteroid injection
Cutaneous lupus erythematosus	Potent to superpotent	Ointment	Variably responsive
Dermatomyositis	Mild to intermediate	Ointment, emollient cream	Atrophic side effects more likely
Lichen planus	Intermediate to superpotent	Ointment, optimized cream	Difficult to control
Lichen sclerosus	Superpotent	Ointment, optimized cream	Only superpotent agents are effective in improving vulvovaginal disease Exception to rule of not applying superpotent agents in intertriginous areas
Vitiligo	Superpotent to potent	Ointment, optimized cream	Frequently not effective Not practical in widespread disease
Alopecia areata	Superpotent	Ointment, optimized cream	Frequently not effective
Patch stage cutaneous T-cell lymphoma	Potent to superpotent	Ointment, cream	Helps symptoms and signs of early-stage disease; not curative
Chronic cutaneous graft versus host disease	Potent to intermediate	Ointment, cream	Helps symptoms
Drug hypersensitivity reactions (not toxic epidermal necrolysis or erythema multiforme)	Potent to intermediate	Ointment, cream	Vasoconstrictive properties help symptoms of burning and itching; does not alter course of eruption Discontinue use when symptoms abate
Insect bites	Superpotent	Ointment, optimized cream	Treat for no more than 2–3 weeks
Pyoderma gangrenosum	Superpotent	Ointment	May be useful under occlusion in limited disease; however, frequently not adequate Rule out infection before implementing treatment
Bullous pemphigoid/ pemphigus vulgaris	Superpotent to potent	Ointment	Often useful in controlling limited disease Can also help while tapering systemic immunosuppressive therapy
Cutaneous sarcoid	Superpotent	Ointment	Frequently not effective
Aphthous ulcers	Superpotent	Water-based gel, ointment	Apply 3–5 times per day Triamcinolone acetonide in benzocaine (Orabase) as well as dexamethasone (Decadron) suspension swish for 5–10 minutes and spit are also effective

plunger of the syringe should be firmly depressed as the needle is slowly withdrawn. Multiple passes may be necessary. Light freezing with liquid nitrogen before treatment may induce lesional edema that can facilitate injection.

Since systemic absorption is expected, intralesional therapy should be limited to 40 to 60 mg total per session. Individual areas should be injected no more frequently than once per month. If presumed inflammatory lesions either do not improve or worsen with intralesional therapy, one should consider biopsy to rule out a cutaneous neoplasm or perform biopsy/cultures to rule out infectious etiologies.

SHORT-COURSE SYSTEMIC THERAPY FOR ACUTE ALLERGIC DERMATITIS

Acute allergic contact dermatitis that is extensive or involves the periorbital area may be best treated with a short course of oral prednisone. In adults, we recommend a 15-day course of prednisone consisting of 60 mg every morning for days 1 to 5, followed by 40 mg every morning for days 6 to 10, then 20 mg for days 11 to 15. Pediatric prednisone dosing guidelines are 1.0 mg/kg for days 1 to 5, 0.5 mg/kg for days 6 to 10, and 0.25 mg/kg for days 11 to 15.

Short-course therapy does not induce the side effects associated with chronic prednisone therapy, such as osteoporotic fractures, central obesity, proximal myopathy, hirsutism, growth retardation, and significant HPA axis suppression. However, the remote possibility of idiosyncratic femoral neck avascular necrosis should be discussed. The complications of short-course therapy include mood alterations, mild and reversible facial edema, derangement of glucose control in diabetic patients, exacerbation of existing peptic ulcer disease, elevation of blood pressure in hypertensive patients, and further immune suppression in immunocompromised hosts.

Prednisone should not be used to treat psoriasis, as rebound flares can be severe and refractory to topical treatment. Systemic therapy should also be avoided in patients with atopic dermatitis; although these patients respond dramatically, they become dependent on systemic therapy and face the side effects of chronic maintenance therapy. The systemic corticosteroid treatment of bullous disorders, refractory cutaneous collagen vascular disease, and neutrophilic dermatoses is beyond the scope of this chapter.

BIBLIOGRAPHY

Aalto-Korte K, Turpeinen M: Pharmacokinetics of topical hydrocortisone at plasma level after applications once or twice daily in patients with widespread dermatitis. Br J Dermatol 1995; 133:259–263.

Arbiser JL, Grossman K, Kaye E, Arndt KA: Use of short-course class I topical glucocorticoid under occlusion for the rapid control of erythrodermic psoriasis. Arch Dermatol 1994; 130:704–706.

Arndt KA: Manual of Dermatologic Therapeutics. 5th ed. Boston: Little, Brown, 1994; pp 299–308.

Arndt KA, Jorizzo JL: Which topical corticosteroid—And when? Patient Care 1992; May, pp 115–134.

Cornell RC, Stoughton RB: Correlation of the vasoconstrictor assay and clinical activity in psoriasis. Arch Dermatol 1985; 121:63–67.

Feldman SR: The biology and clinical application of systemic glucocorticosteroids. Curr Probl Dermatol 1992; 4:207–234.

Hurwitz S: Clinical Pediatric Dermatology. 2nd ed. Philadelphia: WB Saunders, 1993; pp 57–59.

Katz HI: Topical corticosteroids. Dermatol Clin 1995; 4:805–815.

Ling M: The message in the medium. How and why to choose a vehicle. Fitzpatrick's J Clin Dermatol 1995; 3:13–19.

Singh S, Gopal J, Mishra RN, Pandey SS: Topical 0.05% betamethasone dipropionate: Efficacy in psoriasis with once a day vs. twice a day application. Br J Dermatol 1995; 133:497–498.

Stoughton RB: Are generic formulations equivalent to trade name topical glucocorticoids? Arch Dermatol 1987; 123:1312–1314.

SECTION

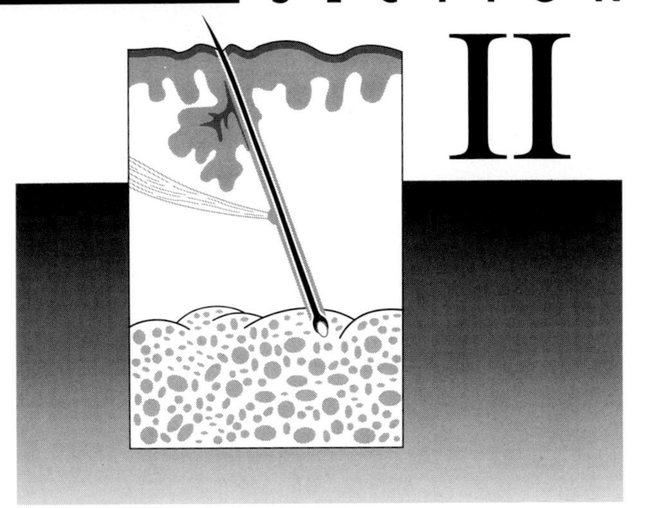

II

What Are the Common Dermatologic Disorders and How Are They Treated?

CHAPTER 5

Abscess

Geetinder Kaus Chattha

CLINICAL APPEARANCE

Definition

An abscess is a localized collection of purulent material in a cavity formed by disintegration or necrosis of tissue.[1] The etiology is infectious in virtually all instances, except in the case of a sterile abscess.

Usual Appearance

The involved area is erythematous, tender, and typically fluctuant, indicating that pus has formed. The overlying skin may be thinned, and a single or multiple pustules may be evident on the surface.

Alternate Forms

Several different conditions may ultimately lead to cutaneous abscess formation. Distinct clinical syndromes include furuncles, carbuncles, hidradenitis suppurtiva, Bartholin's gland abscess, perirectal abscess, pilonidal cyst or sinus with abscess formation, paronychia, breast abscess, inflammatory bowel disease with cutaneous abscess, and dental sinus with cutaneous abscess.[2] Cutaneous abscesses may form as a result of spread from a contiguous focus, such as osteomyelitis, and cervical or thoracic actinomycosis.[3] Bacteremias, including endocarditis, may be complicated by metastatic foci of suppuration such as cutaneous abscesses.[3]

DESCRIPTION

Age/Population/Demographics

In an outpatient study of cutaneous abscesses, the most common locations are axillary, vulvovaginal, perirectal, head and neck, and buttock areas, in decreasing order of incidence in women. In men, the most common locations are head and neck, perirectal, extremity, inguinal, and axillary areas, in decreasing order of incidence.[4] Bacteria were recovered from 96% of abscesses, with the remainder being sterile.[4] Significantly, one third of these sterile abscesses occurred in intravenous drug abusers, suggesting that injected chemical irritants resulted in suppuration clinically indistinguishable from bacterial abscesses.[4]

Etiology/Pathogenesis

The infecting agent is determined in large part by the location of the abscess, reflecting the adjacent microflora of the skin and mucous membranes.[4, 5] Cultures from cutaneous abscesses may yield aerobic, anaerobic, or mixed cultures. Abscesses are usually polymicrobial, with fewer than one third yielding pure cultures.[4] When a pure culture is obtained, it is usually *Staphylococcus aureus*.[4] Mixed aerobic and anaerobic cultures can be isolated from any of the anatomic cutaneous sites; however, the highest incidence of mixed cultures occurs in the perirectal area where approximately two thirds of abscesses are infected with mixed aerobic and anaerobic bacteria.[4] The aerobes typically isolated include *S. aureus, Staphylococcus epidermidis,* aerobic streptococci, diphtheroids, *Proteus mirabilis,* and other enterobacteriaceae.[4, 5] Commonly isolated anaerobes include *Bacteroides, Clostridium, Peptostreptococcus, Propionibacterium, Lactobacillus, Eubacterium,* and *Fusobacterium* spp.[4, 5] Abscesses originating on the trunk, axilla, extremity, and hand are predominantly infected with aerobic bacteria, whereas abscesses originating in the perineal region may only contain anaerobes.[4] *S. aureus* is isolated in approximately 25% of abscesses and has been isolated from all *skin* sites, including the perineal region.[4] It is usually isolated in pure culture.[4] *S. aureus* is only rarely isolated from abscesses in the perirectal and vulvovaginal areas because these originate in mucous membranes rather than skin.

TREATMENT: GENERAL CONSIDERATIONS

Cutaneous abscesses should be treated with incision and drainage of pus. Initial Gram's stain, culture, or antibiotic therapy is not necessary when the abscess is localized and uncomplicated.[4] High-risk situations include abscesses of the central face drained by the cavernous sinus, signs of systemic infection, surrounding cellulitis, and underlying immunodeficiency states.[4] Antibiotic therapy guided by Gram's stain and culture is indicated in these circumstances.[4] The author believes that consultation is recommended for abscesses that have connections to deeper structures such as some in the perineal area and those associated with dental infections.

FURUNCLES AND CARBUNCLES

Definition, Clinical Appearance, and Natural History

A furuncle or ''boil'' is an inflammatory nodule that arises from a hair follicle and thus occurs only in hair-bearing parts of the body. Usually, it is a progression from folliculitis, a superficial infection of hair follicles. The head and neck, axillae, buttocks, and groin areas are particularly susceptible because they are moist and subject to friction. The involved area is red and hard and becomes tender and fluctuant over a period of days. It eventually discharges pus and often a central plug of necrotic material followed by resolution of pain. Eventually, the erythema subsides. This process may spread via autoinnoculation.[1–3]

A carbuncle is a deeper, more serious lesion that arises from more than one hair follicle and typically occurs on the neck, thighs, or back. A red, painful, indurated plaque develops studded with multiple pustules draining around multiple hair follicles (see Fig. 5–1 on Color Plate 1). A dull yellow-gray central crater develops that heals with scarring. Systemic symptoms such as fever and malaise are frequently present, and some patients may be acutely ill.[3] A carbuncle may be complicated by cellulitis and bacteremia.[1–3]

When furuncles occur on the central face, such as about the nose or upper lip, infection may drain via veins to the cavernous sinus, resulting in cavernous sinus thrombosis or meningitis.[3]

Demographics/Etiology/Pathogenesis

The infecting organism is *S. aureus* in nearly all cases.[2, 3] Friction, moisture, or dermatitis compromises the integrity of the skin allowing a portal of entry for *S. aureus.* Furuncles usually occur in healthy individuals; however, underlying conditions such as obesity, immunosuppression, or colonization of *S. aureus* may predispose to infection.[2, 3] Rarely, recurrent furuncles of the skin may occur as part of an underlying immune disorder; hyperimmunoglobulin E syndrome is characterized by dermatitis, immune defects, and recurrent staphylococcal abscesses of the skin.[2]

Treatment

The early stage of the furuncle may be treated with warm compresses, which promotes localization and drainage of the process. If the lesion is large and fluctuant, incision and drainage should be performed and the cavity packed with sterile gauze. When fever or evidence of surrounding cellulitis develops, an antistaphylococcal antibiotic such as dicloxicillin, 250 mg orally every 6 hours, should be added to the measures previously discussed. Alternative therapy for the penicillin-allergic patient is erythromycin, 250 to 500 mg orally every 6 hours, or clindamycin, 150 to 300 mg orally every 6 hours.[3] Antibiotic therapy should continue until systemic symptoms and local signs of erythema and swelling have resolved.

Special attention must be given to furuncles of the central face because of the risk of spread of infection to the brain, as mentioned previously. Warm compresses and prompt antibiotics should be employed. Incision should not be made unless infection does not respond to the aforementioned modalities.[3]

Pitfalls and Problems

Complications include spread of infection via the blood stream and recurrence. Rarely, bacteremic spread of infection may result in ''metastatic'' foci of infection including endocarditis, osteomyelitis, or brain abscess.[2]

When furuncles occur on the central face, such as about the nose or upper lip, infection may drain via veins to the cavernous sinus, resulting in cavernous sinus thrombosis or meningitis.[3] Recurrent furunculosis is thought to occur in individuals who are colonized with *S. aureus.* These patients frequently recolonize after each course of systemic antibiotics and develop clinical recurrence of furuncles.[6] General skin care including daily cleansing with an antimicrobial such as chlorhexidine (4%) solution may decrease skin colonization. The patient's towels should remain separate and should be washed frequently to minimize autoinnoculation of infection in the patient and to prevent spread to other family members. Further measures include attempts to eradicate staphylococcal nasal carriage. Mupirocin ointment applied daily to the anterior nares for 5 days may eliminate *S. aureus* for 3 months.[7] Rifampin, at a dose of 600 mg daily for 10 days, has been shown to eradicate nasal carriage of *S. aureus* for up to 3 months[3, 8] however, rifampin-resistant strains of staphylococci may emerge when it is given as a single agent.[3] For patients with recurrent furunculosis who have failed several courses of systemic antibiotics, a nasal culture should be obtained to confirm staphylococcal carriage. If the patient is colonized, a 14-day course of rifampin (300 mg twice daily) plus an oral antistaphylococcal antibiotic such as dicloxacillin, 250 mg orally every 6 hours, may be employed.[9]

OTHER ABSCESSES

Injection Site Abscesses

Subcutaneous and intramuscular abscesses may develop following therapeutic injections or attempts at intravenous injection by drug addicts. Abscesses in intravenous drug users are common; sharing needles, licking needles, and general lack of aseptic technique are predisposing factors.[10] The forearm is the most common location in this group.[10, 11] *S. aureus,* streptococci, and oral anaerobes are the most common infecting organisms in intravenous drug users.[11] Appropriate management is incision and drainage of pus and antibiotic therapy. A first-generation cephalosporin such as cefazolin sodium (Kefzol) in conjunction with penicillin will provide coverage for gram-positive organisms and oral anaerobes.[10] Complications include necrotizing fasciitis and osteomyelitis.[10] This author believes consultation is advised.

Sterile Abscesses

A subcutaneous abscess may occur when foreign material is introduced into the skin. The material may be identified by examination of biopsy specimens with polarizing microscopy.[3]

Infected Epidermal Cysts

Epidermal follicular cysts are sacs lined by proliferating epidermal cells, and these may occur on the head, neck, trunk, extremities, and perineal areas. They may become inflamed or, on occasion, infected, with resultant abscess formation.[3] Management of epidermal cysts is discussed in Chapter 29: Inflamed Epidermal Cysts.

REFERENCES

1. Champion RH, Burton JL: Diagnosis of skin diseases. *In* Champion RH, Burton JL, Ebling FJG (eds): Textbook of Dermatology. 5th ed. Oxford, Boston: Blackwell Scientific, 1992, p 161.
2. Swartz MN, Weinberg AN: Infections due to gram-positive bacteria. *In* Fitzpatrick TB, Eisen AZ, Wolff K, et al (eds): Dermatology in General Medicine. 4th ed. New York: McGraw-Hill, 1993; pp 2309–2333.
3. Swartz MN: Skin and soft tissue infections. *In* Mandell GL, Douglas RG, Bennet JE (eds): Principles and Practice of Infectious Diseases. 4th ed. New York, Edinburgh: Churchill Livingstone, 1995; pp 909–928.
4. Meislin HW, Lerner SA, Graves MH, et al: Cutaneous abscesses: Anaerobic and aerobic bacteriology and outpatient management. Ann Intern Med 1977; 87:145–149.
5. Brook I, Frazier EH: Aerobic and anaerobic bacteriology of wounds and cutaneous abscesses. Arch Surg 1990; 125:1445–1451.
6. Wheat LJ, Kohler RB, White A: Treatment of nasal carriers of coagulase-positive staphylococci. *In* Maibach H, Aly R (eds): Skin Microbiology: Relevance to Clinical Infection. New York: Springer-Verlag, 1981; pp 50–58.
7. Reagan DR, Doebbeling BN, Pfaller AM, et al: Elimination of coincident *Staphylococcus aureus* nasal and hand carriage with intranasal application of mupirocin calcium ointment. Ann Intern Med 1991; 114:101.
8. Wheat LJ, Kohler RB, Luft FC, et al: Long-term studies of the effect of rifampin on nasal carriage of coagulase-positive staphylococci. Rev Infect Dis 1983; 5:459S.
9. Hoss DM, Feder HM. Addition of rifampin to conventional therapy for recurrent furunculosis. Arch Dermatol 1995; 131:647–648.
10. Gonzalez MH, Garst J, Nourbash P, et al: Abscesses of the upper extremity from drug abuse by injection. J Hand Surg 1993; 18A:868–870.
11. Summanen PH, Talan DA, Strong C, et al: Bacteriology of skin and soft-tissue infections: Comparison of infections in intravenous drug users and individuals with no history of intravenous drug use. Clin Infect Dis 1995; 20(Suppl 2):S279–282.

CHAPTER 6

Acne

Diane M. Thiboutot

CLINICAL APPEARANCE

Definition

Acne is the most common chronic skin disease of adolescents and young adults. It affects the pilosebaceous unit (the hair follicle and sebaceous gland) and is characterized by noninflammatory and inflammatory lesions that most commonly involve the face, chest, and back. Although acne is not a life-threatening condition, it can result in permanent scarring and significant psychologic morbidity. The treatment of acne can be both challenging and rewarding.

Typical Lesions and Symptoms

Recognition of the various types of acne lesions is essential in order to design a successful treatment plan. Typical lesions of acne are comedones, papules, pustules, nodules, cysts, and scars. Open and closed comedones are noninflammatory lesions (see Fig. 6–1 on Color Plate 1). An open comedone (blackhead) appears as a dilated follicular orifice containing a keratinous plug that is black owing to melanin deposition. Closed comedones (whiteheads) are 1-mm flesh-colored follicular papules. Inflammatory lesions of acne consist of papules, pustules, nodules, and cysts. Papules and pustules of acne are erythematous and range from 1 to 5 mm in diameter (see Fig. 6–2 on Color Plate 1). An acne pustule is characterized by a collection of white blood cells within a hair follicle. Inflammatory nodules are larger than 0.5 mm in diameter and are indurated (firm) and tender. Cysts are fluid-filled, erythematous, and tender (see Fig. 6–3 on Color Plate 1). Sequelae to severe inflammatory acne include hyperpigmented macules and scarring (see Fig. 6–4 on Color Plate 1).

Atypical Presentation or Alternative Forms

Steroid-Induced Acne and Acneiform Eruptions

Acneiform eruptions can be induced by drugs such as corticosteroids, phenytoin, lithium, isonicotinic acid hydrazide (INH), psoralen plus ultraviolet A (PUVA), phenobarbital, thiourea, thiouracil, iodides, bromides, disulfiram, quinine, and azathioprine. The eruptions are sudden in onset, characterized by inflammatory papules and pustules, and generally monomorphous in their appearance. In contrast, the lesions of acne vulgaris are a mixture of comedones, papules, and pustules. Acneiform eruptions due to systemic corticosteroids most commonly occur on the chest and back of hospitalized patients receiving intravenous dexamethasone, but they also occur in patients receiving high doses of oral glucocorticoids. The use of topical steroids on the face can cause acneiform eruptions. Corticosteroid-induced facial acne (like corticosteroid-induced rosacea) often develops as a secondary phenomenon during treatment of facial conditions such as eczematous or seborrheic dermatitis with topical steroids. It presents as an increase in facial erythema and the development of inflammatory papules and pustules and is usually localized to discrete regions where the corticosteroids were applied. Drug-induced acneiform eruptions resolve spontaneously following removal of the offending agent.

Acne Fulminans

Acne fulminans is a very severe form of inflammatory acne associated with systemic signs and symptoms including fever, circulating immune complexes, arthralgias, leukocytosis, elevated erythrocyte sedimentation rate, proteinuria, and osteolytic lesions of the clavicles or ribs. It usually occurs in boys aged 13 to 16 years and can be rather sudden in its onset. Clinically, acne fulminans is characterized by multiple intensely inflamed nodules, cysts, and plaques. Large nodules can ulcerate, drain, and necrose. Hemorrhagic crusting is common. The etiology of acne fulminans is unknown. Patients with this disorder should be referred to a dermatologist for management with systemic corticosteroids and isotretinoin.

Chloracne

Chloracne is caused by exposure to halogenated hydrocarbons by either ingestion, inhalation, or contact with the skin. The majority of cases have been reported as a result of accidental industrial exposure, ingestion of contaminated food products, chemical warfare, or exposure to herbicides. Implicated chemicals include polyhalogenated naphthalenes, biphenyls, dibenzofurans, dioxins, and azobenzenes. Chloracne is characterized by the development of dense collections of comedones on the face, retroauricular skin, neck, axillae, and scrotum. Comedones can eventually develop into tender, inflamed cysts. Outbreaks of severe inflammatory lesions that heal with scarring can occur for years following exposure to the offending agent. Treatments include topical tretinoin and systemic isotretinoin.

DESCRIPTION OF DISEASE

Age/Natural History

Acne affects persons of all ages, including neonates, infants, prepubescent children, adolescents, and adults. Neonatal acne is characterized by the development of comedones and inflammatory papules and pustules that generally affect the cheeks. It is thought to result from the production of androgens by the fetal adrenal gland and testes. Neonatal acne usually resolves within the first 3 months of life, but it can persist for up to a year. Acne then becomes active again at the time of adrenarche, generally around 8 to 10 years of age. The onset of acne in this period has been associated with elevated levels of dehydroepiandrosterone sulfate (DHEAS), a weak adrenal androgen. Most prepubertal acne is characterized by the presence of comedones and few inflammatory lesions. Acne is most prevalent and most severe during adolescence. Estimates of the prevalence of acne in the adolescent age group approach 100%. For this reason, it has been termed *physiologic* in this age group. Most acne resolves after adolescence, but for many individuals, it can persist into adulthood. The reasons for the eventual decline in the prevalence of acne with age are not known but are thought to possibly relate to the decline in serum DHEAS levels associated with the aging process. Acne can even affect postmenopausal women, in whom it is thought to result from unopposed androgen secretion by the ovaries.

Etiology/Pathogenesis

The pathophysiology of acne centers on the interplay of follicular hyperkeratinization, the presence of *Propionibacterium acnes* within the follicle, sebum production by the sebaceous gland, and inflammation.[1] Follicular hyperkeratinization is manifested by increased cell division of follicular keratinocytes and increased cohesiveness of the corneocytes lining the follicular lumen. This process has also been referred to as *follicular plugging,* although complete occlusion of the follicular lumen does not occur, as evidenced by the fact that sebum still flows from follicles affected with acne. The cause of follicular hyperkeratinization is not known but may relate to a local deficiency of linoleic acid, production of interleukin-2 within the follicle, or possibly, the effects of androgens on follicular keratinization. Once sebum production begins at adrenarche, sebaceous follicles become colonized with *P. acnes*. This bacterium utilizes sebaceous lipids as a nutrient source and hydrolyzes the triglycerides found in sebum into free fatty acids and glycerol. The free fatty acids are an irritant to the follicular wall and can lead to rupture of the follicle, with subsequent release of keratin and sebum into the dermis. This process intensifies the inflammation associated with acne. Sebum production and sebaceous gland growth are under the control of androgens. Dihydrotestosterone is thought to be the androgen responsible for sebum production, although a possible role of testosterone in this process has not been excluded.

The precursor lesion of acne is the microcomedone that forms as a result of hyperkeratinization of the cells lining the orifice of sebaceous follicles of the face, scalp, chest, or back. A microcomedone is not visible but can be identified by a technique of follicular biopsy using cyanoacrylate glue applied to a glass microscope slide. As hyperkeratinization progresses, a microcomedone develops into either an open or a closed comedone. It generally takes approximately 8 weeks for a micro-

PITFALLS AND PROBLEMS OF DIAGNOSIS AND THERAPY

Differential Diagnosis

The differential diagnosis of acne includes acneiform drug eruptions, rosacea, pyoderma faciale, gram-negative folliculitis, and perioral dermatitis. Rosacea occurs most commonly in adults with fair skin and light hair and eye color. Comedones are notably absent. Pyoderma faciale may represent an explosive form of rosacea, analogous to acne fulminans. This disorder occurs most commonly in young women with a phenotype typical of rosacea patients. Gram-negative folliculitis is characterized by the sudden development of superficial pustules in patients who have been treated for acne with antibiotics. It may seem to represent a flare of the underlying acne, but it actually is a folliculitis caused by gram-negative bacteria. Cultures of pustules should be obtained. If gram-negative organisms are present, the patient should be referred to a dermatologist for consultation regarding treatment with isotretinoin. Perioral dermatitis is characterized by erythema, scaling, and small papules and pustules occurring most commonly around the mouth and on the chin. It often occurs in adult women. Clinically, it behaves as both acne and eczematous dermatitis and can be treated with agents effective for both conditions.

Antibiotic Resistance in Acne

Prior to 1976, there were very few reports of resistance of *P. acnes* to antibiotics. Since that time, however, this bacterium has developed resistance to many of the antibiotics used to treat acne. In a study of 468 treated acne patients, 178 (38%) carried strains of *P. acnes* resistant to one or more antibiotics.[5] Resistance is reported most frequently to erythromycin, followed by tetracycline and doxycycline. Although minocycline was thought to be the only antibiotic to which *P. acnes* had not acquired resistance, recent evidence suggests that this may no longer be true. Rather than testing sensitivities of *P. acnes*, most clinicians advocate switching to an alternate antibiotic when treatment resistance is noted. Additional recommendations to avoid the development of resistant strains of *P. acnes* within an individual patient are outlined in Table 6–4.

TABLE 6–4

Recommendations Regarding Antibiotic Use in Acne

Oral antibiotics should not be used when topical preparations will suffice.
Continue antibiotic treatment for no longer than is necessary.
If further treatment is required after an antibiotic has been discontinued, reuse the original antibiotic whenever possible.
Avoid concomitant oral and topical therapy with chemically dissimilar antibiotics to reduce the risk of developing resistance to both.

Data from Eady EA, Jones CE, Tipper JL, et al: Antibiotic-resistant *Propionibacteria* in acne: Need for policies to modify antibiotic usage. Br Med J 1993; 306:555–556.

Dry/Sensitive Skin

Most topical acne treatments will cause some degree of erythema, dryness, and scaling of the skin. Excessive dryness of the skin is one of the leading reasons that patients discontinue treatment. For this reason, recommendations regarding effective ways of managing facial dryness should be an integral part of any acne treatment plan. Many patients are reluctant to use facial moisturizers because they are concerned that moisturizers might worsen their acne. Nowadays, the majority of moisturizers from reputable companies are clinically tested for comedogenicity in clinical trials and are labeled *noncomedogenic*. Moisturizers are available as creams, lotions, and ointments. Most patients prefer to use lotions because they are easy to apply and do not feel greasy. Lotions containing sunscreens should be recommended, particularly in patients using tretinoin. For recalcitrant dry areas, a heavier cream or ointment may be needed. The regular use of moisturizers is especially important for patients on isotretinoin who are at risk of developing fissuring of the skin with secondary infection. Use of moisturizers and lip balm will help prevent these complications of isotretinoin therapy. Artificial tears can be used for xerostomia associated with isotretinoin.

Hormonal Causes of Acne

A possible endocrine disorder should be suspected in cases of female acne that are associated with hirsutism or irregular menstrual periods, are sudden and severe in their onset, or are resistant to conventional therapy.[2] Screening tests such as serum DHEAS and free and total testosterone can be performed to rule out a possible adrenal or ovarian tumor. Patients with polycystic ovary syndrome may have elevated testosterone, and those with nonclassical adrenal hyperplasia may have elevated levels of DHEAS. Referral to a dermatologist or endocrinologist should be considered for patients in whom acne is associated with a possible endocrine disorder. Agents that can be used in these patients include spironolactone, oral contraceptives, or low-dose glucocorticoids, depending on the disorder.

Postinflammatory Hyperpigmentation and Scarring

In some patients, particularly those with dark skin, hyperpigmented macules may persist following resolution of inflammatory lesions. Postinflammatory hyperpigmentation generally resolves slowly with time but may take up to a year or longer in many cases. The best solution to the problem of acne scarring is to institute appropriate therapy early in the course of acne to avoid this complication. Attention should be paid to any family history of scarring acne, as these patients may have an increased risk of developing acne scars. Dermabrasion or other resurfacing procedures can be used to improve facial acne scars. This procedure should be performed only after the patient's acne is no longer active. Often, a waiting period of 1 to 2 years is recommended before proceeding with dermabrasion following treatment with isotretinoin. Hypertrophic scars are another complication of acne. These occur most often on the chest and back of young patients with severe cystic acne. Referral to a dermatologist should be considered for a consultation regarding the possible use of intralesional injection with triamcinolone or treatment with Silastic gel sheeting or laser excision.

REFERRAL AND CONSULTATION GUIDELINES

Referral or consultation may be considered for

1. Patients who may require treatment with isotretinoin for acne fulminans; severe inflammatory, cystic, or scarring acne; recalcitrant comedonal acne; or gram-negative folliculitis
2. Female patients whose acne may be associated with an endocrine disorder
3. Patients with acne scarring
4. Pregnant patients with acne

REFERENCES

1. Leyden JJ: New understandings of the pathogenesis of acne. J Am Acad Dermatol 1995; 5(3):S15–S25.
2. Thiboutot DM: An overview of acne and its treatment. Cutis 1996; 57(1S):8–12.
3. Maibach H: Second-generation tetracyclines, a dermatology overview: Clinical uses and pharmacology. Cutis 1991; 48(5):411–417.
4. Berson DS, Shalita AR: The treatment of acne: The role of combination therapies. J Am Acad Dermatol 1995; 5(3):S31–S41.
5. Eady EA, Jones CE, Tipper JL, et al: Antibiotic-resistant *Propionibacteria* in acne: Need for policies to modify antibiotic usage. Br Med J 1993; 306:555–556.

CHAPTER 7

Actinic Keratosis

Clark C. Otley

CLINICAL APPEARANCE

Definition

Actinic keratoses (solar keratoses) are premalignant, keratinocytic neoplasms induced by cumulative solar radiation on the sun-exposed areas of fair-skinned patients. These lesions have a low but real potential for malignant transformation into squamous cell carcinoma, and they identify patients with advanced actinic damage who are at increased risk for cutaneous malignancy. The presence of actinic keratoses is an indication for thorough and regular full-skin examination and sun protection education.

Typical Lesions and Symptoms

Arising solely on sun-exposed surfaces, actinic keratoses appear as 2- to 30-mm adherent, white, yellow, pink, or red, compact hyperkeratotic papules (see Fig. 7–1 on Color Plate 2) or rough erythematous patches that may be more readily appreciated by palpation than by visualization (see Fig. 7–2 on Color Plate 2). They may be grouped or isolated, hypertrophic or atrophic, white or pigmented. In patients with severe photodamage, actinic keratoses may tend toward confluence. Actinic keratoses are usually asymptomatic but may have symptoms of burning, pruritus, or pain.

Atypical or Alternative Forms

Confluent actinic keratoses of the lower lip, manifested as chronic, rough scaling, is termed *actinic cheilitis.* Actinic keratoses are one of the many benign and malignant processes that can eventuate in a cutaneous horn—a compact, white, hornlike, protuberant growth, occasionally seen in elderly patients. Other processes that can appear clinically as a cutaneous horn include seborrheic keratosis, squamous and basal cell carcinoma, wart, and rarely, sebaceous carcinoma, granular cell tumor, Kaposi's sarcoma, and metastatic renal cell carcinoma. Actinic keratoses with underlying inflammation can appear as lichenoid keratoses, resembling lichen planus. Other variants include superficial pigmented and hypertrophic actinic keratoses.

DESCRIPTION OF DISEASE

Age/Population/Demographics

Extensive, cumulative photodamage in a genetically susceptible individual is required for the development of actinic keratoses, leading to a predominance of these premalignant lesions in individuals 30 years or older of Phototypes I to III (poor to fair tanning potential). Approximately 17% of Americans develop actinic keratoses during their lifetime, whereas 57% of individuals over the age of 40 years in Victoria, Australia, have similar lesions.

Natural History of Disease

Actinic keratoses often enlarge during the summer months and may regress during the winter. Once present, they usually persist and slowly enlarge, although isolated lesions may undergo spontaneous regression. Actinic keratoses typically evolve over months to years, although aggressive lesions may progress within weeks. Irritated actinic keratoses may bleed, avulse, or become inflamed. After the superficial scale is picked off, actinic keratoses tend to regrow.

Estimates regarding the risk of progression to frank squamous cell carcinoma from an untreated actinic keratosis range from 1:10 to 1:1000 per lesion per year. The risk of metastasis to regional lymph nodes from an actinically induced squamous cell carcinoma has been estimated to be 2 to 6% despite surgical treatment, contrary to earlier estimates of 0.5%.[1]

Pathology

Partial-thickness, epidermal keratinocytic atypia without full progression to squamous cell carcinoma is characteristic of actinic keratoses.

Etiology/Pathogenesis

Prolonged exposure to ultraviolet B (290 to 320 nm) radiation by genetically susceptible people is considered the most important etiologic factor for the development of actinic keratoses.[2] Therapeutic ultraviolet radiation in the form of psoralen plus ultraviolet A (PUVA), a treatment for severe psoriasis, has been associated with the development of actinic keratoses as well. A significant time interval, on the order of years to decades, exists between the acquisition of solar damage and the manifestation as actinic keratosis.

Epidemiologic risk factors for actinic keratoses include older age, childhood freckling, blue eyes, southern latitude, extensive solar exposure through occupation or recreation, and immunosuppression.[3] Immunosuppressed patients have a greatly increased risk of developing premalignant and malignant cutaneous neoplasms, suggesting that host immune defense plays a critical role in the containment of actinically induced atypia. A recent study concluded that significant restriction of dietary fat may reduce the incidence of actinic keratoses in fair-skinned patients with a history of nonmelanoma skin cancer.[4]

Diagnosis

Frequently, the diagnosis of actinic keratosis is made based on clinical features in a fair-skinned patient with evidence of photodamage. Occasionally, a biopsy is necessary to differentiate an actinic keratosis from other cutaneous growths or to exclude squamous cell carcinoma. Features suggestive of squamous cell carcinoma include thick scale, large size, induration, tenderness, rapid growth, bleeding, and recurrence after prior treatment. Full-thickness punch biopsy may be preferred over shave biopsy, as critical information is lost if the deep epidermis is not sampled. The differential diagnosis of actinic keratosis includes squamous cell carcinoma, basal cell carcinoma, seborrheic keratosis, lichen planus, xerosis, seborrheic dermatitis, discoid lupus erythematosus, and lentigo.

TREATMENT

General Therapeutic Expectations

The best therapy for patients with actinic keratoses is protection from excessive sun exposure in the future with protective clothing, use of sunscreens with a sun protection factor of at least 15, and avoidance of exposure during times of peak sun intensity (10 A.M. to 2 P.M.).[5] This strategy may induce regression of preexisting lesions as well as prevent further accumulation of photodamage. Individual actinic keratoses can be easily treated, whereas extensive lesions require more sophisticated measures. Because the squamous cell carcinomas that arise from actinic keratoses have a low but real (2 to 6%) metastatic potential, treatment of these lesions at the premalignant stage is optimal preventive medicine. However, regular follow-up in reliable patients may permit early actinic keratoses to be observed without treatment.

First-Line Therapy

Isolated actinic keratoses may be effectively managed with a 4- to 15-second spray of liquid nitrogen or a 10- to 20-second application with a cotton-tipped applicator, which will induce swelling, vesiculation, and eventual necrosis of the affected epidermis, with subsequent regrowth of normal epidermis in 10 to 14 days.[6] Warn patients of the possibility of associated oozing and edema, especially after treatment of facial lesions.

Recurrent lesions should be considered for consultation or histologic examination. All patients with premalignant or malignant cutaneous neoplasms should have a regular complete cutaneous examination by a physician skilled in the management of these neoplasms.

Age Considerations

The appearance of actinic keratoses in a patient under 30 years of age should prompt consideration of an underlying photosensitive or immunosuppressive disorder, such as xeroderma pigmentosum.

Alternative Therapeutic Options

There are several other effective therapies for actinic keratosis. Lesions may be removed by curettage and electrodesiccation with the patient under local anesthesia. Monsel's solution (ferric subsulfate) or aluminum chloride may be used instead of electrosurgery for hemostasis. Shave excision is sufficient to remove isolated lesions. Individual keratoses may be treated with mild acids such as 30 to 50% trichloracetic acid, and widespread disease can be treated successfully with chemexfoliation with the same agents. Individual lesions and widespread lesions may also be treated with topical chemotherapy using 5-fluorouracil. When using 5-fluorouracil for facial lesions, the usual course is 1 to 5% cream applied twice daily for 2 to 4 weeks. This agent leads to an excellent clinical result, but the intense inflammation it induces during therapy inhibits good patient compliance. Masoprocol is another topical chemotherapeutic agent that may be effective, but it carries with it considerable risk of inducing an allergic contact dermatitis. Other approaches to widespread cutaneous lesions include dermabrasion or laser resurfacing. Actinic cheilitis is best managed with low-char carbon dioxide laser treatments, but rarely vermilionectomy. Excision is almost always unnecessary in treatment of actinic keratoses.

PITFALLS AND PROBLEMS

The evaluation and management of patients with moderate to severe actinic damage or frank cutaneous carcinoma require experience. The greatest risk to the patient occurs when a malignant neoplasm is managed as if it is premalignant. Opportunities for error exist in the failure to diagnose or adequately sample a potential neoplasm and in the failure to adequately treat a neoplasm, resulting in recurrence or metastasis. Cutaneous neoplasms of an uncertain nature should be evaluated with histologic confirmation.

Because the treatment of premalignant neoplasms must be more vigorous than that of benign growths, the potential for adverse effects, such as scarring, ulceration, infection, or pigmentary abnormalities, is increased. Cryotherapy on the face can be associated with significant edema. An index of suspicion for an underlying photosensitive disorder or immunosuppression should be maintained in patients with early-onset or extensive premalignant changes.

REFERRAL AND CONSULTATION GUIDELINES

Cutaneous neoplasms of an indeterminate nature should be further investigated with consultative opinion or biopsy confirmation, or both. Lesions that do not respond typically to standard treatment must be carefully reevaluated. Dermatologists can be helpful in evaluating suspicious growths and avoiding unnecessary biopsies.

REFERENCES

1. Salasche SJ, Cheney ML, Varvares MA: Recognition and management of the high-risk cutaneous squamous cell carcinoma. Curr Probl Dermatol 1993; 5:141–192.
2. Fitzpatrick TB, Sober AJ: Sunlight and skin cancer. N Engl J Med 1985; 313:818.
3. Marks R: Solar keratoses. Br J Dermatol 1990; 122(Suppl 35):49.
4. Black HS, Herd JA, Goldberg LH, et al: Effect of a low-fat diet on the incidence of actinic keratosis. N Engl J Med 1994; 330:1272–1275.
5. Thompson SC, Jolley D, Marks R: Reduction of solar keratoses by regular sunscreen use. N Engl J Med 1993; 329:1147.
6. Lubritz RR, Smolewski SA: Cryosurgical cure rate of actinic keratoses. J Am Acad Dermatol 1982; 7:631.

CHAPTER 8

Alopecia Areata

Virginia C. Fiedler and Samar Alaiti

CLINICAL CHARACTERISTICS

Alopecia areata (AA) is a common disorder characterized by a single or multiple areas of nonscarring hair loss that can affect any hair-bearing surface.

Onset of hair loss may be accompanied by obvious increased hair shedding, or it may be slow and insidious. The classic lesion is round or oval. The skin surface is usually normal, but it may appear pink and occasionally is scaling. Lesions may be asymptomatic or may be associated with itching, tingling, burning, or painful sensations that precede or occur simultaneously with the hair loss.

Exclamation-mark hairs (hairs in which the proximal hair shaft shows gradual tapering and loss of pigment) are pathognomonic when present and may be seen at the expanding edge of active lesions.

The extent of involvement varies from patchy localized alopecia (AA) (see Fig. 8–1 on Color Plate 2) to total scalp hair loss (alopecia totalis) (see Fig. 8–2 on Color Plate 2) or total body hair loss (alopecia universalis). Occasionally, AA causes a diffuse nonscarring alopecia over the scalp mimicking other patterns of diffuse scalp hair loss (see Fig. 8–3 on Color Plate 3). AA may involve the nails, in which case nail pitting is the most common change.

DESCRIPTION

AA begins at any age and affects both sexes equally. The overall lifetime incidence is approximately 1.7%; the prevalence is estimated to be about 0.1%.[1] These numbers may be an underestimate because the incidence rate reflects only those cases brought to medical attention, and milder cases in the community may go undetected. Family history of AA is present in about 30% of patients.[2]

Natural History

The course of AA in any single patient is difficult to predict; spontaneous remissions and relapses are common, often with new patches appearing as old ones resolve. Children, in general, tend to have a prolonged chronic or chronic-intermittent course. Other poor prognostic signs are multiple episodes, hair loss along the scalp margin (ophiasis), very extensive scalp or body hair loss, duration of current episode of more than 2 years, and association with atopy.[2]

Pathology

AA is characterized microscopically by a dense accumulation of T cells, monocytes, and Langerhans' cells surrounding and invading the bulb area of the follicles, which become miniaturized. Helper T cells predominate at the sites of active loss.[3]

Etiology/Pathogenesis

The etiology and pathogenesis of AA are still unknown; however, it is thought to be an autoimmune disease. Emotional stress has been cited as a precipitating factor, but such an association is uncommon. No microbial agents have ever been identified in the lesions. Defects in immunoregulatory mechanisms leading to autoimmunity have been suggested but not clearly proved.[2] Various autoantibodies have been reported in patients with AA (gastric parietal cell, thyroid, smooth muscle, mitochondrial, reticulin, rheumatoid, and antinuclear antibodies [ANA]). It was recently reported that 24% of 29 AA patients studied were ANA-positive by enzyme-linked immunosorbent assay (ELISA), most commonly to single-stranded DNA (ssDNA) antibodies at low titers (<1:320). Positive ANA did not predict the development of lupus erythematosus in AA patients;[4] in fact, the overall incidence of lupus erythematosus in AA patients is low (<1%).[5] Positive ANA did not correlate with any other clinical parameters except that 25% of AA patients with positive ssDNA antibodies had Hashimoto's thyroiditis.[4]

TREATMENT

Treatments for AA may elicit cosmetically good hair regrowth; however, there is no good evidence to suggest that drug-induced remissions occur or that therapy alters the ultimate course of the disease. The goal of treatment is to achieve cosmetically adequate hair regrowth over the scalp. Chronic treatment may be required to maintain regrowth until the disease enters a spontaneous remission.

Topical Steroids

Our general approach to treating mild disease (defined as stable patchy hair loss of 25% or less of the scalp surface) is to have the patient use betamethasone dipropionate 0.05% cream in a nonoptimized vehicle (Diprosone) twice daily on the patches and on 1 inch of adjacent scalp skin and shampoo once daily.[2] For individuals with widespread or actively flaring disease, treatment of the entire scalp seems to be most effective to elicit and maintain cosmetically adequate hair growth.[2] This regimen works particularly well in children (even in some with 100% hair loss); it can also be beneficial in adults.[2] At least 3 months of uninterrupted treatment is necessary to evaluate for early hair regrowth. Cosmetically adequate regrowth may take many months to achieve. Hair loss may flare despite maintenance therapy but usually appears to be minimized when compared with the severity of previous untreated episodes of loss.

When used twice daily on the entire scalp, a 45-g tube of betamethasone dipropionate should last 3 to 4 weeks. The generic product by Fougera costs approximately $15.90 (the brand name costs approximately $43.90; these are approximate costs for 1996) and can be substituted for the brand name.[2]

Topical Anthralin

Anthralin is the only irritant substance generally agreed to induce hair regrowth in AA. Our general therapeutic regimen for anthralin is to have the patient use the 1.0% cream (Drithocreme) for short contact (20 to 60 minutes) followed by shampooing. For the first 2 weeks, treatment is applied on alternate days, and then, if tolerated, daily applications are instituted. Patients are instructed to apply the medication to the entire scalp if the disease is widespread or actively flaring. Patients are cautioned to wash their hands after applying anthralin and to avoid touching any fabric with their treated scalp until after they have shampooed. A 3-month trial of therapy is necessary to determine whether the patient will respond to anthralin, and cosmetic regrowth may take many months. Anthralin may be successfully combined with topical minoxidil, but usually it is not successfully combined with topical or intralesional steroids.[2]

Topical Minoxidil

Topical minoxidil may be effective in AA, especially when used in the 5% concentration that is available only on a study protocol basis. The lower concentrations (2%, Rogaine) are primarily effective in mild patchy AA. The mean time to response with topical minoxidil is 2 to 3 months. The time to maximal response in more severe disease is generally about 1 year, although it may be longer. As with other treatments, cosmetic response to minoxidil is not necessarily associated with 100% regrowth, and small patches may periodically develop and, usually, regrow with fair rapidity during maintenance treatment applied to the entire scalp.[2]

Intralesional Steroids

Intralesional steroids are a common form of treatment for AA. They are useful in stable mild patchy disease, but they are generally ineffective in extensive or actively flaring disease. Repeated injections at approximately monthly intervals may be necessary to elicit and maintain regrowth.[2]

Other Alternative Therapies

Other alternative therapies for AA include systemic glucocorticosteroids, topical sensitizers, and cyclosporine. Both single and combination therapies have been tried for AA, with variable results.[2]

PITFALLS AND PROBLEMS

Differential Diagnosis

It is important to differentiate AA from trichotillomania and tinea capitis. Trichotillomania is characterized by irregular patches of alopecia in unusual shapes. Hairs are broken off at different lengths. It can affect any area of the scalp as well as the eyebrows, eyelashes, and pubic hairs. Trichotillomania in children often represents a temporary reaction to severe stress; however, in adults, it is frequently a manifestation of a severe underlying psychiatric disorder. Tinea capitis is characterized by patchy areas of alopecia that may be accompanied by erythema and scaling. It can affect any part of the scalp. Microscopic examination and culture of plucked hairs or scales make the definitive diagnosis.

Side Effects of Topical Steroids

These consist most commonly of local folliculitis and, occasionally, acneiform facial lesions. Daily shampooing and sparing applications to the scalp seem to markedly diminish the occurrence and severity of these effects. The use of superhigh-potency topical steroids may lead to enhanced systemic steroid absorption and frequently to telangiectasia formation and local atrophy, which limit their applicability as potential long-term maintenance treatments. In 15 years of utilizing topical betamethasone dipropionate 0.05% in the nonoptimized vehicle twice daily as outlined, we have not seen any evidence of systemic side effects even in children as young as 2 years of age who have received long-term maintenance therapy. Despite the absence of side effects, careful monitoring of the growth curve in children as a marker for hypothalamic-pituitary-adrenal axis suppression is advisable.

Side Effects of Topical Anthralin

These are commonly pruritus, erythema, and scaling; occasionally folliculitis, local pyoderma, and regional lymphoadenopathy may occur. The common reactions are minimized and the occasional reactions are usually prevented with sparing applications and prompt shampooing. Reactions resolve quickly if treatment is withheld for a few days. If anthralin is then reinstituted for shorter times, it is usually well tolerated.

Side Effects of Topical Minoxidil

These are usually minimal and involve mild local irritation. Rarely, patients can develop allergic contact dermatitis to minoxidil or to the propylene glycol in the vehicle (VCF, unpublished observation). Very rarely, photoallergic contact dermatitis has been reported. Systemic absorption of minoxidil is minimal even at the 5% concentration. No systemic side effects of topical minoxidil have been reported. Mild hypertrichosis, especially of the face, is sometimes reported.[2]

Side Effects of Intralesional Steroids

These include minimal transient atrophy and, rarely, persistent, more severe atrophy with local follicular destruction. Pain is the most frequent complaint expressed by patients, and it is a significant drawback in children treated with this approach.[2]

ELISA-Positive ANA

This has been reported to be present in 24% of 29 AA patients studied, as noted.[4]

Other Diseases Associated With AA

These include autoimmune diseases such as Hashimoto's thyroiditis, as discussed previously, vitiligo, Crohn's disease, lupus erythematosus, lichen planus, and pernicious anemia. Atopy is a commonly associated finding in AA patients. Down's syndrome and cataracts have been reported in association with AA.

REFERRAL

Referral to a dermatologist is advised for extensive disease, rapidly progressive disease, treatment-resistant disease, or AA requiring chronic treatment. Children under 2 years of age are probably best left untreated because they are psychologically unaware of the hair loss, they are difficult to treat, and the safety of treatments has not been established in this age group.

REFERENCES

1. Safavi KH, Muller SA, Sumon VJ, et al: Incidence of alopecia areata in Olmstead County, Minnesota, 1975 through 1989. Mayo Clin Proc 1995; 70:628–633.
2. Fiedler VC: Alopecia areata. Arch Dermatol 1992; 128:1519–1529.
3. Perret C, Wiesner-Menzel L, Happle R: Immunohistochemical analysis of T cell subsets in the peribulbar and intrabulbar infiltrates of alopecia areata. Acta Derm Venereol 1984; 64:26–30.
4. Alaiti S, Fiedler VC, Ulyanov G, et al: Positive antinuclear antibodies associated with alopecia areata. J Invest Dermatol 1995; 104(4):661.
5. Muller SA, Winkelmann RK: Alopecia areata. Arch Dermatol 1963; 88:290–297.

CHAPTER 9

Anogenital Pruritus

Kathryn E. Bowers

CLINICAL APPEARANCE

Individuals with anogenital pruritus experience localized itching of the vulva (pruritus vulvae), scrotum (pruritus scroti), perineal skin, or anus (pruritus ani). The onset of the pruritus may be sudden, related to one trigger factor, or gradual. Once the itch-scratch cycle is well established, it is very difficult to break. The localized itching or rubbing may be intense, almost pleasurable, and can interfere with daily activities. Paroxysms of severe pruritus occur in a background of low-grade pruritus. There may be evidence of a primary dermatologic disease or secondary changes may predominate, including maceration, lichenification, excoriation, erosions, or fissures (Table 9–1). Essential or idiopathic anogenital pruritus has no visible cutaneous changes.

TABLE 9-1

Causes of Anogenital Pruritus

Idiopathic
Inflammatory: atopic dermatitis, lichen simplex chronicus, seborrheic dermatitis, psoriasis, irritant dermatitis, contact dermatitis, lichen sclerosus, lichen planus, Fox-Fordyce disease, fixed drug eruptions
Infections: candidiasis, dermatophyte, erythrasma, impetigo, condyloma accuminata, condyloma lata, vulvitis (trichomonas, bacterial vaginosis, cytolytic, or Doderlein's vaginosis)
Infestations: scabies, lice, pinworms
Mechanical factors: hemorrhoids, anal fissures
Neoplasia: squamous cell carcinoma, vulvar intraepithelial neoplasia, extramammary Paget's disease, bowenoid papulosis
Miscellaneous: Darier's disease, Hailey-Hailey disease

DESCRIPTION OF DISEASE

Demographics

Anogenital pruritus is very common. Pruritus ani is more common in middle-aged, middle-class white men, outnumbering women 4:1.

Natural History

The pruritus may have started insidiously or at a specific time. It is usually mild during the day, with the symptoms worsening in the evening and at night. Patients will often scratch during their sleep, awakening bed partners and noticing blood stains on the bedclothes in the morning. The itch-scratch cycle is usually very well established at presentation. Multiple over-the-counter remedies have often been tried; some products may make the process worse, as many preparations may be potential irritants or induce a secondary contact dermatitis. Anogenital pruritus, even when treated with appropriate measures, tends to have a high relapse rate and should be considered a chronic disease.

Pathology

The histologic features reflect the presence of a primary dermatologic process or the secondary changes from scratching or rubbing. The changes may be nonspecific. Any individual with longstanding anogenital pruritus that is resistant to therapy should undergo a biopsy to establish the diagnosis. The possibility of an underlying carcinoma such as squamous cell carcinoma or extramammary Paget's disease must be taken into consideration.

Etiology

The etiology of anogenital pruritus is multifactorial and is also somewhat site-dependent, although there is a great deal of overlap between men and women. The underlying cause can be determined in approximately 60% of men and 30% of women. Many of the patients may be atopic, with a genetic predisposition for pruritic disorders.

One of the primary reasons for genital pruritus is the irritancy of stool in the anogenital area. Fecal material contains bacteria, allergens, and bacterial endopeptidases that cause inflammation and pruritus. In general, the anogenital region has a lower irritancy threshold because it is an intertriginous site with multiple folds and thin, more permeable skin.

Obesity, poor ventilation, maceration, improper cleaning, anatomy, increased body hair, and poor hygiene are all contributing factors. Primary or secondary candidiasis, bacterial superinfection, sweat retention, and overzealous cleansing can contribute to difficulty in resolving the problem. The role of psychologic factors is controversial; some investigators have noted anxious, obsessive, or depressive traits in patients with anogenital pruritus.

TREATMENT

One of the primary goals of treatment is to eliminate or control potential trigger factors.

Environmental Factors

1. Reduce retention of sweat; use air conditioning when possible.
2. Wear loose cotton clothes.
3. Avoid sitting for long periods on leather or vinyl upholstery.
4. Avoid overuse of hot water; a warm sitz bath can be very soothing.
5. Avoid excessive washing; use a mild, nonfragranced soap or nonsoap skin cleanser and a soft cotton cloth.
6. Clean well after defecation and urination; dry thoroughly, even using a hair dryer (on low) to eliminate all moisture. Avoid fragranced or colored toilet paper.
7. Use tampons instead of sanitary pads; avoid scented panty liners.
8. Avoid spicy or irritating foods (e.g., coffee, tea, beer, cola, chocolate, tomatoes, pickles, curries).
9. Practice relaxation techniques: for example, yoga, meditation, biofeedback, self-hypnosis.

Nonprescription Products

1. If the skin is dry or cracked, lubricate the area with a bland topical emollient (e.g., petrolatum [Vaseline] jelly, hydrated petrolatum, shortening [Crisco]) after defecation and at bedtime.
2. Use cleansing pads (witch hazel and glycerin [Tucks], hamamelis water, glycerin, and alcohol [Fleet Medicated Wipes], or propylene glycol [Preparation H cleansing tissues]) to cleanse the perineal skin after defecation or to moisten dry, irritated skin.
3. Mineral oil and lanolin (Balneol) lipid perineal cleanser is a topical agent to be used after defecation and to aid in keeping moist areas dry.
4. Pramoxine hydrochloride is a topical anesthetic found in products by the names Prax lotion, Caladryl Clear lotion, and Itch-X gel and spray. This can be applied safely every 4 hours.
5. If the problem is acute, Burow's solution (prepackaged aluminum sulfate and calcium acetate) can be used as a compress for 10 to 15 minutes two or three times daily.

Prescription Products

1. Nonfluorinated topical steroids: Hydrocortisone 1 to 2.5%, cream or ointment, twice daily. Ointment-based steroids can be less irritating to the perineal skin, as they are preservative-free. The steroid preparation should be used twice daily for a week beyond the time when symptoms are under control, then tapered off. Resume application twice daily at the first signs of pruritus.
2. Hydrocortisone and iodoquinol (Vytone) cream and hydrocortisone and clioquinol (Vioform-Hydrocortisone) are a combination of 1% hydrocortisone and an iodine-based product used twice daily. These agents have anti-inflammatory, antibacterial, and antifungal properties. The iodine component may stain clothing or skin and may induce a contact allergy.
3. Analgesics: 5% Lidocaine ointment or 2.5% lidocaine and 2.5% prilocaine (EMLA) cream can be applied every 4 hours in addition to topical steroids if the pruritus continues.
4. Antipruritics: Pramosone, PrameGel (contain 1 to

2.5% hydrocortisone plus pramoxine—a topical anesthetic) and are applied two or three times daily.

5. Topical antihistamines: Doxepin (Zonalon) cream is a new topical antihistamine that is a helpful adjunct to topical steroids for eczematous disorders. The cream is applied sparingly twice daily; patients should be warned regarding possible sedative effects from systemic absorption. Topical diphenhydramine hydrochloride (Benadryl) is a less-potent antihistamine, and cases of contact dermatitis have been reported.

6. Systemic antihistamines: Diphenhydramine hydrochloride, hydroxyzine, and doxepin can be used for both their antihistamine and their sedative effects. These agents can be particularly helpful to decrease nocturnal scratching.

PITFALLS AND PROBLEMS

Males with extensive pruritus of the scrotum and the development of erythematous nodules in this region should be evaluated for the presence of scabies.

Biopsy of recalcitrant anogenital pruritus should be considered. Vulvar pruritus is the most common symptom of vulvar intraepithelial neoplasia. Extramammary Paget's disease usually occurs in the elderly. The majority of cases are in the anogenital region (65% vulva, 20% anal and perianal). Lesions are often present for years before the diagnosis is made.

CONSULTATION GUIDELINES

Patients with refractory anogenital pruritus should be considered for referral for consultation regarding other therapeutic maneuvers and for biopsy to rule out an underlying carcinoma.

BIBLIOGRAPHY

Alexander-Williams J: Pruritus ani. Br Med J 1983; 287:159–160.

Hanno R, Murphy P: Pruritus ani: Classification and management. Dermatol Clin 1987; 5:811–816.

Kantor GR: What to do about pruritus scroti. Postgrad Med 1990; 88(6):95–102.

Lynch PJ, Edwards L: Anogenital Pruritus in Genital Dermatology. New York: Churchill Livingstone, 1994; pp 229–236.

Pincus SH: Vulvar dermatoses and pruritus vulvae. Dermatol Clin 1992; 10:297–308.

Verbov J: Pruritus ani and its management. A study and reappraisal. Clin Exp Dermatol 1984; 9:46–52.

CHAPTER 10

Atopic Dermatitis

Marti Jill Rothe and Jane M. Grant-Kels

CLINICAL APPEARANCE

Definition

Atopic dermatitis is an eczematous skin disease often associated with respiratory atopy in the patient or first-degree relatives. The term *dermatitis* connotes inflammation of the skin. The term *eczema* connotes redness, oozing, superficial blistering, and crusting of the skin acutely and thickening and hyperpigmentation of the skin chronically. Diagnostic criteria for atopic dermatitis have been delineated by Hanifin and Rajka (Table 10–1).

Typical Lesions and Symptoms

Pruritus is the hallmark of atopic dermatitis, and many believe that scratching leads to the formation of characteristic acute and chronic lesions, giving rise to the expression ''atopic dermatitis is the itch that rashes.''

Acute lesions are erythematous and edematous papules and plaques often showing microvesiculation, exudation, crusting, and excoriation. Chronic lesions are characterized by lichenification, hyperpigmentation, skin thickening, and accentuation of skin markings. Follicular papules may be a prominent feature in dark-complected individuals.

Infantile atopic dermatitis may be generalized but usually affects the cheeks of the face and the extensor extremities (see Fig. 10–1 on Color Plate 3). Scaling of the scalp resembling seborrheic dermatitis is common.

Atopic dermatitis in children, adolescents, and adults may be generalized but most commonly affects the flexor extremities—antecubital and popliteal fossae—as well as the dorsal hands, face, and neck (see Fig. 10–2 on Color Plate 3).

Other Forms

In some patients, dermatitis localized to the hands or eyelids is a manifestation of atopic dermatitis.

DESCRIPTION OF DISEASE

Age/Natural History

Atopic dermatitis is typically a disease of childhood, improving and remitting with time; for example, in one study of children aged 11 to 13 years who had been previously treated for generalized dermatitis as infants, dermatitis had resolved in nearly 20% and was less severe in 65%. However, atopic dermatitis and its variants can persist into adolescence and adulthood or have a late age of onset. Another study showed that nearly 75% of young adults who had been diagnosed with atopic dermatitis by age 2 years still showed signs of active disease.

Demographics

The frequency of atopic dermatitis in the general population appears to be increasing; for example, an epidemiologic study of Swedish schoolchildren found a prevalence of 7% in 1979 and 18% in 1991. The increased frequency of atopic dermatitis may be related to multiple factors including increased exposure to allergens such as pollutants, house dust mites, and food additives;

TABLE 10-1

Major and Minor Diagnostic Criteria for Atopic Dermatitis

Major Criteria (Must Have Three or More)
Pruritus
Typical morphology and distribution
Chronic or relapsing dermatitis
Personal or family history of atopy
Minor Criteria (Must Have Three or More)
Xerosis
Ichthyosis, keratosis pilaris, palmar hyperlinearity
Type I skin test reactivity
Elevated serum immunoglobulin E
Early age of onset
Tendency toward cutaneous infections, impaired cell-mediated immunity
Nipple eczema
Cheilitis
Recurrent conjunctivitis
Dennie-Morgan infraorbital fold
Keratoconus
Anterior subcapsular cataracts
Orbital darkening
Facial pallor/facial erythema
Pityriasis alba
Anterior neck folds
Itch when sweating
Intolerance to wool and lipid solvents
Perifollicular accentuation
Food intolerance
Course influenced by environmental/emotional factors
White dermatographism/delayed blanch

Adapted from Hanifin JM, Rajka G: Diagnostic features of atopic dermatitis. Acta Derm Venereol Suppl (Stockh) 1980; 92:44–47.

decline in breast feeding; and heightened parental and clinician awareness of atopic dermatitis.

Epidemiologic studies draw inconsistent conclusions regarding whether certain racial or ethnic groups are more commonly affected by atopic dermatitis. The prevalence of atopic dermatitis has been shown to correlate with socioeconomic class, increasing as socioeconomic class increases.

Approximately 50 to 60% of children of a parent with atopic dermatitis will develop atopic dermatitis. Nearly 80% of children of two parents with atopic dermatitis will develop atopic dermatitis.

Pathology

Although pathologic examination is usually not necessary for the diagnosis or management, the pathology is well described and shows intercellular edema (spongiosis), thickening of the epidermis (acanthosis), retention of nuclei in the stratum corneum (parakeratosis), edema in the superficial dermis, and a superficial perivascular infiltrate predominantly of lymphocytes and occasionally of eosinophils in acute lesions. Chronic rubbing of the skin leads clinically to lichenification or thickening of the skin, which on biopsy shows epidermal and dermal hyperplasia, vertically oriented coarse collagen, dilated blood vessels in the superficial dermis, and a superficial lymphohistiocytic infiltrate. Scratching is evident on pathology as partial or complete loss of the epidermis (erosions) or even part of the underlying dermis (ulcerations).

Pathogenesis/Etiology

The pathogenesis of atopic dermatitis is not precisely delineated, but recent investigation has focused on immunologic features of atopic dermatitis: increased T-lymphocyte activation, hyperstimulation of the antigen-presenting Langerhans' cells, abnormal cell-mediated immunity, and overproduction of immunoglobulin E.

Genetically predisposed individuals seem to develop phenotypic evidence of atopic dermatitis in response to multiple triggering factors: contact irritants and allergens, aeroallergens, foods, microorganisms, hormones, stress, and climate.

Individuals with atopic dermatitis are more prone to irritation from water, soap, solvents, and wool and to contact allergy from nickel, fragrances, and neomycin. Atopics are also more susceptible to newly recognized allergens—latex (Type I hypersensitivity) and topical corticosteroids.

Dust mites, pollen, molds, dander, cow's milk, and other foods may trigger atopic dermatitis.

Evidence that *Staphylococcus aureus* provokes atopic dermatitis includes its presence as the major microorganism in dermatitic lesions, induction of dermatitis in normal skin by *S. aureus* superantigen, and clinical improvement of atopy after treatment with antibiotics. *Pityrosporum ovale* and *Candida albicans* may also play a role in the development of atopic dermatitis.

Hormonally related exacerbations and remissions are seen in response to menses, pregnancy, and menopause. Atopic dermatitis can flare with heightened stress, anxiety, and depression. Most patients will describe worsening of dermatitis during cold, dry seasons and improvement during hot, humid weather.

TREATMENT

Therapeutic Expectations

Atopic dermatitis usually requires long-term preventive measures and repeated therapeutic interventions to treat flares.

First-Line Therapy

Long-term preventive measures are at the core of first-line therapy of atopic dermatitis. Minimizing skin irritants is essential and requires avoidance of clothes made of wool and other coarse fabrics; avoidance of harsh soaps, such as Ivory and antibacterial soaps, and prolonged hot baths or showers; and avoidance of or protection from wet-work at home and in the workplace. Patients should wear loose fitting and soft fabrics such as cotton. Lukewarm baths or showers with moisturizing soaps such as Dove, Basis, colloidal oatmeal (Aveeno), or Cetaphil should be followed by blotting the skin dry and applying moisturizer while the skin is still damp. Soap substitutes such as Cetaphil and Aquanil can be applied as cleansers and removed with a soft cloth to avoid excessive exposure to water; these are especially useful for patients prone to hand or facial dermatitis. Wet-work activities in the home such as dishwashing or diaper changing should be performed with white cotton gloves under rubber. Protective cotton-lined gloves are ideal for health care professionals, hairdressers, and machinists, but such protective measures are often impractical.

First-line topical and oral therapies are directed toward decreasing inflammation, controlling pruritus, and treating secondary bacterial colonization and infection.

Topical corticosteroids are commonly prescribed to suppress erythema and inflammation and decrease pruritus; as well, topical steroids alone can decrease colonization of *S. aureus*. Nonfluorinated, low-potency topical corticosteroids should be prescribed for facial and intertriginous dermatitis. Usually, patients tolerate creams and lotions better than ointments in these areas. Acute flares of nonfacial and nonintertriginous dermatitis can be treated with high-potency to ultrapotent topical corticosteroids in older children, adolescents, and adults. Medium- to high-potency topical corticosteroids can be prescribed for acute flares in younger children. More chronic dermatitis is best treated with the least-potent topical corticosteroid that achieves benefit. Creams are well tolerated in flexural areas of the antecubital and popliteal fossae. Ointments, although somewhat messy, are typically more moisturizing, better tolerated, and useful on extensor surfaces. Patients and parents need to be advised of the potential side effects of topical corticosteroid therapy: adrenal suppression with extensive and prolonged use; epidermal atrophy with thin, paper-like skin and dilated vessels; and dermal atrophy with striae formation. Prolonged and extensive use of topical corticosteroids has been linked to growth arrest, but growth resumes after discontinuation of therapy.

Topical and oral antipruritics are commonly prescribed to treat atopic dermatitis, but these are often of modest benefit. Mentholated lotions such as Sarna or 0.025% menthol compounded in Aquaphor or a topical steroid may be helpful. The topical anesthetic pramoxine can be used alone or with hydrocortisone for itching in products such as Aveeno Anti-Itch, new Caladryl, PrameGel, Epifoam, and Pramosone. Unlike benzocaine, pramoxine does not appear to have the potential to cause allergic contact dermatitis. The new topical antihistamine Zonalon (topical doxepin) may be prescribed for the pruritus of atopic dermatitis; patients occasionally experience drowsiness, especially if Zonalon is applied to a mucosal surface, and there have been reports of contact dermatitis. Topical diphenhydramine (Benadryl) should always be avoided because of the high potential for allergic sensitization. First-generation oral antihistamines such as diphenhydramine and hydroxyzine (Atarax) can be prescribed at recommended pediatric and adult doses, but often the patient will tolerate and require much higher doses. Second-generation nonsedating antihistamines such as astemizole (Hismanal), terfenadine (Seldane), and fexofenadine (Allegra, a Seldane metabolite) can be prescribed to patients 12 years and older. The nonsedating antihistamine loratadine (Claritin) is also available in a pediatric syrup for children aged 6 and older. These are especially useful for daytime use in combination with sedating antihistamines at bedtime. Patients and parents must be cautioned to avoid concomitant use of ketoconazole, itraconazole, and erythromycin with Seldane and Hismanal because of potential cardiac toxicity. The hydroxyzine metabolite cetirizine (Zyrtec) may be prescribed for patients 6 years and older and when given as a once-daily dose is relatively nonsedating. Oral doxepin can be prescribed to adults and is 800 times more powerful an antihistamine than Benadryl. Generally, doxepin is given as a single bedtime dose ranging from 10 to 75 mg.

Topical and oral antibiotics are prescribed for both secondary colonization and frank pyoderma. Patients with widespread excoriations, malodor, and yellow crusting often will have dramatic improvement of their skin lesions when treated with oral antibiotics such as erythromycin (pediatric dose: 30 to 100 mg/kg/day), dicloxacillin (pediatric dose: 12.5 to 50 mg/kg/day), and cephalexin (pediatric dose: 25 to 50 mg/kg/day) with activity against skin flora. Topical antibacterial ointments including bacitracin, polysporin, and mupirocin (Bactroban) can be applied to excoriations and crusted areas. Neomycin-containing topical antibacterial ointments are sensitizers and need to be avoided.

Oatmeal (Aveeno) baths are palliative for itching and inflammation and helpful during acute flares of dermatitis. Use wet dressings with tap water or Burow's solution three times a day for 10 to 15 minutes for exudative lesions, followed by application of topical antibacterial ointments.

Alternative Therapeutic Options

Systemic corticosteroids can be helpful in arresting severe, acute flares of atopic dermatitis. However, recurrence or flare of disease after discontinuation of systemic corticosteroids is common. Both ultraviolet B and psoralen plus ultraviolet A (PUVA) are useful for refractory disease but are appropriate only for adults, adolescents, and children approximately 10 years or older. Systemic corticosteroids are useful in quieting an acute flare as patients initiate ultraviolet light therapy. Corticosteroids can be gradually tapered during the course of ultraviolet therapy.

Less conventional alternative therapies for atopic dermatitis include:

1. Dust mite and other aeroallergen avoidance
2. Dietary restrictions and supplementation
3. Chinese herbal therapy
4. Cyclosporine
5. Interferon
6. Thymic peptides
7. Psychotherapy
8. Hypnotherapy

PITFALLS AND PROBLEMS

Atopic dermatitis can be seen as a feature of inherited immunodeficiencies such as Wiskott-Aldrich syndrome, ataxia telangiectasia, and chronic granulomatous disease. Atopic dermatitis should be distinguished from other dermatoses: atopic dermatitis localized to the face and neck should be distinguished from airborne contact dermatitis; atopic dermatitis localized to the face, neck, and dorsal hands should be distinguished from photosensitive eruptions; widespread, refractory atopic dermatitis in an adult should be distinguished from cutaneous T-cell lymphoma.

Atopic dermatitis can be complicated not only by secondary bacterial infection but also by herpes simplex infection, which can disseminate. Eczema herpeticum requires prompt recognition and treatment with oral or intravenous acyclovir. Eczema herpeticum is characterized by punched-out–appearing grouped and disseminated crusted erosions and ulcerations. Facial involvement with dissemination to the trunk and extremities is common. Occasionally, suppressive therapy with daily acyclovir is needed to prevent recurrences of eczema herpeticum.

Atopic dermatitis refractory to treatment may be complicated by allergic contact dermatitis, especially to topicals applied in the treatment of the atopy. Vehicles, preservatives, fragrances, topical corticosteroids, and neomycin should be suspected.

REFERRAL AND CONSULTATION GUIDELINES

Referral to a dermatologist is appropriate in cases of atopic dermatitis refractory to first-line measures, in cases complicated by secondary herpes simplex infection, or when allergic contact dermatitis is suspected.

Referral to an allergist/immunologist is appropriate in cases of atopic dermatitis associated with underlying congenital immunodeficiency, in cases associated with significant respiratory atopy, or when allergies to dust mites, pollens, dander, or foods are suspected.

BIBLIOGRAPHY

Aberg N, Hesselmar B, Aberg B, et al: Increase of asthma, allergic rhinitis and eczema in Swedish schoolchildren between 1979 and 1991. Clin Exp Allergy 1995; 25:815–819.

Cooper KD: Atopic dermatitis: Recent trends in pathogenesis and therapy. J Invest Dermatol 1994; 120:128–137.

Hanifin JM, Rajka G: Diagnostic features of atopic dermatitis. Acta Derm Venereol Suppl (Stockh) 1980; 92:44–47.

Kissling S, Wuthrich B: Dermatitis in young adults. Personal follow-up 20 years after diagnosis in childhood. Hautarzt 1994; 45:368–371.

Linna O, Kokkonen J, Lahtela P, et al: Ten-year prognosis for generalized infantile eczema. Acta Paediatr 1992; 81:1013–1016.

Morren MA, Przybilla B, Bamielis M, et al: Atopic dermatitis: Triggering factors. J Am Acad Dermatol 1994; 31:467–473.

Rothe MJ, Grant-Kels JM: Atopic dermatitis: An update. J Am Acad Dermatol 1996; 35:1–13.

Uehara M, Kimura C: Descendant family history of atopic dermatitis. Acta Derm Venereol (Stockh) 1993; 73:62–63.

CHAPTER 11

Balding and Hair Loss

Maria K. Hordinsky

BALDING

CLINICAL APPEARANCE[1, 2]

Definition

Androgenetic alopecia, also known as hereditary balding or male and female pattern alopecia, is an inherited, androgen-dependent hair disorder. The development of androgenetic alopecia is related to a genetic predisposition to balding, and an increased reduction of testosterone to dihydrotestosterone by the enzyme 5-α-reductase in the skin.

Typical Lesions

Pattern baldness is commonly described, in men, using the Hamilton-Norwood classification system and, in women, the Ludwig classification. Patients with Type I Hamilton balding present with bitemporal recession. This can progress to midfrontal and vertex recession to the point where the two areas of baldness become confluent—Type V Hamilton. In women, the "male" pattern of androgenetic alopecia does occur, but more commonly, a widening of the part width, associated with a decrease in hair density on the crown, and hairs of varying length are present. In both men and women, the development of androgenetic alopecia is associated with a shortened anagen (growth) phase and an increase in the number of finer, shorter, thinner hairs.

Atypical Presentations or Alternative Forms

Not all individuals predisposed to balding present with the classic Hamilton-Norwood or Ludwig patterns of hair loss. Some individuals experience diffuse scalp hair loss for months to years before their pattern balding process becomes apparent. Such individuals may be misdiagnosed as having chronic telogen effluvium hair loss.

DESCRIPTION OF DISEASE

Androgenetic alopecia affects millions of men and women. It is considered to be an autosomal trait with variable expression or a polygenic trait. In predisposed males, balding is initiated with exposure to androgens at puberty. In women, the same may happen, but in 30% to 40% of affected women, a systemic endocrine problem is present. In contrast to female androgenetic alopecia, the histopathology of male androgenetic alopecia has been well studied. In the early stages, the density of follicular units (about one follicle per mm^2), and the number of terminal anagen follicles per follicular unit (about two or three) remain normal or near normal. As the extent and duration of the condition progress, hair shaft and follicular diameters become reduced, the fraction of anagen hairs present decreases, and the numbers of normal telogen hairs and telogen terminal units increase. An inflammatory infiltrate is commonly present at the bulge region, the postulated site of hair follicle stem cells. The role of this inflammatory infiltrate in androgenetic alopecia is not known.

TREATMENT

If no menstrual irregularities, hirsutism, cystic acne, infertility, or galactorrhea is present, comprehensive endocrine evaluation is usually not necessary. When clinically indicated, free and total testosterone, dehydroepiandrosterone (DHEA-S) and prolactin levels should be measured. If an underlying adrenal or ovarian abnormality is detected and treated, hair density may improve. Drugs commonly prescribed for the treatment of androgenetic alopecia are presented in Table 11–1.

Therapeutic Expectations

As balding is mediated by both genes and hormones, successful treatment requires ongoing therapy.

First-Line Therapy

The first line of therapy is 2% topical minoxidil, which works best in those with mild to moderate balding. Antiandrogens may be indicated in some situations.

The goals of therapy are to decrease further hair thinning and hair loss and to promote hair regrowth. Topical application of 2% minoxidil, 1 ml twice daily, is effective in treating both men and women with mild to moderate androgenetic alopecia. This drug is the only drug approved by the Food and Drug Administration in the United States for the therapy of baldness. In patients who are not completely bald, drug delivery can be enhanced if the topical preparation is applied with a dropper applicator. This minimizes unnecessary drug deposition on the hair fiber. Hair growth typically peaks at 1 year, and discontinuing treatment is associated with loss of hair gained within 4 to 6 months after stopping drug application.

Antiandrogens may be administered topically, intralesionally, or orally to retard hair loss. Antiandrogens either inhibit the conversion of testosterone to dihydrotestosterone by 5-α-reductase or inhibit dihydrotestosterone binding to the steroid receptor. The nonsteroidal drugs flutamide and cimetidine are also antiandrogens and have been used to treat androgenetic alopecia. Flutamide is an androgen receptor blocker and cimetidine competes with dihydrotestosterone. Cosmetic techniques that can be recommended include the use of hair dyes, hair cosmetics, and cosmetic camouflage. Use of full or partial hair prostheses, integration pieces, or hair weaving may also be of benefit to some patients.

TABLE 11–1

Drugs to Treat Balding

Treatment	Dose
Approved by the U.S. Food and Drug Administration	
Topical minoxidil (Rogaine)	1 ml bid
Commonly Used	
Spironolactone	100–200 mg po qd
Flutamide	250 mg po tid
Cimetidine	300 mg 5 times/day
Dexamethasone	0.25–0.75 mg/night
Oral contraceptives	Varied
Brand Names in the United States (Selected and Listed from Least to More Androgenic)	
Desogestrel	Desogen, Ortho-Cept
Norgestimate	Ortho-Cyclen, Ortho Tri-Cyclen
Norethindrone	Micronor, Brevicon, Modicon, Ortho-Novum 7/7/7, Ortho-Novum 10/11, Tri-Norinyl, Norinyl, Ortho
Ethynodiol diacetate	Demulen 1/35
Levonorgestrel	Triphasil, Tri-Levlen, Nordette
Norgestrel	Lo/Ovral, Ovral
Norethindrone acetate	Loestrin 1/20, Loestrin 1.5/30
Future Treatments	
5% topical minoxidil	
Oral 5-α-reductase inhibitors	
Topical androgen-receptor blocking agents	

PITFALLS AND PROBLEMS

Male and female androgenetic alopecia are easily diagnosed when the classic Hamilton types or Ludwig grades are present. The hair disorder is more difficult to diagnose if the onset of the classic balding patterns is preceded by a period of diffuse scalp hair shedding.

HAIR LOSS

Hair loss may occur for several reasons. In this section, three major causes of hair loss are discussed—telogen effluvium hair loss, hair breakage, and the scarring alopecias.

TELOGEN EFFLUVIUM—CLINICAL APPEARANCE[3]

Definition

On the scalp, approximately 10 to 15% of hair follicles are in the telogen stage at any one time. During this stage, the hair follicle releases the hair fiber, and an average daily loss of approximately 100 telogen hairs is considered to be acceptable. In telogen effluvium hair loss, hair follicles move from the active growing stage, called anagen, to the telogen stage, and the number of hair follicles in telogen frequently exceeds 20%. Patients frequently describe their hair as falling out by the ''roots.''

Typical Lesions

Diffuse scalp hair loss is present, and patients are asymptomatic. Examination of the scalp is unremarkable. Light hair pull tests (six or more hairs easily extracted by their telogen ''roots'') may be positive if the disease is active at the time of examination.

DESCRIPTION OF DISEASE

Telogen effluvium hair loss can affect both sexes at any age. The etiology of the hair loss may be attributed to use of certain drugs, physiologic stress, high fevers, the postpartum period, or even travel from low-daylight to high-daylight areas. Although commonly called telogen effluvium hair loss, hair loss may be triggered by different factors that affect different stages of the hair cycle, all of which ultimately cause telogen effluvium hair loss. For example, immediate anagen release is commonly seen with the use of drugs, high fever, or other physiologic stress, whereas delayed anagen release is characteristic of the postpartum period. Some drugs such as minoxidil are associated with a shortened telogen stage and the initiation of anagen. In some patients, increased hair shedding may occur after a period of decreased shedding. This has been called delayed telogen release and characterizes seasonal hair loss.

TREATMENT

Therapeutic Expectations

In general, no treatment is required, and the prognosis is good for normal scalp hair regrowth. However, patients should be cautioned that their hair density may not necessarily return to the full density present prior to their episode of telogen effluvium hair loss. Some individuals may see a greater change in hair density in androgen-dependent areas, such as the crown, where hair regrowth may be more sparse and of varying lengths.

PITFALLS AND PROBLEMS

When a patient presents with the chief complaint of diffuse scalp hair loss and hair falling out by the ''roots,'' the correct diagnosis will be telogen effluvium hair loss most of the time. However, diffuse, active alopecia areata may appear like telogen effluvium hair loss. When in doubt, histopathologic examination of a scalp biopsy specimen is recommended. The patient with telogen effluvium hair loss is counseled that his or her hair will grow back, whereas the patient with alopecia areata will be told he or she has an immune-mediated disease that can recur.

HAIR BREAKAGE—CLINICAL APPEARANCE[4]

Definition

When a patient complains of diffuse scalp hair loss, it is important to differentiate whether the hair loss is coming from the ''roots'' or whether the hair fiber is breaking because of acquired or inherited structural abnormalities.

Typical Lesions

Patients with structural hair abnormalities typically present with short hair. Parents of children with such hair will frequently bring the child to clinic with the chief complaint that their child's hair does not grow.

DESCRIPTION OF DISEASE

The normal hair fiber or shaft consists of three major parts—the cuticle, cortex, and medulla. Physical or chemical trauma to the hair fiber is frequently associated with alterations in the hair cuticle and cortex, resulting in hair fracturing or breaking. Some hair fractures as well as other structural hair abnormalities can be inherited, as seen in patients with monilethrix or trichothiodystrophy.

Laboratory analysis of cut hair fibers provides useful information about the hair fiber and helps delineate where the structural abnormality is present. The most common test is to cut hair fibers in the affected area at the proximal end. Hairs should not be pulled, as the hair fiber will typically break at weak points. Hairs are then mounted in parallel on glass slides with a mounting medium such as Permount and examined under the light microscope.

TREATMENT

Treatment of hair breakage includes identifying whether the hair fiber is breaking because of a genetic defect or whether the hair fragility is related to physical or chemical injury. Treatment consists of informing the patient about the etiology of his or her hair breakage and, if necessary, altering hair care habits. The use of hair conditioners and gentle combing and brushing should be encouraged.

SCARRING ALOPECIAS—CLINICAL APPEARANCE[5]

Definition

Patients develop permanent hair loss for many reasons. Destruction of hair follicles can occur secondary to trauma, infections, immune-mediated diseases such as lupus erythematosus or scleroderma, or with infiltrative processes such as sarcoidosis or tumors. There are also diseases that are unique to the hair follicle that result in a scarring alopecia. Examples include lichen planopilaris (LPP) and pseudopelade. The remainder of this section focuses on these two diseases.

Typical Lesions and Symptoms

Pseudopelade is characterized by small, glistening white patches of alopecia that look like "footprints in the snow." In contrast to the early stages, no erythema or scale is present in the late stages of pseudopelade. LPP is characterized by atrophic, circumscribed patches with hyperkeratotic follicular areas and scale. Pustules may be present.

DESCRIPTION OF DISEASE

Follicular lichen planus usually occurs between 30 and 70 years of age, and a 2:1 female predominance has been noted. Pruritus, perifollicular spines, and erythema are usually present. Shed hairs are unique in that their roots are covered in translucent material consisting of keratinous matter and internal and external root sheaths. Lichen planus of the scalp typically progresses slowly.

Many authorities postulate that pseudopelade represents the final stage of several diseases such as LPP, chronic discoid lupus erythematosus, scleroderma, or folliculitis decalvans. Others consider pseudopelade to be its own entity. In the late stages of this disease, patients are relatively asymptomatic.

TREATMENT

Therapeutic Expectations

The course of pseudopelade is progressive, and treatment is difficult. Anti-inflammatory drugs such as topical, intralesional, or oral steroids can be prescribed prior to the development of scarring. Scarred areas can be surgically removed if appropriate. LPP may also be very difficult to treat.

First-Line Therapy

Patients with LPP or active pseudopelade may require oral anti-inflammatory therapy. Drugs commonly prescribed include prednisone or hydroxychloroquine sulfate (Plaquenil). If *Staphylococcus aureus* is cultured from the pustules, antibiotic treatment may be required for weeks. In both conditions, scalp hygiene should be addressed. To reduce superficial inflammation, the use of antiseborrheic shampoos should be encouraged. Many patients also find relief from their scalp symptoms with the application of midpotency or suprapotency topical steroids. After the inflammatory process subsides, surgical removal of any scarred areas may benefit some patients.

PITFALLS AND PROBLEMS

The scarring alopecias can usually be diagnosed by histologic examination of scalp biopsy specimens. It is sometimes difficult to differentiate between pseudopelade and alopecia areata. Therefore, if the patient is suspected to have patchy alopecia areata but does not respond to the usual anti-inflammatory therapies, examination of a scalp biopsy may be helpful in differentiating between a scarring process such as pseudopelade and alopecia areata.

REFERRAL OF PATIENTS WITH BALDING OR HAIR LOSS

Androgenetic balding is usually easily diagnosed on the basis of history and clinical findings. The differential diagnosis of hair loss is far more complex, and early intervention in cases of scarring alopecia may prevent permanent hair loss and will certainly put the patient at ease. For this reason, referral to a hair specialist is reasonable if the clinician is not certain of the presenting diagnosis.

REFERENCES

1. Sawaya ME, Hordinsky MK: The antiandrogens. Dermatol Clin 1993; 11:65–72.
2. Kaufman KD: Androgen metabolism as it affects hair growth in androgenetic alopecia. Dermatol Clin 1996; 14:697–712.
3. Headington JT: Telogen effluvium. Arch Dermatol 1993; 129:356–363.
4. Price VH: Structural anomalies of the hair shaft. In Orfanos CE, Happle R (eds): Hair and Hair Diseases. Berlin: Springer-Verlag, 1990; pp 363–422.
5. Sperling LC: Evaluation of hair loss. Curr Probl Dermatol 1996; 7:97–136.

CHAPTER 12

Candidiasis

Agnes M. Lynch and Matthew J. Stiller

CLINICAL APPEARANCE

Definition

Candida spp. are opportunistic organisms capable of causing superficial infections of the skin, nails, and oral and genital mucosa. *Candida albicans* may inhabit the flora of the mouth, intestine, and vagina, without any signs or symptoms of disease. Therefore, in patients with candidiasis, it is important to be aware of underlying disease (e.g., human immunodeficiency virus [HIV] infection or diabetes mellitus), as host defense mechanisms may play a greater role in the pathogenicity than the virulence of the organism.

Many terms are used interchangeably to describe candidal infections. In the United States, *candidiasis* is the term used most often, whereas in France, Italy, Canada, and the United Kingdom, the preferred term is *candidosis.* Other synonyms include *moniliasis, thrush, dermatocandidiasis,* and *muguet.* Many species of *Candida* are capable of acting as pathogens, including *C. parapsilosis* (important in paronychias), *C. tropicalis* (vaginitis), *C. krusei,* and *C. zeylanoides. C. albicans* is the most prevalent and most virulent of all candidal species.

Typical Lesions and Symptoms

The clinical appearance of candidal infections varies at different anatomic sites and may vary within a single site. Three broad clinical categories of candidal infection are important in primary care dermatology: oral candidiasis, genital candidiasis, and cutaneous candidiasis. Less common subtypes of candidiasis are candidal folliculitis, nail infections, and chronic mucocutaneous candidiasis (CMC).

Oral Candidiasis

Oral candidiasis, pseudomembranous candidiasis, or thrush appears as a white layer of variable thickness resembling curdled milk. It may cover the entire tongue as a single continuous layer or may appear as scattered thick, white patches. The buccal mucosa and palate are often involved, as is the gingiva. Removal of the easily scraped white layer reveals a tender, inflamed base. Two other subtypes of oral candidiasis are angular cheiltis (perlèche) and erythematous candidiasis. Cheilitis, which may be quite painful, occurs bilaterally in the corners of the mouth and is characterized by erythema, dryness, and cracking or fissuring. Erythematous oral candidiasis appears on the tongue as a circinate, shiny, bright red patch lacking papillae. Unlike with thrush, there is no exudate on patches of erythematous candidiasis. The aforementioned subtypes of oral candidiasis may coexist, and it is not uncommon for a single patient to exhibit symptoms of two or three subtypes.

Black hairy tongue, which may occur following antibiotic administration, is another possible manifestation of oral candidiasis. *Candida* spp. are one of the causes of this disease, which presents with brownish or black hairlike projections of the lingual papillae. Predisposing factors include smoking and use of oxidizing agents (e.g., beta carotene, vitamin C, vitamin E, and selenium).[1]

Genital Candidiasis

Vaginal candidiasis is extremely common, affecting 75% of all women with at least one episode in their lifetime.[2] It presents with a white discharge similar in appearance to that in pseudomembranous candidiasis: thick, white, curdlike, and easily scraped. The vulva and surrounding area are usually inflamed and severely pruritic. The infection frequently spreads to sexual partners, so it is therefore important to treat them to prevent recurrence. Recurrent infections often affect sexual performance owing to pain and psychologic factors. This should be considered in management of vaginal candidiasis.[2] Pregnant women are predisposed, and many women have a first episode during pregnancy. Oral contraceptive pills have been considered a predisposing factor, but data fail to support this conclusion.[2]

Candidal balanitis (balanoposthitis) is characterized by erythema and tenderness often accompanied by papulopustular lesions. Pruritus and burning are common symptoms. Diabetic patients and uncircumcised men are predisposed to infection.

Diaper rash (napkin dermatitis) is another common form of genital candidiasis. Typically appearing in the first week of life and aggravated by wet diapers, it classically resembles candidal intertrigo with erythematous well-demarcated patches, having inconsistently scaly edges, and occasional satellite papules and pustules.

Cutaneous Candidiasis

Intertriginous candidiasis typically has a strikingly bright red-orange color. Candidal intertrigo is usually not shiny, may be scaly peripherally, or may be surrounded by satellite papules and pustules. Areas with friction between contiguous surfaces, such as the axillae, submammary area (see Fig. 12–1*A* on Color Plate 4), inguinal region, and perianal regions, and in obese people, between tissue folds (especially preumbilically), are affected. Infection generally starts at a site of friction (tissue fold) extending outward, to form hallmark satellite lesions. Pruritus is common, and scratching may contribute to spread of the infection.

Interdigital candidiasis (erosio interdigitale blastomycetica) is characterized by macerated skin in finger (or toe) webs. When fissuring occurs, pain and tenderness are frequently present. The web between the middle digit and the ring finger is the most common site (see Fig. 12–1*B* on Color Plate 4). Chronic exposure to water, as seen in bartenders, waitresses, waiters, and dishwashers, is the usual precipitating factor.[1]

Other Forms of Candidiasis

Other forms of candidiasis include nail infection, paronychia, CMC, and candidal folliculitis. *Paronychia,* an infection of the nail fold, occurs in individuals who routinely immerse their hands in water.[1] It usually presents as a tender, painful, purulent inflammation of the nail folds. If the nail plate becomes infected (onychomycosis), transverse ridges may form. Another identifying feature is brownish discoloration of the lateral edges of the nail plate, which may help to distinguish candidiasis from other types of onychomycosis. When evaluating dystrophic, discolored, onychomycotic nails, it is important to identify the pathogen before initiating treatment. In cases of paronychia, the clinician must realize that bacterial infection of the nail fold can be a contributing factor.

Candidal folliculitis in the beard area is characterized by perioral scabs and pustules. This uncommon form of cutaneous candidiasis resembles tinea barbae.

The term *chronic mucocutaneous candidiasis* refers to a set of disorders caused by defects in cell-mediated immunity and other immunologic abnormalities, which predispose patients to chronic, recurrent candidal infections of the skin, nails (see Fig. 12–1*C* on Color Plate 4), and mucous membranes. Severity, location of infection, and age of onset are important in characterizing the subgroup of CMC to which a patient belongs and ultimately in determining the best treatment. Endocrinopathies, thymoma, and autoimmune disease are associated with CMC, and their presence helps to identify their specific subgroup.[1]

Correction of the immune defect is the best treatment, followed by treatment with oral antifungal agents, such as ketoconazole and fluconazole. In treating patients with CMC, it is important to look for infection by other organisms such as bacteria, herpesviruses, and other fungi, which are seen in 20% of patients (Table 4–1).[3]

DESCRIPTION OF DISEASE

Age is a predisposing factor in candidal infections. Frequent targets are newborns and the elderly. Pregnant women with vaginal candidiasis often give birth to infants with thrush. Diaper rash is common in neonates, as the napkin area is a favorable environment for yeast. Candidal infections are also common in the geriatric population, particularly in denture wearers. Up to 60% of those over the age of 60 years with dentures have some form of oral candidiasis.[1] Oral candidiasis in denture wearers may have a distinctive morphology. Unlike thrush, the shiny, white affected areas cannot be easily scraped, sometimes making it difficult to obtain a speci-

TABLE 12-1

Differential Diagnosis of Candidal Infections

Intertriginous Candidiasis	Candidal Nail Infections and Paronychia
Toe Webs	Dermatophytosis
Tinea pedis	Nondermatophyte fungi (aspergillus, scopulariopsis)
Erythrasma	Psoriasis
Groin	Acrodermatitis continua of Halopeau
Hailey-Hailey disease	Dermatitis repens
Tinea cruris	**Oral Mucocutaneous Candidiasis**
Inverse psoriasis	Oral hairy leukoplakia
Seborrheic dermatitis	Lichen planus
Erythrasma	Leukoplakia
Axillae	**Candidal Balanitis**
Inverse psoriasis	Psoriasis
Seborrheic dermatitis	Lichen planus
Tinea corporis	Contact dermatitis
Erythrasma	Erythroplasia of Queryat
Contact dermatitis	Fixed drug eruption
Submammary	Zoon's plasma cell balanitis
Inverse psoriasis	
Seborrheic dermatitis	
Tinea corporis	
Intertrigo	

men for mycologic evaluation. Good oral hygiene and disinfection of the dentures are usually curative.

One of the highest risk groups for oral candidiasis is HIV-positive patients, 90% of whom become infected with *Candida* during their lives. Treatment of this subpopulation is especially difficult.[3]

Immunosuppression owing to other factors including diabetes, systemic malignancy, or chemotherapeutic drugs also increases the risk of candidal infections. Other predisposing factors are obesity, large pendulous breasts, hyperhidrosis, other endocrine disorders (including Cushing's syndrome), and chronic systemic use of glucocorticoids or antibiotics.

In addition to mucocutaneous infections, *Candida* may cause life-threatening systemic involvement including meningitis, endocarditis, and bronchopulmonary infections. The presence of oral candidiasis does not appear to be increase the risk of systemic infection.

A diagnosis of mucocutaneous candidiasis can be made clinically if classic signs and symptoms are present. A combination of yeast and pseudomycelia organisms revealed by microscopic examination of a potassium hydroxide wet mount from infected skin or mucosae is highly suggestive of candidiasis (see Fig. 12–2*A* on Color Plate 4). Each ovoid yeast cell is 5 to 7 μm in diameter. Modified Sabouraud's agar with antibiotics (e.g., Mycosel) is the best laboratory medium for isolating *Candida*. Colonies grow rapidly at 25° C and are creamy, smooth, beige to ivory-colored after 3 days (see Fig. 12–2*B* on Color Plate 4), becoming waxy or pasty after several weeks. Speciation of *Candida* requires sophisticated laboratory tests such as formation of chlamydoconidia (see Fig. 12–2*C* on Color Plate 4) or germ tubes on special media.[4]

TREATMENT (Tables 12–2 through 12–4)

Treatment of candidiasis varies with location, duration of infection, recurrence rate, and immunocompetence of the host. HIV-positive individuals are one of the most complicated groups to treat.

Vaginal and oral infections are easily treated with topical formulations. The imidazoles, azoles, and polyenes are all very effective in treating candidal infections, and most are available in a wide variety of formulations—creams, ointments, powders, and oral suspensions. A consideration in treatment of oral candidiasis is taste of medication. A common complaint with pastilles, lozenges, and troches is the poor taste, as many of these must be held in the mouth for a while. Some preparations are available without prescription for treatment of vaginal and cutaneous infections. It is worth considering whether a patient has time to apply a topical medication twice daily. Many single-dose therapies are available. If a patient is unwilling to use a medication daily or twice daily for a week or two, it may be beneficial to opt for single-dose therapy. In most cases, resolution of symptoms takes 7 to 14 days.

Formulation is important with regard to treatment location. Macerated lesions respond better to powders than to ointments. Powders may also be less irritating in treating some types of infections. Other important treatment considerations are cost, ease of application, and potential patient compliance.

Oral ketoconazole, fluconazole, and itraconazole are usually efficacious in the treatment of resistant mucocutaneous infections. It is important to carefully monitor patients on oral agents, adjusting dosages when laboratory abnormalities occur or when patients are treated concomitantly with other interacting drugs. With recurring oral infections, or when treating an HIV-infected individual, oral agents are preferred. Fluconazole has been used successfully in treating HIV-associated oral candidiasis, but it is not effective against a few resistant strains.[3]

TABLE 12–2

Treatments for Vaginal Candidiasis

Topical

Drug	*How Supplied*	*AWP Cost**	*Average Dose*	*Duration of Treatment*	*Pregnancy Precautions†*
Butoconazole nitrate					
Femstat	2% cream‡	$20.16	5 g	3 days	Level C
Clotrimazole					
Lotrimin	1% cream‡	$16.25	5 g	7 days	Level B
Mycelex-G	Suppository	$12.71	500 mg	Once	
Econazole nitrate					
Spectazole	2% cream‡	$37.56	5 g	7 days	Level C
Gentian violet	5-mg tampons	NA	5 mg	12 days	Level C
Miconazole nitrate	1% cream†	$12.48	5 g	3 days	Level C
Monistat 3	Suppository	$24.36	200 mg	3 days	
Nystatin vaginal tablet	Suppository	$ 7.43	100,000 units	14 days	Level A
Terconazole					
Terazol 3	0.8% cream‡	$23.34	5 g	7 days	Level C
Terazol 7	Suppository	$23.34	80 mg	7 days	
	0.4% cream‡	$23.34	80 mg	7 days	
Tioconazole					
Vagistat 1	6.5% ointment	$24.20	4.6 g	Once	Level C

Oral

Drug	*How Supplied*	*AWP Cost**	*Average Dose*	*Duration of Treatment*	*Interactions*
Fluconazole Diflucan	Tablet	$12.75	150 mg	Once	Hydrochlorothiazide, cimetidine, rifampin, warfarin, phenytoin, terfenadine, astemizole, loratadine, ketoconazole, itraconazole, terbinafine, cyclosporine, tolbutamide, chlorpropamide, glipizide, glyburide, tolazamide
Itraconazole Sporanox	Tablet	$10.80	200 mg	Once	Antacids, anticholinergics, H_2 blockers, rifampin, isoniazid

Abbreviations: AWP, average wholesale price, 1996; NA, not available.
*Cost is based on one full course of treatment using the AWP.
†Pregnancy level is based on the U.S. Food and Drug Administration codes for safety during pregnancy.
‡Cream formulations come with applicator; one applicator-full is approximately 5 g.

PITFALLS AND PROBLEMS

Cutaneous candidal infections often resemble dermatophytoses. Clinically, tinea pedis and tinea cruris are similar in appearance to intertriginous candidiasis. Candida intertrigo of toe webs needs to be distinguished from interdigital tinea pedis and erythrasma. In the inguinal area, candida intertrigo can mimic tinea cruris, inverse psoriasis, seborrheic dermatitis, erythrasma, Hailey-Hailey disease, intertrigo, and flexural Darier's disease.

Vaginal candidiasis, which can sometimes be diagnosed by symptoms of pruritus and vaginal discharge, must be distinguished from trichomoniasis, bacterial vaginosis, and chlamydial and gonococcal infection. Allergic contact dermatitis and herpes simplex may present with pruritus and be confused with candidiasis.[2] Bacteria may coexist with *Candida,* either as the primary pathogen or secondarily. Classic ''satellite'' papules and pustules are important in distinguishing candidiasis from other dermatoses. Oral candidiasis may resemble oral hairy leukoplakia, lichen planus, and leukoplakia (Table 12–4).

REFERRAL GUIDELINES

Most candidal infections can be diagnosed easily and treated by a primary care physician. One exception is CMC. Other difficult groups to treat are adults with

TABLE 12-3

Treatments for Cutaneous Candidiasis

Drug	Formulation	AWP Cost	Frequency	Duration
Ciclopirox olamine Loprox	2% cream	$10.18	q.d.	14 days
Clotrimazole Lotrimin	1% cream	$ 7.85	b.i.d.	3 days
Econazole Spectazole	1% cream	$11.46	b.i.d.	14 days
Ketoconazole Nizoral	2% cream	$13.46	q.d.	14 days
Miconazole Monistat-Derm	2% cream	$12.48	q.d.	14 days
Oxiconazole nitrate Oxistat	1% cream	$12.41	q.d.-b.i.d.	14 days
Sulconazole nitrate Exelderm	1% cream	$ 9.34	b.i.d.	21 days
Terbinafine hydrochloride Lamisil	1% cream	$24.06	b.i.d.	7 days
Amphotericin B Fungizone	3% cream 3% lotion	$29.21 $40.07	b.i.d.-q.i.d. b.i.d.-q.i.d.	14 days
Gentian violet	1% 2%	$ 7.50	b.i.d.-t.i.d. b.i.d.-t.i.d.	3 days
Nystatin Mycostatin	100,000 units/g Powder Ointment Cream	 $27.50 $ 1.46 $ 1.46	 b.i.d.-t.i.d. b.i.d. b.i.d.	 14 days

Abbreviations: AWP, average wholesale price, 1995; q.d., every day; b.i.d., twice daily; q.i.d., four times daily; t.i.d., three times daily.

TABLE 12-4

Treatments for Oral Candidiasis

Drug	Form	AWP Cost	Dose	Frequency	Duration	Interactions
Amphotericin B Fungilin	Lozenge	NA	10 mg	q.i.d.	7–14 days	Corticosteroids, digitalis, glycosides, other nephrotoxic drugs
Clotrimazole Mycelex	Troche	$52.59	10 mg	5 times/day	14 days	None significant
Fluconazole Diflucan	Tablet	$12.75	150 mg	Once	Once	Hydrochlorothiazide, cimetidine, rifampin, warfarin, phenytoin, terfenadine, astemizole, loratadine, ketoconazole, itraconazole, terbinafine, cyclosporine, tolbutamide, chlorpropamide, glipizide, glyburide, tolazamide
Ketoconazole Nizoral	Tablet	$ 2.71	200 mg	Once	Once	Antacids, anticholinergics, H_2 blockers, rifampin, isoniazid
Nystatin						
Mycostatin	Pastille	$56.00	200,000 units/ml	q.d.	14 days	None significant
Nilstat	Oral suspension	$20.96	100,000 units/ml	q.i.d.	14 days	
Nystex	Oral suspension	$15.73	100,000 units/ml	q.i.d.	14 days	

Abbreviations: AWP, average wholesale price, 1995; NA, not available; q.i.d., four times daily; q.d., every day.

chronic oral candidal infections, HIV-positive patients, and patients with chronic paronychia or onychomycosis. A dermatologist may be best able to advise on current therapies. Treating patients with chronic or recalcitrant mucocutaneous candidal infections may require a team approach. Not only primary care physicians but also specialists in dermatology, infectious disease, endocrinology, otolaryngology, gynecology, immunology, pharmacology, and oral surgery should be consulted when necessary.

REFERENCES

1. Martin AG, Kobayashi GS: Yeast infections: Candidiasis, pityriasis (tinea) versicolor. *In* Fitzpatrick TB, Eisen AZ, Wolff K, et al (eds): Dermatology in General Medicine. 4th ed. New York: McGraw-Hill, 1993; pp 2452–2467.
2. Denning DW: Management of genital candidiasis. Br Med J 1995; 310:2141–2144.
3. Greenspan D: Treatment of oropharyngeal candidiasis in HIV-positive patients. J Am Acad Dermatol 1994; 31:S51–S55.
4. Rippon JW: Medical Mycology: The Pathogenic Fungi and the Pathogenic Actinomycetes. 3rd ed. Philadelphia: WB Saunders, 1988.

CHAPTER 13

Cellulitis

Geetinder Kaus Chattha

CLINICAL APPEARANCE

Definition

Cellulitis is the general term for an acute, spreading inflammation of the dermis and subcutaneous tissue produced by an infective etiology, usually bacterial. Erysipelas, manifested by a distinctive clinical appearance, is confined to the dermis and upper subcutaneous tissue and is thought to be a superficial form of cellulitis.[1, 2]

Clinical Findings

The involved area is red, hot, swollen, and tender.[1, 3, 4] The margins of involvement are diffuse in cellulitis in contrast to the demarcated and elevated margins of erysipelas.[1] A portal of entry can usually be identified, such as a wound, ulcer, or inflammatory lesion.[3] The patient may have systemic symptoms of fever, chills, and malaise. In one study of adults, fever was present in only 26% of patients.[3] The involved area of erythema may develop blisters, bullae, and purpura.[5, 6] However, tissue necrosis, hemorrhagic bullae, and bronze discoloration of the skin may indicate a deeper, necrotizing infection.[5, 7]

Infection may spread via lymphatics and be manifested by reddish streaks extending from the involved area to the local lymph node group, with associated regional lymphadenopathy. Bacteremia and sepsis may occur, indicating the serious nature of cellulitis.[2]

Atypical or Alternate Forms

Cellulitis involving the head or neck area is much less common than that involving an extremity. In a study of children, 16% had facial involvement.[8] Periorbital cellulitis is characterized by erythema and swelling of the periorbital tissues. *Haemophilus influenzae,* often associated with a violaceous hue, is the most common pathogen isolated in children. An upper respiratory infection, otitis media, or sinusitis is present in half of cases. Less commonly, infection with or without associated trauma is the predisposing condition.[9] When the infection involves deeper tissues, proptosis or ophthalmoplegia may be present, indicating orbital cellulitis or abscess.[9] Complications include cerebral abscess formation, meningitis, and cavernous sinus thrombosis.

Perianal streptococcal cellulitis occurs usually in children. It is characterized by perianal erythema associated with tenderness, rectal bleeding, and painful defecation.[1]

DESCRIPTION OF DISEASE

Age/Population/Demographics

Cellulitis occurs in all age groups.[4] The lower extremity is most commonly involved in adults and children (see Fig. 13–1 on Color Plate 5).[3, 8] One study found that the upper extremity is most commonly involved in young adults—a factor that may be explained by intravenous drug abuse in this age group.[4] A portal of entry such as an inflammatory lesion, trauma, or surgical wound is identified in most cases.[2, 3, 4] Underlying disease may be identified in approximately half of the patients, with drug use and alcoholism being the most common.[4] Peripheral venous disease is a common underlying local factor.[4] Recurrent episodes of cellulitis may result in chronic lymphedema, which in turn may predispose to recurrent episodes of cellulitis, necessitating frequent courses of antibiotics.[1, 2] A form of cellulitis occurs in the lower extremities of patients following saphenous vein harvesting for coronary artery bypass surgery.[1, 2, 10] Cellulitis is thought to occur in this setting because of venous insufficiency. An associated tinea pedis in many of the described patients is thought to be the portal of entry.[1, 2, 10]

Etiology/Pathogenesis

Group A streptococci and *Staphylococcus aureus* alone or combined are the causative agents in most cases.[1, 2] Cellulitis caused by group B streptococci, also referred to as puerperal sepsis, may occur in mother or child around the time of delivery.[2] Gram-negative bacteria such as *Pseudomonas aeruginosa* and fungi such as *Cryptococcus neoformans* may cause cellulitis in immunocompromised patients.[1, 2] *Vibrio* spp. may cause cellulitis following ingestion of undercooked seafood in patients with diabetes or cirrhosis. This is an example of cellulitis caused by a primary bacteremia with secondary involvement of the skin.[1, 2]

Following a break in skin integrity, infection occurs in the dermis and subcutaneous tissue.[2, 11] Paradoxically, despite the low density of invading organisms, the clinical picture is dramatic, suggesting that inflammatory mediators and lymphatic failure play a major role in the observed findings.[2, 6]

Diagnosis

Cellulitis is diagnosed by the typical clinical findings. However, it is sometimes important to identify the etiologic agent. This agent may be confirmed by Gram's stain and cultures obtained from the affected site and from blood. Specimens may be obtained from the likely portal of entry, if present, or may be obtained from the drainage in blisters or bullae. When the involved skin is intact, specimens for culture may also be obtained by needle aspiration.[1–3, 5, 6, 8, 12] The skin is first disinfected with povidone-iodine or other disinfectant. A 21- or 22-gauge needle is then inserted into the skin at the leading margin of involvement, and an attempt is made to aspirate fluid. If no fluid is obtained, then the procedure is repeated using 1 ml of nonbacteriostatic saline solution injected into the subcutaneous tissue, followed by immediate aspiration. This fluid is then sent for bacterial culture. The yield for this procedure is variable.[3, 5, 6, 8, 12, 13] Positive cultures were more likely when this technique was employed in the setting of underlying diabetes mellitus or malignancy in adults.[13] A prospective study of children with cellulitis yielded a pathogen in almost half the cases with needle aspiration.[8] Specimens for stains and culture may also be obtained from biopsy of the involved skin.[6]

Pathology

Although skin biopsy is often unnecessary, it may be helpful in the evaluation of cellulitis. Noninfectious inflammatory diseases such as erythema nodosum and vasculitis may be excluded. Frozen sections of incisional biopsy specimens may expediently distinguish necrotizing fasciitis from cellulitis.[2]

TREATMENT

Treatment should be based on the clinical setting. Initial treatment should cover streptococci and staphylococci in all cases and *H. influenzae* in the setting of facial infections in young children. Intravenous penicillin is the treatment of choice for infections presumed to be a result of streptococci, such as erysipelas.[1, 14] When both streptococci and staphylococci are considered or the etiology is unclear, parenteral administration of a penicillanase-resistant penicillin, such as nafcillin, 1.0 to 1.5 g intravenously every 4 hours, is appropriate therapy.[1, 14] Mild early infection may be treated with an oral penicillinase-resistant penicillin, such as dicloxacillin, 0.25 to 0.5 g orally every 6 hours.[1, 14] An alternative therapy covering both streptococci and staphylococci is use of a first-generation cephalosporin, such as cephalexin, 0.25 to 0.5 g orally every 6 hours, for mild infection.[14] An intravenous first-generation cephalosporin, such as cefazolin, may be used as an alternative for severe infection.[14] Alternative therapy for severely penicillin-allergic patients is erythromycin, 0.5 g orally every 6 hours, for mild infection and vancomycin, 1.0 to 1.5 g/day intravenously, for severe infection.[1, 14] When infection with *H. influenzae* is suspected, a third-generation cephalosporin, such as cefotaxime or ceftriaxone, is the first choice for treatment. A special consideration should be made when evaluating cellulitis in immunocompromised and possibly neutropenic patients. Because of the risk of pseudomonal infection in this setting, a broader-spectrum antibiotic regimen such as a third-generation cephalosporin (e.g., ceftazidime) or an antipseudomonas penicillin (e.g., ticarcillin, mezlocillin, or piperacillin) each in conjunction with an aminoglycoside (e.g., gentamicin, tobramycin, or amikacin) should be employed until the pathogen is confirmed.[2, 14]

Patients with severe infection initially begun on parenteral therapy may be switched to an oral antibiotic when systemic symptoms such as fever and chills have resolved and significant local clinical improvement has taken place. Treatment should be continued until all signs and symptoms have resolved, typically 10 days for uncomplicated infections. Adjunctive measures include bedrest, elevation of the involved extremity, and marking the margins of involvement with pen in order to follow progression or regression of the involved area.[1, 2]

PITFALLS AND PROBLEMS

Signs of devitalized tissue such as cyanosis, blistering, or bronzing of the skin, poor response to antibiotics, or significant systemic symptoms may indicate an underlying necrotizing soft tissue infection.[7] Antimicrobial therapy is not sufficient treatment. Surgical débridement of all necrotic tissue is mandatory.[2, 7] Distinguishing between necrotizing cellulitis and necrotizing fasciitis is critical in order determine the extent for débridement because the skin findings may be identical. Direct surgical inspection of the involved tissues with the use of an instrument probe to determine the extent of undermining allows the surgeon to distinguish between necrotizing cellulitis, fasciitis, and myositis. When the diagnosis is uncertain, as mentioned earlier, frozen sections of incisional biopsy specimens may rapidly provide information about the condition of the soft tissues prior to surgical exploration.[2] Necrotizing cellulitis does not involve the fascia; therefore, involvement is limited to the margins of overlying skin changes. Necrotizing fasciitis, however, rapidly spreads along fascial lines and is characterized by significant undermining of devitalized tissue, systemic toxicity, and high mortality.[2, 7]

REFERRAL/CONSULTATION GUIDELINES

Other conditions such as vasculitis, erythema nodosum, stasis dermatitis, and thrombophlebitis may mimic the signs of cellulitis and require specialized therapy. Cellulitis that does not respond to initial therapy or shows signs of a necrotizing soft tissue infection warrants consultation.

REFERENCES

1. Swartz MN: Skin and soft tissue infections. *In* Mandell GL, Douglas RG, Bennet JE (eds): Principles and Practice of Infectious Diseases. 4th ed. New York: Churchill Livingstone, 1995; pp 909–928.
2. Johnson RA: The compleat dermatologist's guide to cellulitis. Fitzpatrick's J Clin Dermatol 1994; 6:12–23.
3. Hook EW III, Hooton TM, Horton CA, et al: Microbiologic evaluation of cutaneous cellulitis in adults. Arch Intern Med 1986; 146:295–297.
4. Ginsberg MB: Cellulitis: Analysis of 101 cases and review of the literature. South Med J 1981; 74:530–533.
5. Sachs MK: The optimum use of needle aspiration in the bacteriologic diagnosis of cellulitis in adults. Arch Intern Med 1990; 150:1907–1912.
6. Duvanel T, Auckenthaler R, Rohner P, et al: Quantitative cultures of biopsy specimens from cutaneous cellulitis. Arch Intern Med 1989; 149:293–296.
7. Arhenholtz DH: Necrotizing soft tissue infections. Surg Clin North Am 1988, 68:199–214.
8. Fleisher G, Ludwig S, Camos J: Cellulitis: Bacterial etiology, clinical features, and laboratory findings. J Pediatr 1980; 97:591–593.
9. Israele V, Nelson JD: Periorbital and orbital cellulitis. Pediatr Infect Dis J 1987; 6:404–410.
10. Hurwitz RM, Tisserand ME: Streptococcal cellulitis proved by skin biopsy in a coronary artery bypass graft patient. Arch Dermatol 1985; 121:908–909.
11. Finch R: Skin and soft-tissue infections. Lancet 1988; 2:164–167.
12. Uman SJ, Kunin CM: Needle aspiration in the diagnosis of soft-tissue infections. Arch Intern Med 1975; 135:959–962.
13. Kielhofner MA, Brown B, Dall L: Influence of underlying disease process on the utility of cellulitis needle aspirates. Arch Intern Med 1988; 148:2451–2452.
14. The choice of antibacterial drugs. Med Lett Drugs Ther 1994; 36:53–60.

CHAPTER 14

Varicella

Toby A. Maurer and Timothy G. Berger

CLINICAL APPEARANCE

Varicella is characterized by a vesicular eruption consisting of delicate "teardrop" vesicles on an erythematous base (see Fig. 14–1 on Color Plate 5). The eruption starts with faint macules that develop rapidly into vesicles within 24 hours. Successive fresh crops of vesicles appear for a few days, mainly on the trunk, the face, and the oral mucosa. The vesicles quickly become pustular, umbilicated, then crusted. Lesions tend not to scar, but larger lesions, and those that become secondarily infected, may heal with a characteristic round, depressed scar.

Varicella can be extremely severe and even fatal in immunosuppressed patients, especially those with impaired cell-mediated immunity. The skin lesions in the immunosuppressed host are usually identical to varicella in the healthy host; however, the lesions may be numerous. In the setting of immunosuppression, the lesions more frequently become necrotic and ulceration may occur. Even if the lesions are few, the size of the lesion may be large (up to several centimeters), and necrosis of the full thickness of the dermis may occur. In patients with human immunodeficiency virus (HIV) infection, varicella may be severe and fatal. Atypical cases of a few scattered lesions but without a dermatomal distribution usually represent reactivation of disease with dissemination. Chronic varicella may complicate HIV infection, resulting in ulcerative (ecthymatous) or hyperkeratotic (verrucous) lesions. These patterns of infection may be associated with acyclovir resistance.[1]

The congenital varicella syndrome is characterized by a series of anomalies including hypoplastic limbs (usually unilateral and lower extremity), cutaneous scars, and ocular and central nervous system disease. The overall risk for this syndrome is between 1 and 2%. The highest risk (about 2%) is when the mother is infected between weeks 13 and 20. Infection of the fetus in utero may result in zoster occurring postnatally, often in the first 2 years of life. This occurs in about 1% of varicella-complicated pregnancies, and the risk for this complication is greatest in varicella occurring in weeks 25 to 36 of gestation. If the mother develops varicella between 5 days before and 2 days after delivery, neonatal varicella can occur and be severe. These neonates develop varicella at 5 to 10 days of age.[2]

DESCRIPTION OF DISEASE

Varicella, commonly known as chickenpox, is primary infection with the varicella-zoster virus. In temperate regions, 90% of cases occur in children less than 10 years of age. In tropical countries, however, it tends to be a disease of teenagers.

The incubation period is 14 to 21 days. Transmission is via the respiratory route, with initial viral replication in the nasopharynx and conjunctiva. There is an initial viremia between days 4 and 6, seeding the liver, spleen, lungs, and perhaps other organs.

A secondary viremia occurs at days 11 to 20, resulting in infection of the epidermis and the appearance of the characteristic skin lesions. Individuals are infectious for at least 4 days before and 5 days after the appearance of the exanthem. Low-grade fever, malaise, and headache are usually present but slight. The severity of the disease is age-dependent, with adults having more severe disease and a greater risk of visceral disease. In healthy children, the death rate from varicella is 1.4 per 100,000 cases, and in adults, 30.9 deaths per 100,000 cases. As with most viral infections, immunosuppression may worsen the course of the disease.

The diagnosis is easily made clinically. In atypical cases, a Tzanck smear from the floor of a vesicle will usually show typical multinucleate giant cells, as in herpes zoster or simplex. If needed, the most useful clinical test is a direct fluorescent antibody test, which is rapid and will both confirm the infection and type the virus. Biopsy will show findings typical of a viral vesicle but is not diagnostic of varicella-zoster virus infection.

TREATMENT

Both immunocompetent children and adults with varicella benefit from acyclovir therapy if it is started early (within 24 hours of the appearance of the eruption). Therapy does not appear to alter the development of adequate immunity to reinfection.

Since the complications of varicella are infrequent in children, routine treatment is not recommended; rather, therapeutic decisions are made on a case by case basis.[3] Acyclovir therapy seems to benefit most secondary cases within a household, probably since therapy is instituted earlier. Therapy does not, however, return children to school sooner. The dose is 20 mg/kg (maximum 800 mg/dose) four times daily for 5 days.[4] The newer antivirals, valacyclovir and famciclovir, are as effective as or superior to acyclovir, probably because of better absorption and higher blood levels. They are as safe as acyclovir and, if not contraindicated, are preferred. Aspirin and other salicylates should not be used as antipyretics in varicella, as they increase the risk of Reye's syndrome. In cases where antiviral treatment is not used, topical antipruritic lotions, oatmeal baths, and dressing the patient in light cool clothing and keeping the environment cool are helpful.

Since varicella is more severe and complications are more common in adults, treatment is recommended in adolescents and adults (13 years of age and older). The dose is 800 mg four or five times daily for 5 days. Severe, fulminant cutaneous disease and visceral complications are treated with intravenous acyclovir 10 mg/kg every 8 hours, adjusted for creatinine clearance.

If a patient is hospitalized for therapy, strict isolation is required. Varicella patients should not be admitted to wards with immunocompromised hosts or on to pediatric wards, but rather are best placed on wards with healthy patients recovering from acute trauma.[5] In such cases, the administration of varicella-zoster immune globulin (VZIG) is warranted, and intravenous acyclovir therapy should be considered.[6]

Varicella Vaccine

In healthy children, the vaccine is very efficacious, with 95% of children remaining free of varicella during a 7-year follow-up. Household exposures resulted in a 12% rate of breakthrough varicella, well below the expected 90%. Many of the breakthrough cases were mild, and many of the skin lesions not vesicular. Antibodies appear to persist for many years, but the duration of immunity is unknown. Long-term studies are being performed following immunized children for up to 15 years.[7–9]

Varicella in Pregnancy and the Neonate

Maternal infection with the varicella-zoster virus during the first 20 weeks of gestation may result in a syndrome of congenital malformations (congenital varicella syndrome) as well as severe illness in the mother. Severe varicella and varicella pneumonia or disseminated disease in pregnancy should be treated with intravenous acyclovir. The value of oral acyclovir in all cases of varicella in pregnancy is unknown. VZIG should not be given once the pregnant woman has developed varicella. It can be given for family (intimate) exposures within the first 72 to 96 hours to prevent or ameliorate maternal varicella. Its use should be limited (owing to its cost and the high rate of asymptomatic infection in the United States) to seronegative women. The lack of a history of prior varicella is associated with seronegativity in only 20% or less of persons from the United States.[10, 11]

Although acyclovir is apparently safe in pregnancy, its efficacy in preventing fetal complications of maternal varicella is unknown.[6]

Varicella in the Immunocompromised

Varicella may be complicated by pneumonia, hepatitis, and encephalitis. Prior varicella does not always protect the immunosuppressed host from recurrent outbreaks.

In a recent case-control study, corticosteroid use, either as short courses or inhaled steroids, did not appear to be a risk factor for the development of severe varicella. In general, special management is not required for persons using these agents who are exposed to varicella.[12] However, the clinician should be aware that severe disease can occur, albeit rarely, and the patient should be counseled to return immediately for treatment if varicella develops.[13]

Ideally, treatment of varicella in the immunocompromised patient would involve prevention through the use of varicella vaccination if possible prior to immunosuppression. Intravenous acyclovir at a dose of 10 mg/kg three times daily is given as soon as the diagnosis is suspected. VZIG may be given if the patient has life-threatening disease and is not responding to intravenous acyclovir. VZIG may also be used to protect immunosuppressed hosts with high-risk exposure, if given within 96 hours of exposure.

In HIV-infected persons, treatment is individualized. Persons with typical varicella should be evaluated for the presence of pneumonia or hepatitis. Oral acyclovir in full doses may be used if no visceral complications are present. Visceral disease mandates intravenous therapy. If there is not a rapid response to oral acyclovir, intravenous acyclovir should be instituted. Atypical disseminated cases must be treated aggressively until all lesions resolve. If inadequate doses of acyclovir are given initially, relapse may occur, with the subsequent development of acyclovir resistance. The diagnosis of acyclovir-resistant varicella-zoster virus is difficult. These acyclovir-resistant strains may be difficult to grow, and sensitivity testing is still not standardized or readily available for varicella-zoster virus. Acyclovir-resistant varicella is treated with foscarnet.[14]

PITFALLS AND PROBLEMS

Secondary bacterial infection is the most common complication. Other complications are rare. Pneumonia (uncommon in normal children but seen in 1 in 400 adults with varicella), encephalitis, and glomerulonephritis are those most frequently seen. Carditis, hepatitis, keratitis, vesicular conjunctivitis, orchitis, Reye's syndrome, arthritis, cerebellar ataxia, myelitis, optic neuritis, pancreatitis, and splenic hemorrhage with rupture have also been reported. Symptomatic thrombocytopenia, with purpura and bleeding into mucous membranes, is a rare manifestation of varicella. Purpura fulminans represents a form of disseminated intravascular coagulation, with the clinical findings secondary to widespread arterial thrombosis. Lasting immunity follows varicella. Zoster typically occurs some years after varicella.

REFERRAL/CONSULTATION GUIDELINES

Varicella in nonimmunocompromised children and adults is best managed by the primary care provider. Because of the complications of varicella in pregnancy and neonates as well as in the immunocompromised host, consultation with persons who have experience in these areas may be of benefit.

REFERENCES

1. Alessi E, Cusini M, Zerboni R, et al: Unusual varicella zoster virus infection in patients with AIDS. Arch Dermatol 1988; 124:1011.
2. Prober CG, Gershon AA, Grose C, et al: Consensus: Varicella-zoster infections in pregnancy and the perinatal period. Pediatr Infect Dis J 1990; 9:865.
3. Dunkle LM, Arvin AM, Whitley RJ, et al: A controlled trial of acyclovir for chickenpox in normal children. N Engl J Med 1991; 325:1539.
4. Balfour HH Jr, Kelly JM, Suarez CS, et al: Acyclovir treatment of varicella in otherwise healthy children. J Pediatr 1990; 116:633.
5. Felder HM: Treatment of adult chickenpox with oral acyclovir. Arch Intern Med 1990; 150:2061.
6. Boyd K, Walker E: Acyclovir treatment of varicella in pregnancy. Br Med J 1988; 296:393.
7. Gershon AA, LaRussa P, Hardy I, et al: Varicella vaccine: The American experience. J Infect Dis 1992; 166:S63.
8. Krause PR, Klinman DM: Efficacy, immunogenicity, safety, and use of live attenuated chickenpox vaccine. J Pediatr 1995; 127:518.
9. Weibel RE, Neff BJ, Kuter BJ, et al: Live attenuated varicella virus vaccine: Efficacy in healthy children. N Engl J Med 1984; 310:1410.
10. Brunell PA: Varicella in pregnancy, the fetus, and the newborn: Problems in management. J Infect Dis 1992; 166:S42.
11. Enders G, Miller E, Cradock-Watson J, et al: Consequences of varicella and herpes zoster in pregnancy: Prospective study of 1739 cases. Lancet 1994; 343:1548.
12. Patel H, MacArthur C, Johnson D: Recent corticosteroid use and the risk of complicated varicella in otherwise immunocompetent children. Arch Pediatr Adolesc Med 1996; 150:409.
13. Dowell SF, Bresee JS: Severe varicella associated with steroid use. Pediatrics 1993; 92:223.
14. Janier M, Hillon B, Baccard M, et al: Chronic varicella zoster infection in AIDS. J Am Acad Dermatol 1988; 18:584.

CHAPTER 15

Common Skin Cancers (Basal Cell and Squamous Cell)

S. Teri McGillis

Basal cell and squamous cell carcinomas are the most common neoplasms affecting the skin. Approximately 1 million Americans develop these "nonmelanoma" cancers each year. Despite their potential for morbidity, early detection and treatment result in high cure rates. Although they share several features in common, it is important for the clinician to distinguish between these two leading skin cancer types.

BASAL CELL CARCINOMA

CLINICAL APPEARANCE

Basal cell carcinoma (BCC) is the most common cancer of the skin. Close to 800,000 Americans will be diagnosed with a BCC in 1996. Basal cell epithelioma, rodent ulcer, and Jacob's ulcer are other names for this malignancy.

Chronic sun exposure plays a major role in their development, so it is not surprising that most BCCs occur on areas of high visibility. The face, head, neck, and in men, the trunk are common sites of predilection. Any body area, however, can be involved, making it imperative to fully examine any patient with a prior history of skin cancer or who evidences chronic sun exposure.

No single characteristic consistently identifies a BCC. They present as solitary or multiple lesions that are nonhealing for several months. Although many are asymptomatic, a tendency to easy bleeding or pruritus is not unusual. There are six clinical variants: noduloulcerative, superficial, pigmented, morpheaform, metatypical, and premalignant fibroepithelioma.

BCC CLINICAL VARIANTS*

Noduloulcerative BCC (Fig. 15–1*A* and *C*)

This is the most common type, accounting for approximately 60% of all primary BCCs. These begin as *pearly, translucent papules* with overlying *telangiectasias.* Allowed to enlarge, *ulceration* and *crusting* occur, and the lesion may present as an *erosion* or *ulcer* with a *pearly, rolled margin.* Left unrecognized, they continue a slow growth pattern and can eventually erode through subcutaneous tissues including cartilage and bone. The term *rodent ulcer* was coined to describe the large areas of destruction created by neglected tumors.

Superficial BCC

This type is found most often on the *trunk* and *extremities.* It is typically *flat, erythematous,* and *scaly.* It varies in size from a few millimeters to several centimeters in diameter. To the untrained eye, this type can be mis-

*Key features are set in italics.

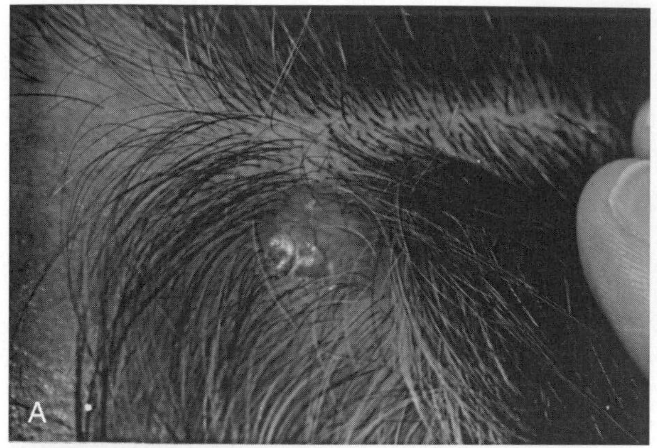

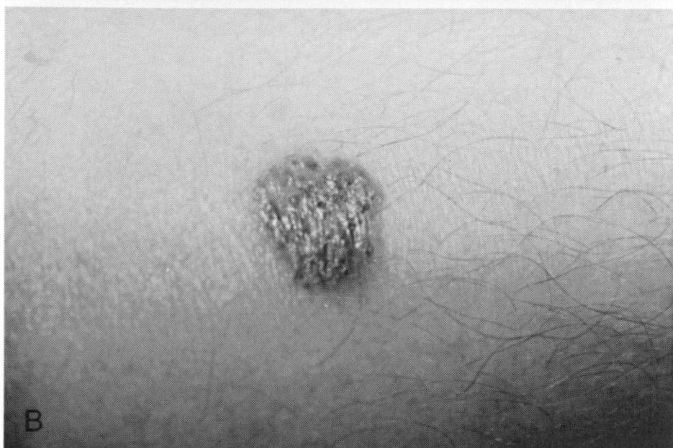

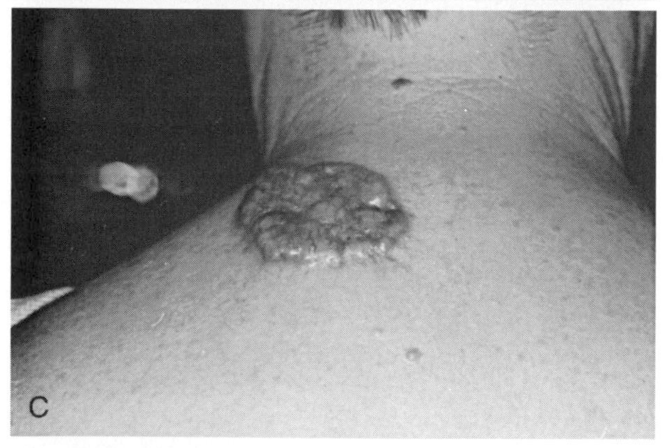

FIGURE 15–1

A, Noduloulcerative basal cell carcinoma (BCC) on the scalp. Note the pearly quality and overlying telangiectasias. *B,* Pigmented BCC of the forearm. Brownish-black pigment is noted throughout the lesion. *C,* Large noduloulcerative BCC of the upper trunk.

taken for psoriasis, eczema, or tinea corporis. This type of BCC is the least aggressive.

Pigmented BCC (Fig. 15–1*B*)

This variant resembles a *noduloulcerative* lesion but has varying degrees of *blue, black,* or *brown pigment.* It is most often seen in darker-skinned persons. It is not unusual for these BCC types to be mistaken for severely dysplastic nevi or even for malignant melanomas.

Morpheaform BCC

This variant derives its name from its resemblance to *morphea* (localized scleroderma). It is also known as a sclerotic BCC and can appear as *scar tissue.* It commonly presents as a *pink, yellow,* or *ivory plaque* with little or *no ulceration.* This type responds poorly to most treatment modalities because it is embedded in a thick stroma. It *exhibits high recurrence rates.*

Metatypical BCC

No distinct clinical feature typifies this variant. On histologic examination, however, these BCCs *resemble squamous cell carcinomas (SCCs).* In fact, they behave more like an SCC in that they are more aggressive.

Premalignant Fibroepithelioma

Also known as *fibroepithelioma of Pinkus,* this variant occurs as a *smooth, firm, erythematous nodule.* It is most often found on the thighs, lower back, and groin. It is very rare.

ATYPICAL FORMS

Albinism, xeroderma pigmentosa, and the basal cell nevus syndrome are conditions in which many skin cancers arise at an early age. Patients with albinism lack the photoprotective effects of melanin. Persons with xeroderma pigmentosa lack the ability to repair cellular DNA damage induced by ultraviolet light. Basal cell nevus syndrome is a rare, inherited disease characterized by multiple BCCs. Other associated abnormalities of this syndrome include palmar pitting, bifid ribs, mandibular cysts, and cranial calcifications.

DESCRIPTION OF DISEASE

The risk of developing a BCC increases with patient age. Although most are diagnosed between the ages of 40 and 70 years, an increase in outdoor lifestyles, suntan parlor usage, and earlier sun exposure make diagnosis in younger individuals more common. BCC is rare in children.

BCC development is strongly correlated with cumulative sunlight exposure. Fair-skinned individuals (those that burn easily, tan poorly), those with blue/green eyes, as well as blonds and redheads are at highest risk. This is due to a lack of natural melanocytic protection. Likewise, BCCs are rare among blacks living in the United States.

Additional risk factors include having a family history of skin cancer, engaging in outdoor occupations or pastimes, and living in geographic regions where year-round sun exposure is the norm. Individuals with histories of ionizing radiation (as in the treatment of acne) or with burn scars are also at increased risk.

Epidermal DNA damage is felt to promote BCC development. Sunlight in the ultraviolet B UVB range (290 to 320 nm) causes such damage. UVB exposure may also be locally immunosuppressive. These effects together inhibit the ability to repair cellular injury and thus initiate tumor growth.

PATHOLOGY

Histologic variants of BCC are as diverse as their clinical presentations. All BCCs share the presence of darkly staining basaloid cells arranged in a variety of patterns (such as cords, strands, or nodules). Retraction spaces are commonly seen around tumor islands. Many BCCs demonstrate attachment to the overlying epidermis or to hair follicle structures from which they evolve.

TREATMENT

(See "Treatment of Basal Cell and Squamous Cell Carcinomas," later in this chapter.)

METASTASIS RATE

Fortunately, metastasis is a rare occurrence for BCCs and is estimated at less than 0.2%. Spread via both hematogenous and lymphatic pathways has been documented.[1]

FOLLOW-UP GUIDELINES

Meticulous follow-up is important. Half of all patients with a primary BCC will subsequently develop a second primary lesion.

Recurrences of previously treated lesions are generally detected within 2 to 5 years postoperatively. Frequency of follow-up visits must be individualized. Those patients with an isolated primary lesion may be followed yearly after careful postoperative evaluation. Patients with a history of aggressive tumors, rare tumor variants, chronic sun damage, or multiple tumors, as well as those with basal cell nevus syndrome or immunosuppression, will need more frequent examinations.

Follow-up visits should include not only a careful cutaneous examination but also appropriate patient education in sun protection, sunscreen use, tumor recognition, and self–skin examinations.

PITFALLS IN DIAGNOSIS

Delays in diagnosis are detrimental. BCCs can present with a wide array of clinical appearances and, as discussed earlier, can mimic several benign lesions such as eczema, psoriasis, or nevi. If any doubt exists as to the etiology of a nonhealing lesion, a biopsy should be done.

REFERRAL GUIDELINES

Recurrent lesions or those occurring in areas of high risk for recurrence should be referred. Lesions over 2 cm in diameter should be treated by those with expertise in cutaneous oncology.

SQUAMOUS CELL CARCINOMA

CLINICAL APPEARANCE

SCC is less common than BCC. Approximately 200,000 SCCs are diagnosed yearly in the United States. Unlike BCCs, these tumors can metastasize. They account for the majority of nonmelanoma skin cancer deaths.

Since SCC is a neoplasm arising from stratified epithelium, it can be located anywhere on the skin and mucous membranes. In general, SCCs of the mucous membranes and those that arise de novo have higher potentials for metastasis than those arising from precursor lesions such as actinic keratoses.

No single feature typifies an SCC. Any slow-growing keratotic papule or plaque that persists for several months is suspect. Tumors that are in situ differ from those that are invasive.

Squamous cell carcinomas in situ refer to lesions that demonstrate full-thickness dysplasia of the epidermis without invasion of the deeper dermis. SCCs of this type commonly appear as slowly enlarging erythematous macules. There is often associated scaling and crusting, leading to a mistaken diagnosis of psoriasis, eczema, or even fungal lesions (Fig. 15–2*A*). Bowen's disease and erythroplasia of Queyrat are types of in situ SCC.

Bowen's disease is synonymous with in situ SCC. At times, it may involve hair follicle lining, rendering it less amenable to superficial forms of destruction. *Erythroplasia of Queyrat* is SCC in situ of the penis. Even though it is classified as intraepithelial, its mucous membrane location portends more aggressive behavior. Any form of in situ SCC can evolve into an invasive lesion.

Invasive SCCs vary greatly in their clinical presentations. They can appear as indurated papules or plaques or as thickened hyperkeratotic nodules. Likewise, they can occur rapidly with aggressive behaviors or be indolent in their growth phase. Many are ulcerated at the time of presentation. (Figs. 15–2*B* and 15–3*A*).

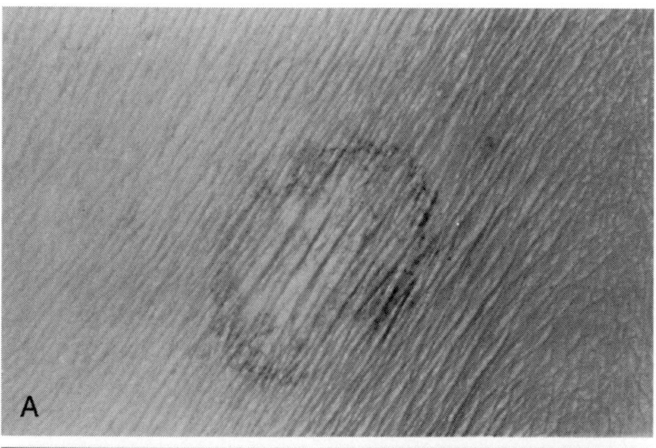

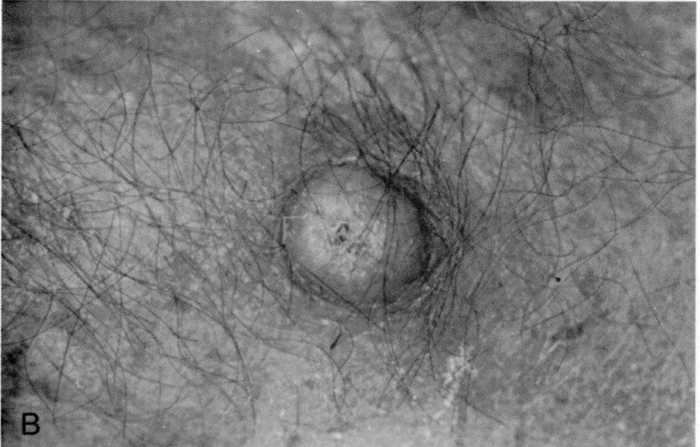

FIGURE 15-2
A, Squamous cell carcinoma (SCC) in situ presenting as an enlarging erythematous macule with crusting at the periphery. *B*, SCC presenting as a firm, keratotic nodule.

SCCs that arise on cutaneous surfaces may differ from those occurring on mucous membranes. Those on cutaneous surfaces tend to be on areas of sun exposure, with 80% occurring on the head and neck. Evidence of chronic sun exposure will often be present, evidenced by freckling, telangiectasias, lentigines, and actinic keratoses. Interestingly, the dorsa of the hands, which receives much sunlight, has a 3:1 higher incidence of developing SCC over BCC.

Mucous membrane SCCs can begin as velvety, erythematous plaques or as moist, thickened, ulcerated nodules. Since metastasis rates are higher with such SCCs, regional lymphadenopathy may be present. The lower lip is involved more frequently than the upper lip, and SCC affects men more often than women. Likewise, SCC of the penis, anus, and scrotum have high morbidity and mortality rates.

Invasive SCCs grow along ''paths of least resistance'' and, if left untreated, can invade muscle, cartilage, and bone. Perineural spread is much more common for SCC than BCC. Patients often remain asymptomatic for years before neurologic symptoms present. Such tumors portend a poor prognosis because they are difficult to treat and often recur (see Fig. 15–3*B*).

Any patient with a suspected SCC should always have regional lymph nodes palpated.

ATYPICAL FORMS

Verrucous carcinoma is a low-grade SCC that affects both cutaneous and mucous membrane surfaces. As its name suggests, these lesions resemble recalcitrant verrucae (warts). They are named for their sites of origin. In the oral cavity, it is called *oral florid papillomatosis,* in the genital region, it is referred to as *giant condyloma* of *Buschke* and *Lowenstein,* whereas on the plantar surface, verrucous carcinoma is known as *epithelioma coniculatum.* Unlike invasive SCC, radiation therapy is believed to cause malignant transformation of verrucous carcinoma and should be avoided.

Keratoacanthoma is considered a benign cutaneous tumor that morphologically resembles SCC. It typically occurs rapidly, often in a matter of weeks. It appears as a dome-shaped nodule with a keratin-filled center. Controversy exists as to its true nature and etiology. Complete removal is advised even though spontaneous regression is known to occur.

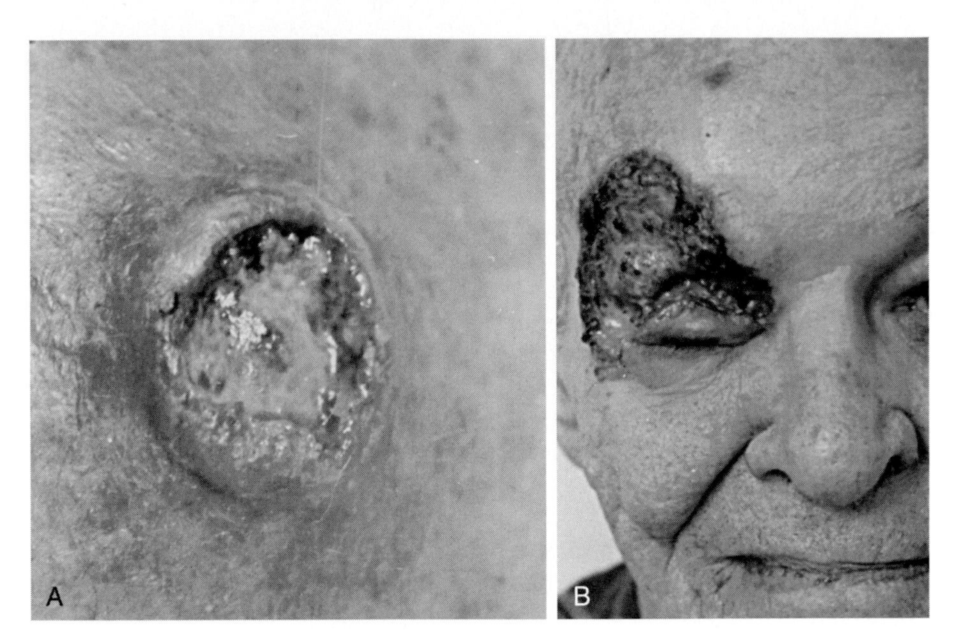

FIGURE 15-3
A, Ulcerated SCC arising on sun-damaged skin. *B,* Neglected SCC of the periorbital region. Such lesions demonstrate high morbidity and mortality.

DESCRIPTION OF DISEASE

Like BCC, the major predisposing factor for SCC occurrence is ultraviolet damage. Those individuals at most risk have fair skin types, blue/green eyes, and blond or red hair. The mean age of onset for SCC is older than that for BCC.

The incidence of solar-induced SCC is rising. This is in part due to a reduction in the earth's protective ozone layer. The National Academy of Sciences estimates that a 16.5% depletion of the ozone layer could lead to a 30% increase in UVB exposure, which, in turn, could cause skin cancer rates to increase as much as 50%.[2]

Other factors play a role in SCC development and, in fact, may serve as malignant transforming events. These include chronic scarring, human papillomavirus infection, immunosuppression, arsenic exposure, and contact with industrial chemicals.

Patients with chronic scarring, ulcers, or burn scars may develop SCC in the scar bed. Known as *Marjolin's ulcers,* these have a poor prognosis and a higher incidence of metastasis.

Human papillomavirus types 16, 18, 31, 33, and 35 are implicated in genital, oral, and periungal SCCs. Routine testing of SCCs for viral proteins is not recommended except in selected cases.

Chronic immunosuppression appears to promote SCC development, especially on sun-exposed areas. Organ-transplant patients or those on drugs such as cyclosporine or azothioprine are at risk. Such medications may potentiate the carcinogenic effects of ultraviolet light. A latency of 8 to 10 years seems to occur between exposure and tumor development.

Exposure to arsenic is known to initiate cancer of the skin. Arsenic is found in contaminated well water as well as in some pesticides. Arsenical keratoses of the palms and soles can occur and are precursors to tumor growth.

Industrial chemicals such as tar, coal, fuel oils, and soot may induce SCC. Chimney sweeps, for example, have high incidences of scrotal SCC, presumably from chemical exposure.

PATHOLOGY

SCC appears as irregular nests and cords of epidermal cells invading the dermis. In situ forms are limited to the epidermis. SCC is graded according to degree of differentiation. In general, a well-differentiated or low-grade SCC is less aggressive than a poorly differentiated, high-grade tumor. Squamous "pearls" are areas of incomplete keratinization and are pale staining. They are seen in lower-grade SCCs.

TREATMENT

(See "Treatment of Basal Cell and Squamous Cell Carcinomas," later in this chapter.)

METASTASIS RATE

Rates of metastasis are lower for SCCs arising on sun-exposed skin (0.3 to 3.7%) when compared with those occurring on mucous membranes (3.0 to 29.0%).[3] Metastatic potential is only partially defined by anatomic size, histologic features, prior treatment, and tumor etiology. Even an innocuous SCC that has been declared "cured" can, at times, metastasize.

All patients with SCC should have regional nodes palpated. Metastatic nodes tend to be very firm. In addition to regional spread, distant metastases occur via hematogenous and lymphatic channels.

FOLLOW-UP GUIDELINES

The aggressive potential of SCC cannot be emphasized enough. The first 5 years following diagnosis and treatment is a critical period, as the majority of local recurrences are detected within 2 years. Metastases often develop within 5 years. Those patients with high-risk lesions including perineural tumors are at significant risk for recurrence and metastasis and should be followed carefully.

Patient evaluation must be individualized. Patients with invasive SCC should be seen every 3 months for the first year; then every 3 to 6 months for the following 2 years. If no further skin cancer is detected, yearly follow-up visits may suffice.

Follow-up visits must include a full skin examination and lymph node palpation. Also, patient education including information on sunscreen use and cancer prevention must be a part of every examination.

PITFALLS IN DIAGNOSIS

A delay in diagnosis can be detrimental. In situ SCCs can mimic psoriasis or eczema and, if left untreated, may evolve into more invasive tumors. Invasive lesions may likewise be misinterpreted as verrucae, ulcers, or scars. A prompt biopsy should be done for any nonresolving or rapidly evolving lesion.

REFERRAL GUIDELINES

Patients with advanced disease including evidence of lymphadenopathy or neural symptoms must be referred. Additionally, those with mucous membrane lesions, recurrent tumors, or lesions greater than 2 cm are best treated by a skin cancer specialist.

TREATMENT OF BASAL CELL AND SQUAMOUS CELL CARCINOMAS

The primary goal of skin cancer treatment is complete eradication of the tumor at the outset. If the tumor recurs or is incompletely excised, morbidity will be increased. The secondary goal is a good cosmetic result.

Biopsy confirmation of the tumor is necessary to help define optimal treatment. Therapy must then be individualized according to tumor type, location, and patient status. Options for treatment include electrodesiccation, cryosurgery, radiation therapy, excision, and Mohs' micrographic surgery (Table 15–1).

High-risk areas for local recurrence include the central zone of the face, ear canals, periorbital regions, and postauricular sulci (Fig. 15–4). Tumors in these areas can extend subclinically along perichondrium, cartilage, or embryonic fusion planes. This can result in gross underestimation of tumor size and subsequently result in incomplete tumor removal.[4] Tumors in these areas should be identified as candidates for Mohs' micrographic surgery.

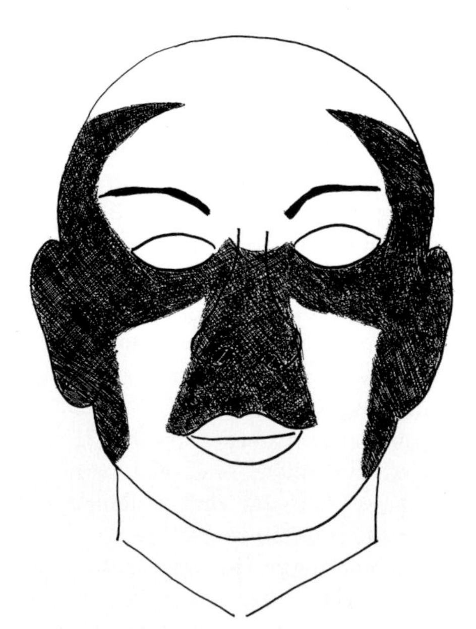

FIGURE 15–4
Tumors occurring in the "H-zone" of the face may exhibit subclinical extension and higher rates of recurrence.

TABLE 15-1

Common Treatment Options for Basal and Squamous Cell Carcinomas

Technique	Indications	Advantages	Disadvantages
ED&C	Low-risk tumors Superficial/nodular BCCs In situ SCCs Good for truncal lesions	Quick No suturing needed Can treat multiple lesions	No pathology specimen High recurrence rates if not adequately treated, especially on head and neck Poor cosmesis May bury tumor
Cryosurgery	Same as for ED&C Best for well-circumscribed lesions Morpheaform, scalp, and aggressive tumors should *not* be treated	Similar to those for ED&C	Painful Must train to do technique properly No specimen Cosmesis similar to that of ED&C
Radiation therapy	Adjunct to surgery Palliative for inoperable lesions *Not* for tumors in areas of prior radiation	Good for patients unable to undergo surgery Preserves tissue Good cosmesis initially, deteriorates with time	Radiation dermatitis Repeated trips necessary Special equipment and training necessary Not for young patients
5-Fluorouracil	In situ SCCs Superficial BCCs Actinic keratoses (superficial lesions only!)	Nonsurgical Inexpensive Excellent cosmesis	May delay diagnosis or mask more aggressive lesions Treatment can be uncomfortable
Excision	Good for large or small BCCs/SCCs	Specimen available to confirm clearance Good cosmesis	Need expertise May miss tumor areas, in which case, Mohs' may be needed Time consuming
Mohs' micrographic surgery	Recurrent tumors Incompletely excised tumors Those with aggressive histology Tumors in high-risk locations Poorly demarcated margins	Maximal cure rate Preserves normal tissue	Time consuming Special training and equipment necessary Expensive
Laser vaporization (CO_2)	Superficial lesions only SCCs in situ Superficial BCCs	Seals vessels, reduces bleeding Good for patients with pacemakers Good for multiple lesions	May miss tumor areas Cosmesis similar to that of ED&C Must be well skilled in laser use

Abbreviations: ED&C, electrodesiccation and curettage; BCCs, basal cell carcinomas; SCCs, squamous cell carcinomas.

ELECTRODESICCATION AND CURETTAGE

TECHNIQUE. Electrodesiccation and curettage (EDGC) involves curetting or ''shelling'' the tumor from the dermis and desiccating the base. It is usually repeated three times. It must be performed properly in order to achieve high cure rates. The obvious disadvantage is that no specimen is available for tissue confirmation following removal.

BCC. ED&C is ideal for small (<1 cm) nodular or superficial tumors. Morpheaform BCCs are poor candidates. It is best for tumors in low-risk regions such as the trunk and extremities. ED&C of tumors in high-risk regions unfortunately can result in recurrence rates as high as 20%. Resulting scars are flat, white, and approximately the surgical defect in size.

SCC. ED&C can successfully treat small lesions in low-risk areas, particularly in situ and superficial lesions.

CRYOSURGERY

TECHNIQUE. Freezing tumors with liquid nitrogen drops their temperature to lethal levels, halting cellular activity. Treating skin cancers with liquid nitrogen differs from treating benign lesions. Special equipment ensures that the base of the tumor reaches a critical −40° C. Cryosurgery is contraindicated in persons with cold intolerance, dysglobulinemias, and with lesions overlying nerves.

BCC. Superficial lesions in low-risk areas are ideal. Morpheaform BCCs and those occurring on the scalp are poor candidates.

SCC. In situ and small superficial lesions can be treated. Cryosurgery is *not* ideal for lesions on mucous membranes.

RADIATION THERAPY

TECHNIQUE. Standard radiation, electron beam, and radionucleotide implants have all been used to treat skin cancer. Radiation treatment is a good alternative to surgery for elderly or debilitated patients. It is also used as palliative therapy delivered in fractional doses. Multiple patient visits are required.

BCC. Radiation is not advised for tumors arising in areas of prior x-ray treatment. Otherwise, it can treat most tumor variants. Tumors extending to bone are at risk for necrosis.

SCC. Radiation treatment should be avoided on mucous membranes. It can be used as palliative therapy or for those in whom perineural or lymphatic involvement is noted at surgery.

FLUOROURACIL

TECHNIQUE. Best reserved for precancerous lesions, this treatment is applied topically, twice a day for 3 to 4 weeks. Fluorouracil blocks production of thymidylic acid necessary for DNA production.

BCC. Fluorouracil may play a role in treating superficial BCCs. Deeper or more aggressive lesions should not be treated. Long-term cure rates for superficial lesions have not been established.

SCC. In situ SCCs that do not involve the follicular epithelium may respond. Any remaining lesions should be biopsied and treated appropriately.

EXCISION

TECHNIQUE. Surgical excision leads to lesion removal and provides good cosmesis. It involves using a scalpel to excise elliptically around the tumor, followed by suturing of the defect. The specimen can then be evaluated for tumor clearance, depth, subtype, and other factors.

BCC. Most tumors of less than 2 cm in diameter can be excised. A margin of 0.4 cm should be taken.

SCC. Small, discrete, primary lesions can be excised successfully.

MOHS' MICROGRAPHIC SURGERY

TECHNIQUE. Mohs' surgery is a specialized excision technique named after Dr. Frederick Mohs. This technique involves excision followed by immediate frozen section analysis. Tumors are excised as thin disks of tissue that are stained and recorded. Tissue is then frozen and sectioned horizontally. Microscopic examination reveals any subclinical tumor extensions that otherwise may have been missed with routine excision or processing. The method is repeated until the tumor is completely removed. This technique provides the highest cure rates for both primary and recurrent lesions.[5]

Recommendations for Mohs' surgery are similar for both BCC and SCC:

- Recurrent tumors or those evolving in old scars
- Lesions that have been incompletely excised
- Tumors with aggressive histology
- Lesions occurring in high-risk areas (see Fig. 15–4)
- Lesions with poorly demarcated margins that may result in incomplete excision
- Lesions occurring in areas where tissue sparing is necessary

CO_2 LASERS

TECHNIQUE. Laser treatment of cancers is relatively new. The CO_2 laser has been used to vaporize cutaneous carcinomas. Since the laser seals small vessels, bleeding is reduced. It is also ideal for patients with pacemakers as well as for those with multiple superficial lesions.

BCC. The CO_2 laser should be used to treat small (<1 cm) and superficial lesions only.

SCC. The CO_2 laser is good for SCC in situ. Up to 0.5-cm margins should be vaporized around the primary tumor site.

OTHER TREATMENTS

As more is understood about tumor biology and behavior, alternative treatments will continue to emerge. Presently, immunotherapy (interferon alfa-2a), and chemotherapy (high-dose retinoids, intralesional fluorouracil) are areas of active investigation. Photodynamic therapy is another evolving area. Tumors are sensitized prior to exposure to specific wavelengths of light. This combination produces cytotoxic changes and tumor destruction. The future holds many promising avenues of improving skin cancer diagnosis and treatment.

REFERENCES

1. Miller SJ: Biology of basal cell carcinoma (Part I). J Am Acad Dermatol 1991; 24:1–13.
2. Fears TR, Scotto J: Estimating increases in skin cancer morbidity due to increases in ultraviolet radiation exposure. Cancer Invest 1983; 1(2):119–126.
3. Kwa RE, Compana K, Moy RL: Biology of cutaneous squamous cell carcinoma. J Am Acad Dermatol 1992; 26(1):1–26.
4. Mora GG, Robins P: Basal cell carcinoma in the center of the face: Special diagnostic, prognostic and therapeutic considerations. J Dermatol Surg Oncol 1978; 4:315–321.
5. Rowe DE, Carroll RJ, Day CL: Mohs surgery is the treatment of choice for recurrent (previously treated) basal cell carcinoma. J Dermatol Surg Oncol 1989; 15(4):424–431.

CHAPTER 16

Contact Dermatitis

Ponciano D. Cruz, Jr.

CLINICAL APPEARANCE

Definition

Contact dermatitis is an eczematous dermatitis caused by exposure to chemicals in the environment. It is an "outside-in" rather than an "inside-out" process, in which skin inflammation may be acute, subacute, or chronic. Contact dermatitis due to irritation should be differentiated from contact dermatitis due to allergy. Patch-testing is the principal method used to confirm the diagnosis of allergic contact dermatitis and to document the offending allergen.

Typical Lesions and Symptoms

The intensity of the dermatitis depends on the concentration of the inciting chemical and, in the case of allergic contact dermatitis, on the sensitivity of the individual to the allergen. Acute inflammation is expressed as erythema, blistering, crusting, or even frank necrosis. Subacute inflammation manifests as erythema, scaling, fissuring, or a parched, scalded appearance (see Figs. 16–1 through 16–3 on Color Plate 5). Chronic inflammation may have less erythema but more skin thickening with accentuated skin markings (lichenification) and excoriation. Itching is a cardinal feature of contact dermatitis, regardless of the severity of inflammation.

Keys to diagnosis are recognition of the eczematous nature of the skin eruption and correlation of the pattern and distribution of the lesions to the shape of the offending substance or the nature of exposure to it. For example, the diagnosis is obvious when inflammation is confined to the area under a watchband or a shoe or on skin sprayed with cologne. The location of the dermatitis also serves as an important clue to the source of the offending chemical. Table 16–1 lists substances that are common causes of contact dermatitis in specific body areas.

Atypical Presentation or Alternative Forms

Although the typical presentation is eczematous, contact dermatitis may occasionally present as urticaria or altered pigmentation (either hyperpigmentation or hypopigmentation). Widespread involvement, particularly of

TABLE 16–1

Common Causes of Contact Dermatitis by Location

Location	Cause
Scalp	Shampoos, hair dyes
Ears	Metal earrings, eyeglasses, hair care products
Eyelids	Nail polish, cosmetics, contact lens solution, airborne allergens
Face	Cosmetics, other topical preparations including sunscreens, airborne allergens
Neck	Necklaces, perfumes, airborne allergens
Trunk	Topical preparations, clothing including metal components and elastic in undergarments
Axillae	Deodorants, clothing
Hands	Soaps and detergents, occupational chemicals, metals including jewelry, topical preparations, rubber gloves
Genitals	Topical preparations, condoms
Anal region	Fecal spillage, topical preparations
Legs	Topical preparations, elastic in socks
Feet	Rubber, leather, synthetic materials in shoes

the face and of body parts unprotected by clothing, should call into consideration contact dermatitis produced by airborne allergens such as plant pollen, sprays, or fumes. Photocontact dermatitis may also have similar diffuse affectation. Rarely, contact dermatitis may become generalized, presenting as exfoliative erythroderma.

DESCRIPTION OF DISEASE

Demographics

Contact dermatitis is the most common skin disease acquired from the workplace, accounting for a considerable proportion of work compensation claims. Although irritant contact dermatitis accounts for the vast majority of these cases, a significant proportion may be due to allergic contact dermatitis.

Contact dermatitis can occur at any age. In infancy, the most common example is diaper dermatitis, which is irritant dermatitis due to prolonged contact with urine or feces, or both; residual soap or detergent in diapers; or friction. Common causes of allergic dermatitis in childhood are poison ivy, nickel (jewelry), rubber (shoe), fragrance, formaldehyde (cosmetics and shampoos), and neomycin (topical antibiotics).

In adults, the most likely sources of contact dermatitis are irritants or allergens peculiar to the individual's occupation or hobbies.

Natural History

Irritant contact dermatitis (especially cases due to strong irritants) may manifest within minutes to hours of contact. By contrast, allergic contact dermatitis may take several hours, days, or even weeks to develop. If left alone, most contact dermatitis will resolve completely. Unfortunately, this ideal situation is almost never realized because the accompanying itch results in scratching and attempts at topical treatment, which in turn lead to spread of the dermatitis, superimposed bacterial or dermatophytic infection, or partial but incomplete treatment, all of which may produce diagnostic confusion.

Pathology

The histopathology of contact dermatitis will typically demonstrate spongiotic inflammation, which distinguishes eczematous dermatitis from noneczematous dermatitis. Because spongiotic inflammation is nonspecific, however, it may not differentiate contact dermatitis from other eczematous dermatitis. Irritant and allergic contact dermatitis may also show similar histology. Skin biopsy is usually not necessary.

Etiology/Pathogenesis

Irritant dermatitis is produced by physical and chemical alteration of the epidermis, resulting in destruction of the normal mechanical barrier of skin. By contrast, allergic dermatitis is a delayed response of the T-cell arm of the immune system against low-molecular-weight haptens that come in contact with the skin. High concentrations of irritant chemicals are usually required to produce a dermatitis. By contrast, in sensitized individuals, very low concentrations of allergens can readily trigger the dermatitis.

TREATMENT

Therapeutic Expectations

Acute forms of contact dermatitis, particularly those involving greater than 20% of total body surface, respond well to systemic steroid treatment. Topical therapy may suffice for less-acute or less-widespread forms of contact dermatitis. Prevention of recurrences depends wholly on avoidance of the offending chemical or protection from it.

First-Line Therapy/Alternative Options

Cold, wet compresses are highly effective during the acute blistering state; they should be used for 15 to 30 minutes several times a day for 1 to 3 days until blistering and severe itching are controlled. Short, cool, tub baths, especially with colloidal oatmeal (Aveeno), are soothing and help to control the acute inflammation. Calamine lotion controls itching, but prolonged use causes excessive dryness. Antihistamine agents are best administered orally; they control itching and encourage sleep.

Short courses of corticosteroids over 2 to 3 weeks are the definitive treatment. As cited previously, acute dermatitis and widespread involvement require systemic administration. This may take the form of a single dose of intramuscular triamcinolone acetonide (Kenalog; maximal dose of 1 mg/kg) or peroral prednisone (initially at a maximal dose of 1 mg/kg, tapered over at least 2 weeks). Less-acute or less-widespread dermatitis

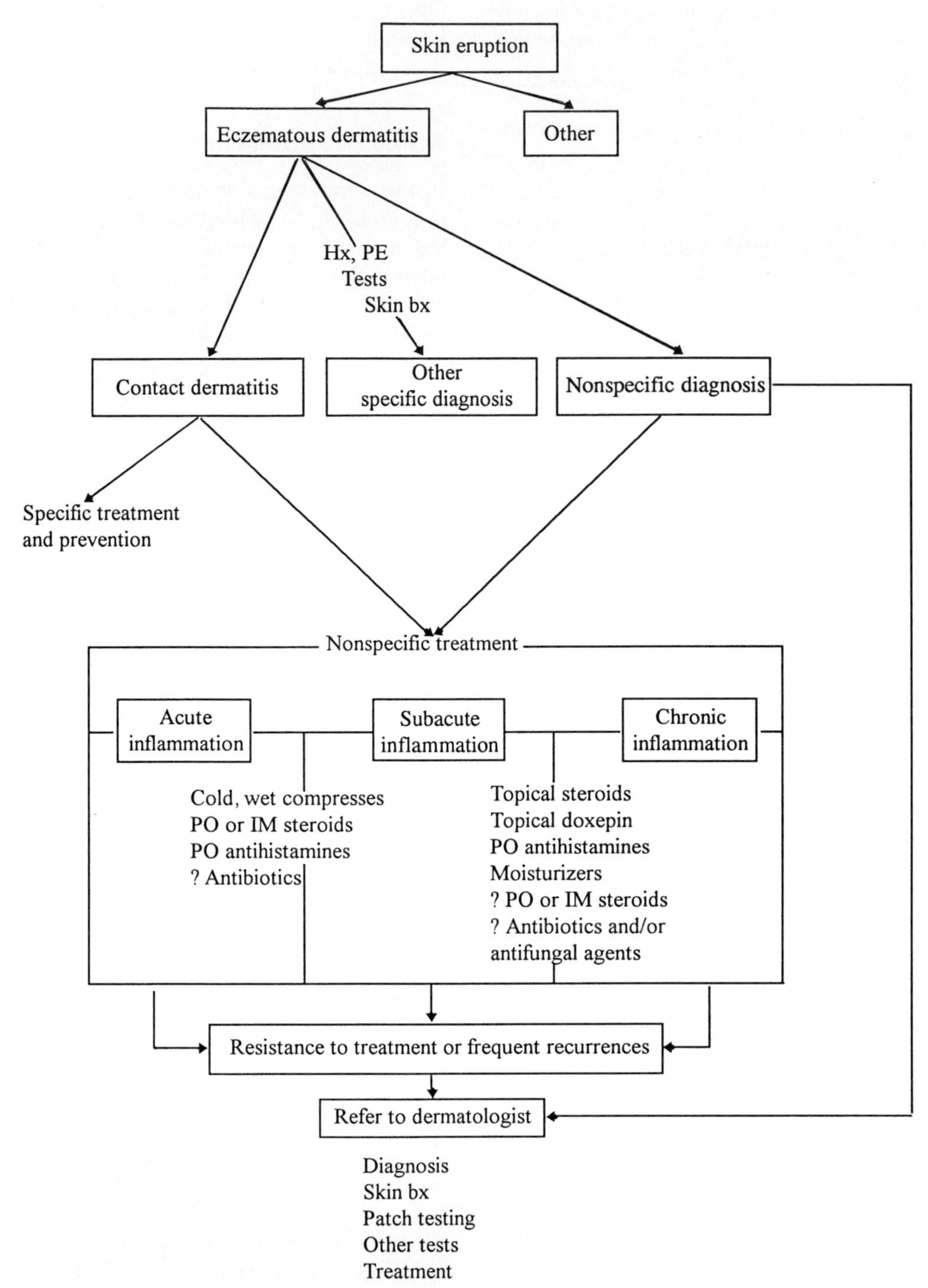

FIGURE 16-4

Algorithmic approach to the diagnosis of contact dermatitis. *Abbreviations:* Hx, history; PE, physical examination; bx, biopsy; PO, per os (orally); IM, intramuscular.

may respond to topical corticosteroids, the strength of which should be tailored to the age of the patient and the body part involved. For example, desonide (DesOwen) cream, ointment, or lotion, or 1 to 2% hydrocortisone cream may be used in infants or on the face and mucous membranes of adults, whereas higher-strength corticosteroids like 0.1% triamcinolone cream or ointment, clidinium bromide and chlordiazepoxide hydrochloride (Lidex) cream, or even augmented betamethasone dipropionate (Diprolene) cream may be used on other areas.

PITFALLS AND PROBLEMS

1. A variety of skin disorders may mimic eczematous dermatitis and thus be mistaken for contact dermatitis. These disorders include tinea, nummular eczema, atopic dermatitis, dyshidrotic eczema, seborrheic dermatitis, psoriasis (especially on intertriginous areas), scabies, and impetigo.
2. Patients may have more than one diagnosis. For example, individuals with atopic dermatitis are prone to develop irritant hand dermatitis, especially if they indulge in wet work. In addition, contact dermatitis may be complicated by superimposed bacterial or dermatophyte infection.
3. Airborne contact dermatitis, photodermatitis, and photocontact dermatitis overlap in their clinical presentations.
4. Recurrent episodes of allergic contact dermatitis mandate identification of the offending allergen. Patch-testing is the only reliable and objective method for documenting the allergic cause.
5. In some cases (e.g., chromate allergy), the dermatitis may persist over an indefinite time period despite avoidance of the inciting chemical.
6. Allergic contact dermatitis to topical corticosteroids is a possibility in patients who exhibit worsening of the dermatitis following use of topical steroids.

REFERRAL AND CONSULTATION GUIDELINES

See Figure 16–4 for an algorithmic approach to the diagnosis of contact dermatitis.

BIBLIOGRAPHY

Adams RM: Hand eczema. Cutis 1993; 52:267–269.
Guin J (ed): Practical Contact Dermatitis. 2nd ed. New York: McGraw-Hill, 1995.
Product information accompanying Allergen Patch Test T.R.U.E. Test distributed in the United States by Glaxo Dermatology, Division of Glaxo, Inc.
Rietschel RL, Fowler JF (eds): Fisher's Contact Dermatitis. 4th ed. Baltimore: Williams & Wilkins, 1995.

CHAPTER 17

Diaper Dermatitis

Ilona J. Frieden

CLINICAL APPEARANCE

Diaper rashes are common. Many are due to the presence of the diaper environment, some are simply exacerbated by the presence of diapers, and still other eruptions develop in this area irrespective of the presence of diapers (Table 17–1). Irritant diaper dermatitis occurs in approximately 50% of infants, but it can also develop in older individuals with urinary or fecal incontinence. This discussion emphasizes the most common forms of diaper dermatitis—irritant, *Candida,* and seborrheic diaper dermatitis—which are usually distinguishable by distribution and morphology.[1]

DESCRIPTION OF DISEASE

Irritant Diaper Dermatitis

The peak age of irritant diaper dermatitis is between 9 and 12 months, and the condition occurs three to four times more often in infants with diarrhea. Erythema with or without scale is present over the convex surfaces of the buttocks, upper thighs, and abdomen, with sparing of the inguinal creases. It varies in severity from mild ''tidewater marks'' to much more severe involvement (see Fig. 17–1 on Color Plate 5). A variety of irritant diaper dermatitis, sometimes seen in older children, is an ulcerative form known as *ammoniacal ulcers* or *Jacquet's erosive dermatitis,* characterized by well-demarcated punched-out ulcers or erosions. Longstanding fecal soiling or urinary incontinence can also result in a condition known as *perianal pseudoverrucous papules and nodules,* characterized by shiny, smooth, moist, flat-topped papules and nodules located in the perianal or pubic area.[2] Irritant diaper dermatitis is thought to be secondary to the interaction of fecal urease and urine raising the pH of the diaper environment, which in turn causes activation of fecal lipases and proteases, leading to increased skin permeability and irritation.[3]

Candida Diaper Dermatitis

Candida albicans is a common cause of diaper dermatitis. The onset may be as early as a few days of life, but it often occurs later in infancy as well, sometimes following oral antibiotic therapy. The eruption is characterized by beefy-red erythematous plaques with satellite papules or pustules, usually involving the inguinal folds (see Fig. 17–2 on Color Plate 6). Occasionally, oral thrush is present. If pustules are present, the diagnosis can usually be confirmed with a potassium hydroxide preparation. *C. albicans* may also act as a secondary invader in many cases of diaper dermatitis and is often present in those cases with a duration of more than 72 hours.[4]

Seborrheic Diaper Dermatitis

Seborrheic dermatitis can affect the scalp, face, and diaper area, with a peak incidence between 1 and 6 months of age. The diaper rash usually consists of well-circumscribed erythematous patches or plaques with variable involvement of the inguinal folds (see Fig. 17–3 on Color Plate 6). The ''greasy scale'' sometimes seen in the scalp is rarely present in the diaper area, and scale itself is uncommonly seen, owing to the hydration

TABLE 17-1

Differential Diagnosis of Diaper Dermatitis

Disease	Usual Age	Morphology	Distribution	Diagnosis
Dermatoses Primarily Related to the Wearing of Diapers				
Irritant contact dermatitis	Peak, 9–12 mo; rare before 1 mo	Erythema ± scale; shallow ulcerations	Convexities—i.e., buttock, thigh, abdomen, and perianal area; spares creases	Clinical
Candidal diaper dermatitis	Any age	Beefy, red, scaly plaques with satellites, papules, and pustules	Usually involves inguinal folds	Clinical; potassium hydroxide
Miliaria (prickly heat)	Any age	Multiple discrete, sterile vesicopustules or erythematous papules	Also lesions on face, neck, axillae, and groin	Clinical; history of fever, sudden warm spell, etc.
Granuloma gluteal infantum	2–8 mo	Reddish-brown to purplish nodules, 0.5–4 cm in diameter	Arises within area of preexisting diaper dermatitis	Clinical and/or skin biopsy
Pseudoverrucous papules and nodules	Any age	Multiple shiny, red, moist, flat-topped papules and/or nodules	Diaper and perianal area	Clinical and/or skin biopsy
Dermatoses Exaggerated by the Wearing of Diapers				
Seborrheic dermatitis	1–6 mo	Well-circumscribed erythematous patches or plaques; occasionally "greasy scale"	Groin ± involvement of folds	Clinical; involvement of scalp, ears, axillae
Atopic dermatitis	≥1 mo	Erythema, papules, lichenification	Convex surfaces; worst area may be adjacent to diaper	Clinical; other areas show atopic dermatitis; history of atopy
Psoriasis	6–18 mo	Well-defined scaly plaques	Convex surfaces, involvement of folds	Clinical; recalcitrant to therapy; family history
Dermatoses in Diaper Area (Whether or Not Diapers Are Worn)				
Bullous impetigo	Usually newborns, but any age possible	Vesicles, pustules, bullae, or crusts	Anywhere, but common at diaper and periumbilical areas	Clinical; Gram's stain and bacterial culture
Langerhans cell histiocytosis	Peak, 1–9 mo	Discrete, yellow-brown scaly papules, often purpuric, atrophic, or ulcerated	"Seborrheic distribution" on scalp, neck, axillae, and groin; usually involves skin folds	Clinical plus skin biopsy; may have associated anemia, lymphadenopathy, hepatosplenomegaly
Acrodermatitis enteropathica	Weeks to months	Sharply dermarcated psoriasiform plaques, vesicles, and bullae	Periorificial and acral	Associated with diarrhea, alopecia, irritability, serum zinc <50 μg/dl
Congenital syphilis	Usually at birth to 2–6 mo	Papulosquamous, reddish-brown lesions; rarely, erosive or bullous	Palms, soles, knees, abdomen, and diaper area	Associated with low birth weight, hepatosplenomegaly, anemia; dark field + syphilis serologies
Molluscum contagiosum	Any age, usually ≥1 yr	Discrete umbilicated papules	Anywhere	Clinical
Scabies	3–4 wk or later	Papules, vesicles, burrows, nodules, and excoriations	Generalized, with predilection at palms and soles, genitalia	Clinical; positive scraping for mites, eggs, or feces
Hand-foot-and-mouth disease	Early childhood	Discrete papules and/or vesicles	Hands, feet, mouth, and diaper area	Clinical
Genital warts	Any age	Verrucous papules	Perineal and perianal area	Clinical
Human immunodeficiency virus (HIV)	≥3 mo	Severe erosions and ulcers	Perineal area, especially gluteal cleft	HIV risk factors, serologies, associated cytomegalovirus, herpes infection

From Singalavanija S, Frieden IJ: Diaper dermatitis. Reproduced by permission of Pediatrics in Review, Vol 16, pp 143–144, 1995.

of the area caused by diapers. The diagnosis is usually made because of an associated eruption on the face or scalp that resembles seborrheic dermatitis as well. The eruption is usually asymptomatic.

TREATMENT

The management of diaper dermatitis includes both specific therapy and measures aimed at minimizing irritation. In most cases, a combination of a low-potency corticosteroid ointment such as hydrocortisone 1% (available over-the-counter) combined with an anticandidal agent such as nystatin ointment or clotrimazole or miconazole cream, applied four times daily with diaper changes, is very effective. Anticandidal agents should be used in any clinically significant diaper dermatitis present for greater than 72 hours, regardless of the morphology, because of the likelihood that *C. albicans* is playing a secondary role in perpetuating the dermatitis. Conversely, the addition of hydrocortisone ointment to typical *Candida* diaper rash may help speed its resolution. Unless ongoing diarrhea or other factors are present, diaper dermatitis usually improves in less than a week.

In addition to specific therapy, the frequency of diaper changes should be increased. Disposable diapers containing absorbable gel matrix may also be helpful in reducing moisture and maintaining a more normal skin pH.[1, 3, 5] Over-the-counter barrier creams and pastes, which usually contain zinc oxide, may be helpful as adjunctive therapy and in preventing recurrences. Diaper wipes containing alcohol or other irritants should be avoided.

Alternative options:

Leave diaper off as long as possible.

1-2-3 Paste: 1 part Burow's solution 1:20, 2 parts Aquaphor, 3 parts zinc oxide paste.

''Butt Balm'': Karaya powder 2.5 ounces, cod liver oil and zinc oxide (Desitin) 1 ounce, nystatin (Nystatin) cream 1 ounce, Eucerin cream 200 g.

PITFALLS AND PROBLEMS

1. Many conditions other than irritant, seborrheic, and *Candida* diaper dermatitis can cause eruptions in this area (see Table 17–1). In atypical cases or those failing to respond to appropriate therapy, the initial diagnosis should be reconsidered. Occasionally, skin biopsy is necessary for diagnosis.

2. The diaper itself acts as an occlusive environment, markedly enhancing local and systemic absorption of topically applied medications. Moreover, the skin of the perineal area is particularly permeable to topically applied substances. Therefore, potent topical corticosteroids such as those found in fixed-combination medications such as triamcinolone acetonide and nystatin (Mycolog-II) and betamethasone dipropionate and clotrimazole (Lotrisone) should be avoided in the diaper area. Iodohydroxyquin (i.e., clioquinol [Vioform], hydrocortisone and iodoquinol [Vytone]) should be avoided because of potential neurotoxicity. Other home or folk remedies such as baking soda (which can cause hypernatremia) and boric acid ointment (which can cause boric acid poisoning) should not be used in the diaper area.

3. Irritant diaper dermatitis is rare in the newborn period. If eruptions occur at this age, infectious etiologies including *C. albicans,* herpes simplex, streptococcal or staphylococcal infection, and scabies; metabolic disorders; and other conditions should be considered (see Table 17–1).

REFERRAL/CONSULTATION GUIDELINES

The differential diagnosis of diaper dermatitis is extensive and includes several unusual conditions, such as Langerhans cell histiocytosis, acrodermatitis enteropathica, and biotin-responsive multiple carboxylase deficiency. Any diaper rash with unusual morphology or that is not responding to the initial therapy outlined previously may require specialized consultation.

REFERENCES

1. Singalavanija S, Frieden IJ: Diaper dermatitis. Pediatr Rev 1995; 16:142–147.
2. Goldberg NS, Esterly NB, Rothman KF, et al: Perianal pseudoverrucous papules and nodules in children. Arch Dermatol 1992; 128:240–242.
3. Berg RW: Etiology and pathophysiology of diaper dermatitis. Adv Dermatol 1988; 3:75–98.
4. Leyden JJ, Kligman AM: The role of microorganisms in diaper dermatitis. Arch Dermatol 1978; 114:56–59.
5. Wong LD, Brantly D, Clutter LB, et al: Diapering choices: A critical review of the issues. Pediatr Nurs 1992; 18:41–54.

CHAPTER 18

Cutaneous Drug Reactions

Robert S. Stern

CLINICAL APPEARANCE

Cutaneous reactions to drugs are drug-induced changes of the skin and mucous membranes. They are frequent and may have associated systemic symptoms and signs including fever and dysfunction of other organs. Although most cutaneous drug reactions are self-limited and are of limited morbidity if the drug is discontinued, some may be serious and even life-threatening. Cutaneous drug reactions vary in their morphology and pathophysiology. The more common types of drug reactions and reactions that are potentially more serious are discussed separately. The etiology and pathogenesis of each type of reaction are noted. Potentially more serious reactions include urticaria, angioedema, anaphylaxis, hypersensitivity syndromes, serum sickness, vasculitis, anticoagulant-induced necrosis, photosensitivity, Stevens-Johnson syndrome, and toxic epidermal necrolysis.

The presence of certain signs, symptoms, and laboratory test results should alert the clinician to the possibility that a patient with a cutaneous eruption thought to be possibly drug induced may have a serious condition. Important clinical signs include confluent erythema, skin pain, blisters, facial edema, palpable purpura, skin necrosis, mucous membrane involvement, and tongue swelling. High fever, enlarged lymph nodes, arthritis, shortness of breath, wheezing, and hypotension are especially worrisome symptoms. Patients with drug-induced eruptions with abnormal liver function tests, eosinophilia, or atypical lymphocytes are also especially likely to have severe eruptions.

Stevens-Johnson syndrome and toxic epidermal necrolysis are discussed in a separate chapter (see Chapter 57). Most other forms of skin reactions, common or serious, that are often caused by drugs are considered herein.

DESCRIPTION OF DISEASE

Demographics

Drug reactions can occur in persons of any age and either sex. The risk of a reaction is highest in the first weeks of drug use. Because of higher utilization of drugs among elderly people, these reactions are most commonly seen in this age group. Even after adjusting for frequency of drug use, patients with certain diseases, especially human immunodeficiency virus (HIV) infection, appear to have an increased risk of these reactions.

Natural History of Disease

The more frequent types of drug reactions, urticaria and morbilliform eruptions, are self-limited and will have limited morbidity if the causative drug is discontinued. If causative drugs are not discontinued, the probability that a more severe reaction will evolve is increased and the duration of symptoms will also increase. Paradoxically, some classic cutaneous drug eruptions will abate even when a patient continues to take the medication that is, in all likelihood, causative. If a drug that caused a previous reaction is reintroduced, the reaction is likely to be more severe and the new reaction can begin within minutes for urticaria/angioedema/anaphylaxis and within hours for other types of reactions.

Overall, morbilliform eruptions account for about

75% of all skin reactions attributed to drugs. Urticaria accounts for an additional 15 to 20% of all reactions. Among the frequently used drugs with the highest risks of causing these skin reactions are the sulfonamides, the penicillins, especially the aminopenicillins, and the cephalosporins.

For certain types of reactions, patients with specific attributes are at increased risk. Fair-skinned individuals are more likely to develop photosensitivity reactions. There appears to be genetic predisposition to the development of hypersensitivity syndromes. Unfortunately, no practical test that predicts the risk of this and other more severe types is available.

For all types of drug reactions, it is important to remember that stopping a drug does not mean that the drug is no longer present in the body. Some drugs have long half-lives (i.e., about 100 hours for phenobarbital in children). Therefore, reactions may persist or even begin long after drug discontinuation. Also, drug metabolites rather than the parent drug may be the cause of the reaction.

Common and Serious Reactions: Morphology, Natural History, Etiology, and Pathogenesis

Urticaria, Angioedema, and Anaphylaxis

Urticaria presents as erythematous papules and plaques that are symmetrically distributed. If there is involvement of the central face, especially tongue and lips, with swelling and edema, this is considered angioedema. An accelerated reaction may include systemic symptoms such as laryngeal edema, nausea, vomiting, and occasionally shock. When this occurs, the reaction is termed *anaphylaxis*; these reactions may be fatal. Individual urticarial lesions (or hives) are blanchable. They are often, but not always, itchy and may range in size from small papules to giant wheals.

In individuals not previously sensitized to a drug, urticaria or angioedema most often begins 1 to 2 weeks after starting a drug. Previously sensitized individuals rapidly develop urticarial lesions as well as associated symptoms. With rechallenge, reactions can be immediate, accelerated, or delayed. Immediate reactions may be fatal unless treated. Withdrawal of the offending drug is essential.

Classically, antibody (immunoglobulin E)–mediated hypersensitivity is often responsible for these conditions. Not all urticarial reactions are, however, a result of a hypersensitivity (i.e., antibody mediated) reaction. Especially important as causes of nonimmune angioedema and urticaria are the angiotensin-converting enzyme inhibitors, nonsteroidal anti-inflammatory drugs, and radiocontrast media.

Morbilliform Reactions

Morbilliform or measles-like reactions are the most common cutaneous reactions to drugs, accounting for about 75% of all drug-induced skin rashes. They consist of symmetric erythematous papules and macules that may coalesce to form plaques. Usually, they are itchy and are blanchable. Mucosal involvement sometimes occurs but is usually limited. Blisters are usually absent except in dependent areas (e.g., lower legs). Low-grade fever may occur, but fever in excess of 101.4° F is unusual.

Morbilliform reactions typically begin on the trunk and spread outward. Because of their timing (longer time to onset with first exposure to a drug and more rapid occurrence with reexposure) and their histopathology, these reactions are thought to be delayed (Type IV) hypersensitivity reactions. The exact mechanism of these reactions is unknown. These reactions usually persist until the drug is withdrawn.

Hypersensitivity Syndromes

A severe eczematous eruption or exfoliative dermatitis, which consists of generalized redness and scaling, may also be associated with more severe hypersensitivity syndromes. Facial swelling is frequent. Sometimes, the eruption may become indurated and have an appearance similar to that of cutaneous T-cell lymphoma. In most cases, hypersensitivity syndromes include fever, lymphadenopathy, and rash. Hepatitis, nephritis, carditis, and eosinophilia are also seen frequently. Circulating atypical lymphocytes may be seen. The aromatic amine anticonvulsants (phenytoin [Dilantin], carbamazepine, and phenobarbital), sulfonamides, and allopurinol are the most frequent causes of this eruption.

Hypersensitivity syndromes tend to begin as morbilliform or exanthematous eruptions, but they often become more inflammatory than typical morbilliform eruptions. Mucous membrane involvement is infrequent. These reactions may occur up to 6 to 8 weeks after a drug is introduced, a longer interval from the beginning of drug therapy than is usual for simple morbilliform eruptions. Patients who develop hypersensitivity syndromes are likely to have a decreased ability to metabolize toxic drug metabolites, and a patient's cells may also be more susceptible to injury from these toxic drug metabolites.

Serum Sickness

Serum sickness often presents as a morbilliform eruption indistinguishable from the usual morbilliform eruption. Urticarial lesions and occasionally purpura may be seen. The presence of fever and arthralgia differentiate serum sickness or serum sickness–like reactions from more common and innocuous morbilliform eruptions. Classic serum sickness is due to immune complex deposition in the skin and other organs. This reaction is most often due to the administration of foreign proteins but has been reported with other types of drugs. Clinically indistinguishable reactions without evidence of immune complex disease may occur, especially among children treated with cephalosporins.

Vasculitis

Palpable purpura, which occurs most often on the legs, is the most frequent cutaneous manifestation of vasculitis. It can be drug induced, but it usually has other causes. In addition to cutaneous lesions and fever, vasculitis of other organs, especially the kidney and gastrointestinal tract, may be seen. Drug-induced vasculitis almost certainly represents an immunologic reaction to a drug, with subsequent inflammation of blood vessels. Drugs should be suspected in a person who has recently begun using drugs and has new onset of otherwise unexplained cutaneous vasculitis. Drug-induced vasculitis is a diagnosis of exclusion.

Anticoagulant-Induced Necrosis

This eruption presents as erythematous, tender plaques that rapidly become purpuric and necrotic. Fatty areas are especially likely to be affected in coumarin necrosis. Affected areas are usually painful. Coumarin and heparin can cause clinically similar but pathologically distinct reactions of this type. Both reactions are probably due to drug-induced hypercoagulable states. Coumarin-induced necrosis usually occurs in persons with protein C or protein S deficiency, but most people with these deficiencies tolerate coumarin without incident. Activation of platelets is probably important for heparin necrosis.

Photosensitivity

Drugs and exposure to appropriate wavelengths of ultraviolet radiation (usually ultraviolet A, 320 to 400 nm) or even visible light can induce an exaggerated sunburn-like reaction, known as a *phototoxic reaction*. These reactions occur in exposed areas. They typically sting and may blister. Occasionally, drugs and ultraviolet radiation can induce a more persistent photoallergic reaction.

Most photosensitivity eruptions are phototoxic. Therefore, their severity is proportional to skin levels of the causative drug, the efficiency of the drug as a photosensitizer, and the amount of exposure to relevant wavelengths of ultraviolet (or visible light) radiation. These reactions can begin as burning or stinging while the patient is still in the sun and typically evolve like sunburns, although sometimes more rapidly or more slowly than a sunburn. First redness and swelling are seen. Blistering may develop, and desquamation is later seen. Among the most potent photosensitizers are the fluoroquinolones, some tetracyclines (especially doxycycline and demethylchlortetracycline), and thiazide diuretics.

Fixed Drug Eruptions

Fixed drug eruptions are characterized by the development of round, edematous or erythematous plaques that resolve, leaving hyperpigmentation. Blisters may occur in these lesions. Genitalia, face, hands, and mucous membranes are especially likely to be affected. Most often, only a small number of lesions occur initially. With reexposure to the drug, previously affected sites will once more become red and new sites are likely to become involved. The timing of the eruption relative to drug use and the prominent lymphocytic infiltrate seen in this eruption suggest that it is a localized form of delayed hypersensitivity. Barbiturates, phenophthalein, sulfonamides, and tetracyclines probably account for the majority of cases.

TREATMENT

The key to the treatment of drug eruptions is the identification and withdrawal of the causative drug. Otherwise, in most cases therapy is oriented toward symptom reduction (e.g., treatment of pruritus and fever). Sometimes, identifying the causative drug can be difficult. To aid in this process, systematically charting the dates of use of all drugs (including over-the-counter drugs, "homeopathic drugs," and drugs used intermittently) is helpful. Recently begun medications (within 2 to 3 weeks) are the most likely causes of most drug-induced skin reactions. For hypersensitivity syndromes, a longer susceptible period should be considered. All suspect drugs that are not medically essential should be discontinued. Patients and their families should be educated about the drugs to which the patient may be sensitive and cautioned to avoid these in the future. Patients should also be made aware of drugs that may cross-react with the suspect agent.

Morbilliform eruptions, which account for about 75% of all drug eruptions, are usually treated symptomatically. Oral antihistamines and soothing baths (colloidal oatmeal [Aveeno]) are useful for treatment of pruritus. Topical antihistamines (doxepin [Zonalon]) may also have some useful effect, as do emollients and antipruritic lotions (white petrolatum in water [Eucerin] and camphor and menthol [Sarna]). Topical corticosteroids can reduce inflammation and may reduce symptoms. Short courses of potent topical steroids are probably most helpful. The beneficial effect of systemic steroids relative to risk is less clear for morbilliform eruptions.

How aggressive the treatment of urticaria or angioedema should be depends on the severity of the reaction and the rate at which it is evolving. In addition to drug withdrawal, for patients with only cutaneous symptoms and without symptoms of angioedema or anaphylaxis, oral antihistamines are usually sufficient. For adults, diphenhydramine (Benadryl), up to 50 mg every 6 hours, or loratadine (Claritin), one or two 10-mg tablets a day, is helpful. Sedation, dry mouth, and urinary retention usually limit the doses of the older H_1 antihistamines that can be used. For patients with anaphylaxis, systemic steroids, sometimes intravenously administered (hydrocortisone, 100 mg every 6 hours intravenously), or prednisone, 30 mg orally, each day may be useful. Epinephrine is often indicated in cases when respiratory or cardiovascular compromise may be occurring (dosage: epinephrine, 0.3 to 0.5 ml of a 1:1000 dilution intramuscularly, every 15 to 30 minutes as needed). Monitoring for cardiovascular side effects is essential, and lower doses of epinephrine may be needed in the elderly.

Although there are no controlled studies, it would appear that systemic steroids (prednisone, 0.5 to 1.0 mg/kg) help reduce both the symptoms and signs and the laboratory evidence of severe hypersensitivity syndromes. Other treatment for these conditions is supportive. It is especially important to recognize that there may be cross-reactivity between the aromatic anticonvulsants (e.g., phenobarbital, phenytoin [Dilantin], and carbamazepine), which, along with sulfonamides, are the most frequent causes of these reactions.

Both serum sickness and vasculitis will usually improve rapidly if the drug is withdrawn. Systemic corticosteroids also seem to benefit these patients.

Coumarin-induced cutaneous necrosis is treated with vitamin K and heparin. Vitamin K (2.5 to 10 mg intravenously) reverses the effects of coumarin. Heparin acts as an anticoagulant. Heparin dosage should be individualized according to clotting time, with a goal of a clotting time of 2.5 to 3 times the normal usual. Treatment with protein C concentrates may also be helpful in individuals with deficiencies of protein C, the predisposing factor for development of these reactions.

Since most phototoxic reactions are due to the interaction of long-wave ultraviolet A radiation and the drug, nonopaque sunscreens are not very effective in blocking reactions. Avoiding exposure to ultraviolet light (sunlight) and treating as one would a sunburn (see Chapter 46) are helpful. Individuals who have severe photosensitive reactions may have enhanced reactions to sunlight for some weeks after their initial phototoxic reaction and, occasionally, may develop photoallergic reactions or persistent sensitivity to light, necessitating long-term avoidance of sun exposure.

PITFALLS AND PROBLEMS

The key to diagnosis and treatment of drug eruptions is to determine the likely etiologic agent and to establish whether this reaction is likely to be serious. Essential to this is a complete drug history that includes nonprescription medications and medications used intermittently. The presence of fever, lymphadenopathy, arthralgias, arthritis, shortness of breath, wheezing, or hypotension, as well as a more extensive eruption, facial edema, and of course purpura, blisters, or mucosal involvement, all suggest more serious reactions. Prompt withdrawal of the drug is the key to proper treatment.

As noted previously, occasionally systemic steroid administration and, in the case of angioedema/anaphylaxis, epinephrine may change the outcome of these reactions. Generally, once the causative drug is withdrawn, more common drug reactions will resolve with supportive therapy alone. In addition to treating the acute reaction, it is essential to be sure that the patient and those who care for the patient are fully informed about the likely cause of the reaction and both the brand and the generic names of the likely causative drug and the drugs that may cross-react with this causative agent.

For some drugs that are extremely important to the patient, desensitization can be carried out. At present, the principal indication for desensitization is for sulfonamide-sensitive HIV-infected persons. For most other drugs, alternative therapy makes this lengthy and sometimes risky process unnecessary.

REFERRAL AND CONSULTATION GUIDELINES

Patients with symptoms of angioedema and anaphylaxis should be immediately seen in a facility that can provide adequate life support, especially if these reactions appear to be worsening or it appears that the patient may be about to suffer respiratory compromise or cardiovascular collapse. Patients with the signs or symptoms of the more severe reactions noted previously or whose reactions are persistent should be seen in consultation with experts. Especially important is ruling out alternative causes of the reaction ascribed to a drug. Blistering reactions to drugs are further considered in the chapter on Stevens-Johnson syndrome and toxic epidermal necrolysis (see Chapter 57).

BIBLIOGRAPHY

Bigby M, Jick S, Jick H, Arndt K: Drug-induced cutaneous reactions: A report from the Boston Collaborative Drug Surveillance Program on 15,438 consecutive inpatients, 1975 to 1982. JAMA 1986; 256:3358–3363.

Coopman SA, Johnson RA, Platt R, Stern RS: Cutaneous disease and drug reactions in HIV infection. N Engl J Med 1993; 328:1670–1674.

Roujeau JC, Stern RS: Severe adverse cutaneous reactions to drugs. N Engl J Med 1994; 331:1271–1285.

Shear NH, Speilberg SP: Anticonvulsant hypersensitivity syndrome: In vitro assessment of risk. J Clin Invest 1988; 82:1826–1832.

CHAPTER 19

Erythema Multiforme

Marcia G. Tonnesen

CLINICAL APPEARANCE

Definition

Erythema multiforme is an acute, self-limited, inflammatory disorder of the skin and mucous membranes with distinctive skin lesions and characteristic histopathology. Currently, the classification of erythema multiforme is evolving as distinct subsets are identified[1] and diagnostic criteria are established. Two clinical forms of erythema multiforme have been designated *erythema multiforme minor* and *erythema multiforme major.*

Erythema multiforme minor is primarily an acral eruption with characteristic target lesions, variably accompanied by oral mucosal involvement, without systemic symptoms. Erythema multiforme major is a severe form with more extensive cutaneous lesions, frequent involvement of more than one mucosal surface, and association with systemic toxicity.

Typical Lesions and Symptoms

Erythema Multiforme Minor

Erythema multiforme minor, comprising the majority of cases of erythema multiforme, is a relatively mild, self-limited cutaneous illness that is frequently recurrent.[2] The typical clinical picture is the sudden onset of a symmetrically distributed erythematous eruption with a predilection for the extensor aspects of the extremities and the presence of target lesions, a clinical hallmark. Mucosal involvement, when present, is usually limited to the oral cavity.

The primary skin lesion is a round, erythematous papule that, over hours to days, may enlarge and develop a central vesicle or bulla. At least some of the lesions evolve with concentric zones of color change to form characteristic target or iris lesions.[1] A classic target lesion has a well-defined border and at least three different zones of color—typically, a central dusky erythematous area surrounded by a pale edematous ring with a peripheral erythematous margin (see Fig. 19–1 on Color Plate 6).[2] The eruption typically appears in successive crops; thus, a variable array of cutaneous lesions at different stages of evolution may be observed.

Individual skin lesions are usually symptomless but may be associated with burning or itching. Oral bullous lesions, when present, usually appear simultaneously with the cutaneous eruption and rapidly become painful, superficial erosions.

Erythema Multiforme Major

Erythema multiforme major, also known as bullous erythema multiforme or Stevens-Johnson syndrome, is a severe, self-limited, variable mucocutaneous illness characterized by an extensive eruption with areas of epidermal detachment and systemic symptoms. Significant involvement of multiple mucosal surfaces often occurs. A prodrome with constitutional symptoms, such as fever, cough, sore throat, myalgias, and malaise, may herald the onset of the eruption.

Skin lesions begin as erythematous macules or papules and may evolve to form raised or flat atypical target lesions, with only two zones of color or a poorly defined border. Central vesiculation may progress to widespread bullae formation and produce limited areas of epidermal necrosis and detachment. The eruption is typically prominent on the trunk.[1] Mucosal involvement, particularly oropharyngeal, labial, and conjunctival, is frequently severe and associated with significant morbidity. Painful, extensive oral mucosal bullae and erosions result in characteristic hemorrhagic crusting of the lips, decreased oral intake, and possible dehydration. Ocular involvement may produce red painful conjunctivae, associated photophobia, and if severe, an erosive, exudative conjunctivitis with residual scarring and lash and lacrimal abnormalities. Permanent visual loss may occur. Balanitis and vulvovaginitis may cause difficulty with micturition and result in scarring and stenosis.

DESCRIPTION OF DISEASE

Especially in its recurrent form, erythema multiforme minor is predominantly a disease of otherwise healthy, young adults, with no clear racial or sexual predilection. Erythema multiforme major primarily occurs in children and young adults and is less common in very early childhood and in the elderly.

Erythema multiforme is uncommon but not rare, with an annual incidence reported to be far less than 1% of dermatology patients. A recent study found erythema multiforme major to be a rare condition with an incidence rate of approximately 6 per million per year.

Erythema multiforme minor is frequently a recurrent disorder. Each episode is self-limited and resolves within 2 to 4 weeks, typically leaving residual postinflammatory hyperpigmentation as the sole sequela.[2] The duration of erythema multiforme major, reflecting more severe mucocutaneous damage, is typically 4 to 6 weeks. Recurrences are infrequent. Erythema multiforme major is associated with significant morbidity; mortality has been reported to be in the range of 1 to 10%.

The histopathology of erythema multiforme is distinctive but not diagnostic. Nevertheless, biopsy of a typical early skin lesion should help to establish the correct diagnosis. Characteristic features include perivascular infiltrate of lymphocytes and edema in the upper dermis, basal vacuolization, epidermal spongiosis, and dyskeratosis with scattered necrotic keratinocytes associated with exocytosis of lymphocytes. Target and bullous lesions demonstrate central epidermal necrosis overlying a subepidermal blister.

Erythema multiforme has been considered to be a hypersensitivity reaction in a host manifesting an immune response to one of a variety of etiologic factors capable of generating foreign antigens, primarily infectious agents or drugs.[2] However, the pathogenic mechanisms involved have not yet been elucidated. Although a myriad of etiologic associations have been suggested over the years, the three best-documented and best-described are recurrent herpes simplex virus (HSV) infection, *Mycoplasma pneumoniae* infection, and drugs.

The majority of cases of classic recurrent erythema multiforme minor are associated with HSV infection (Type 1 or 2) and typically occur 7 to 10 days after the appearance of a recurrent HSV lesion (oral, genital, or other location).[2] The most significant evidence implicating HSV in the pathogenesis of erythema multiforme minor derives from studies localizing HSV antigens and DNA to skin lesions of erythema multiforme. The presence of HSV in skin lesions supports the concept that herpes-associated erythema multiforme may represent a herpes-specific immune response in the skin.

Erythema multiforme major may be triggered by infection, most notably *M. pneumoniae* or, infrequently, HSV. However, erythema multiforme major is most commonly associated with exposure to certain drugs.[3] The major offenders include sulfonamides, systemic (including trimethoprim-sulfamethoxazole) and topical, anticonvulsants (phenytoin and barbiturates), penicillins, cephalosporins, allopurinol, and nonsteroidal anti-inflammatory agents, although many other drugs have been implicated. The mechanism by which a drug precipitates erythema multiforme major is unknown, but it may involve a specific defect in the detoxification of reactive drug metabolites.

TREATMENT

General Therapeutic Expectations

Optimal therapeutic strategies for erythema multiforme have been controversial, since specific pathogenic mechanisms of tissue injury are unknown and since few controlled studies have yet been performed to evaluate the effectiveness of various treatment modalities. A rational therapeutic approach should encompass a diligent search for possible etiologic factors, careful consideration of clinical characteristics—including extent and severity of mucocutaneous lesions and patient discomfort—and assessment of potential complications.

Identification and elimination of any potential etiologic or precipitating factors are critical. Optimal therapy should also combine symptomatic and supportive measures with observation for and treatment of associated complications, depending on the severity of the episode. Frequently, erythema multiforme minor requires only symptomatic care. However, because of the degree and extent of epidermal and mucosal involvement that can occur in erythema multiforme major, careful monitoring is critical, hospitalization is often required, and supportive care is usually necessary.

First-Line Therapy

Identification and Elimination of Etiologic Factors

Because of the well-documented etiologic association between recurrent HSV infection and recurrent erythema multiforme minor, measures taken to attempt to prevent recurrences of HSV should lessen or abort subsequent episodes of erythema multiforme minor. Reduction of ultraviolet light–induced HSV recurrences might be accomplished by sun avoidance utilizing such strategies as minimizing sun exposure at midday, using protective clothing, and applying sunscreens (sun protection factor [SPF] 15 or higher) and sunscreen-containing lip balms. Prophylactic administration of oral acyclovir has been reported to result in abolition of recurrent HSV infections and of ensuing recurrent episodes of erythema multiforme minor, without significant side effects.[4] Therefore, the treatment of choice for patients with frequently recurring and debilitating HSV-associated erythema multiforme minor is daily administration of an antiviral antibiotic such as oral acyclovir for a period of 6 months or longer. The recommended starting dose is 400 mg orally twice daily. After the disease is brought under control, the dose should be tapered to the minimal effective dose for each individual patient. It is advisable to stop the drug periodically and reassess the need for its continuance.

Because of the well-documented etiologic association between drugs and erythema multiforme major,[3] immediate withdrawal and future avoidance of any incriminated, suspected, or unnecessary drug(s) are imperative. *M. pneumoniae* infection, if diagnosed or strongly suspected, should be treated with a course of appropriate systemic antibiotic therapy.

Skin Care

Symptomatic relief for pruritic or painful skin lesions may be provided by the administration of systemic antihistamines or analgesics. For oozing and crusted erosive skin lesions, mild drying, cleansing, and débridement, as well as a soothing antipruritic effect, can be achieved with frequent application of open, wet-to-damp compresses of tepid water or a dilute solution of aluminum acetate, and with frequent bathing in lukewarm to cool water. Topical steroid therapy has not been shown to be beneficial in the treatment of erythema multiforme and may predispose eroded lesions to the development of secondary infection. If close monitoring reveals signs of secondary infection, lesions should be cultured and treatment initiated with the appropriate systemic antibiotic.

Mouth Care

To minimize infection and discomfort associated with extensive, painful mouth erosions, good oral hygiene consisting of mouthwashes, irrigations, and tooth brushing, as tolerated, is essential. Topical anesthetics such as dyclonine, viscous lidocaine, or a mixture of Kaopectate and elixir of diphenhydramine (1:1) may be used as a mouthwash. If secondary bacterial infection develops, associated with purulent, foul-smelling lesions and tender cervical lymphadenopathy, systemic antibiotic therapy should be instituted. A liquid or soft diet is usually better tolerated and thereby contributes to the maintenance of hydration and nutrition. Extensive oral involvement may result in an inability to eat or drink despite the use of topical anesthetics, thus necessitating administration of fluids and electrolytes and parenteral nutrition.

Eye Care

Particularly in cases of erythema multiforme major, careful monitoring and immediate and continuing therapeutic intervention for ocular involvement are essential. Because of the potential for late complications resulting in visual loss, early consultation with an ophthalmologist is strongly recommended. Appropriate therapy might include frequent irrigation and tear replacement, lysis of adhesions, and surveillance cultures with prompt instillation of topical antibiotics if secondary infection occurs. Late surgical intervention may be beneficial to correct lid deformities, lyse scar tissue, or perhaps replace the cornea.

Alternative Therapeutic Options

If extensive, advanced epidermal necrosis occurs (approaching 20% or more total body surface area involvement), management of the patient in a burn unit is strongly advocated. Current recommendations for therapeutic strategies in a burn unit include withdrawal of systemic steroid therapy because of increased risk of sepsis, complications, and adverse effects on wound healing; avoidance of indwelling lines whenever possible; constant monitoring for the development of secondary infection including frequent surveillance cultures of skin, blood, urine, and indwelling lines, and aggressive treatment if sepsis or localized infection occurs; supportive care with pain relief, fluid replacement, parenteral nutrition, and respiratory therapy; and early gentle débridement of appropriate skin lesions followed by application of silver nitrate dressings, biologic dressings, allografts, or porcine xenografts to facilitate rapid reepithelialization.[5]

PITFALLS AND PROBLEMS

The use of systemic glucocorticosteroid therapy in HSV-associated erythema multiforme minor is not recommended. Systemic steroid therapy, although perhaps beneficial in reducing inflammation, might actually be detrimental and contribute to the development of continuous or overlapping episodes.

Since no controlled studies have been conducted to document efficacy, the use of systemic glucocorticosteroids in erythema multiforme major is still highly controversial.[6] Although this treatment is strongly recommended by some, it has been condemned by others, since some retrospective and prospective reports have suggested that patients treated with systemic steroids have an increased incidence of complications, morbidity, and prolonged hospitalization times. In an attempt to minimize the extent of tissue damage, early use of a short course of high-dose systemic steroid (prednisone, 1 to 2 mg/kg/day, or an equivalent drug) in the severe, progressive phase of the disease process may at times be justified. Once disease progression ceases and the wound healing process begins, or if no response is noted within 3 to 5 days, treatment should be abruptly discontinued to minimize risk of associated complications and increased morbidity and mortality.

REFERRAL/CONSULTATION GUIDELINES

For patients with erythema multiforme major, early consultation with an ophthalmologist may be crucial to decrease morbidity. If extensive epidermal detachment occurs, involving as much as 20 to 30% of the total body surface area, surgical intervention and transfer to a burn unit are advisable.

REFERENCES

1. Bastuji-Garin S, Rzany B, Stern RS, et al: Clinical classification of cases of toxic epidermal necrolysis, Stevens-Johnson syndrome, and erythema multiforme. Arch Dermatol 1993; 129:92–96.
2. Huff JC, Weston WL: Recurrent erythema multiforme. Medicine 1989; 68:133–140.
3. Roujeau JC, Kelly JP, Naldi L, et al: Medication use and the risk of Stevens-Johnson syndrome or toxic epidermal necrolysis. N Engl J Med 1995; 333:1600–1607.
4. Lemak MA, Duvic M, Bean SF: Oral acyclovir for the prevention of herpes-associated erythema multiforme. J Am Acad Dermatol 1986; 15:50–54.
5. Halebian PH, Madden MR, Finklestein JL, et al: Improved burn center survival of patients with toxic epidermal necrolysis managed without corticosteroids. Ann Surg 1986; 204:503–512.
6. Esterly NB (ed): Special symposium: Corticosteroids for erythema multiforme? Pediatr Dermatol 1989; 6:229–250.

CHAPTER 20

Folliculitis

A. Paul Kelly

CLINICAL APPEARANCE

Folliculitis is a term that refers to a superficial or deep infection of the hair follicles. Coagulase-positive *Staphylococcus aureus* is the most common pathogen.

Superficial folliculitis (Table 20–1) begins as thin, yellowish-white pustules with a hair in the center and sometimes presents with a narrow red areola around the pustules. It is more common in children and occurs most often on the scalp, buttocks, and extremities (see Fig. 20–1 on Color Plate 6). It generally heals in 7 to 10 days. The lesions may be asymptomatic but are often pruritic and are occasionally tender or painful.

Deep folliculitis (Table 20–2) (furunculosis, boils) occurs when a preceding superficial folliculitis extends deeply into the follicle. This produces a firm, tender, erythematous nodule 1 to 2 cm in diameter, which becomes fluctuant within 24 to 48 hours. At this stage, the lesions are tender and painful; however, spontaneous drainage and healing usually take place. They occur in all ages and are more common in staphylococcal carriers.

One of the major concerns about furunculosis is bacteremic spread of infection and recurrence. Midface lesions raise concern about spread to the cavernous sinus. Boils should never be squeezed because the pressure may cause vascular spread, resulting in acute endocarditis, brain abscess, osteomyelitis, or spread to other foci.

In addition to the conditions listed previously, pustular drug reactions to halogens and corticosteroids must be part of the differential diagnosis of superficial folliculitis. Corticosteroid-induced follicular lesions usually have an abrupt onset several weeks after the institution of high-dose systemic or potent topical preparations. Systemic-induced lesions respond best to topical tretinoin, and topical-induced lesions respond best, although somewhat slowly, to oral tetracyclines.

In contradistinction to the steroid-induced pustules, halogens (iodides and bromides) usually induce nonfollicular pustules. The most common source of the ingested halogens are asthma and thyroid medication and expectorants containing potassium iodide. Removing the halogen is the best way of treating the disorder. Sometimes, topical corticosteroids are beneficial.

DESCRIPTION OF DISEASE

Histopathology

Acute superficial folliculitis is characterized histologically by a subcorneal pustule overlying a hair follicle. The superficial portion of the hair follicle is surrounded by an inflammatory infiltrate composed mostly of neutrophils.

Acute deep folliculitis (furuncles, boils) has an area of perifollicular necrosis that contains an abundance of neutrophils. The distal end of the follicle, in the subcutaneous tissue, usually has a large abscess that contains staphylococci.

TREATMENT (see also Tables 20–1 and 20–2)

The majority of cases encountered by the primary care physician are the result of superficial folliculitis caused

TABLE 20-1

Types of Superficial Folliculitis

Types	Clinical Features	Therapy
Superficial Bockhart's impetigo	Dome-shaped pustules of hair follicles; most common in children and most often on scalp, face, and extremities; maceration and poor hygiene are promoting factors	Soap (antibacterial) and water and topical antibiotics, especially if recurrences
Oil folliculitis (secondary to cutting oils and solvents)	Sterile pustules in hairy areas	Discontinue patient exposure to precipitating chemicals; scrub with soap and water
Gram-negative folliculitis (see Fig. 20–2 on Color Plate 6)	Pustules around the nose associated with *Klebsiella* or *Enterobacter*	Discontinue long-term systemic antibiotic therapy for acne
Tar folliculitis (see Fig. 20–3 on Color Plate 7)	Pustules in hairy areas	Discontinue use of tar products; use topical corticosteroids
Eosinophilic pustular folliculitis (Ofuji's disease)	Recurrent crops of intensely pruritic, grouped follicular pustules and papulopustules, mainly in the seborrheic areas of the skin; they develop in explosive fashion, last approximately 7–10 days, involute, and relapse on an average of every 3 weeks; centrifugal extension and central clearing of the lesions produces annular and serpiginous plaques; they lack systemic symptoms but have intermittent flares with associated eosinophilia and leukocytosis; marked male predominance	Therapy is difficult, although these lesions involute on their own; cold compresses and topical steroids 3 times a day with antihistamine therapy may alleviate the itching; indomethacin has successfully controlled the disease, as has acetylsalicylic acid; systemic steroids, dapsone, and isotretinoin have sometimes been successful
Candida folliculitis	Pruritic satellite pustules surrounding areas of intertriginous candidiasis	Discontinue long-term antibiotic or corticosteroid therapy if possible; keep the patient dry and cool; treat with topical econazole, clotrimazole, ketoconazole, iodoquinol, or iodochlorhydroxyquin; if not responsive, then use systemic ketoconazole
Eosinophilic folliculitis associated with human immunodeficiency virus infection	Chronic dermatosis characterized by discrete, pruritic, folliculocentric papules, usually found on the face, scalp, and upper trunk; histopathology shows mainly lymphocytes and eosinophils	Does not respond to systemic antibiotics; may respond to interferon therapy or metronidazole
Pseudomonas folliculitis—hot tub folliculitis, caused by *Pseudomonas aeruginosa*	Discrete pruritic papules and erythematous papulopustular lesions that appear 6 hours–5 days (usually 2 days) after hot tub or whirlpool use or, less commonly, after using a public swimming pool or water slide; most lesions appear in the areas covered by the bathing suit	Lesions usually abate when the exposure source is withdrawn; inadvertent therapy with corticosteroid may result in rapid spread of the folliculitis, and predisposition to invasive disease may occur
Actinic folliculitis	Numerous follicular pustules on the upper trunk and arms; occurs several hours after sun exposure, is nonpruritic, and spares the face	Sun avoidance; sunscreens do not provide adequate protection
Perforating folliculitis (must rule out keratosis pilaris or Kyrle's disease)	Asymptomatic erythematous follicular papules 2–8 mm in diameter involving the upper thighs, buttocks, and extensor surface of the arms; lesions often have a whitish keratotic plug, which, in turn, may leave a small, bleeding, cratiform lesion when removed	Resistant to most treatment; however, they may respond to topical tretinoin (Retin-A) or 25% urea lotion (Ultra Mide 25)

TABLE 20-2

Types of Deep Folliculitis

Types	Clinical Features	Therapy
Folliculitis decalvans (follicular inflammation that leads to cicatricial loss of scalp hair)	Initial lesions are perifollicular pustules that crust and expand centrifugally, leaving a central area of scarring alopecia with finger-like projection; scars are smooth, shiny, and depressed; men have more severe involvement than women; must rule out tinea capitis via potassium hydroxide examination	Aluminum acetate (Burow's) solution compresses three times daily, followed by application of mupirocin ointment; systemic antibiotics dictated by culture results
Sycosis barbae (deep-seated staphylococcal infection of the beard area in men)	Follicular papules and pustules with perifollicular inflammation; no broken off or loosened hairs as in tinea barbae	Warm saline or aluminum acetate compresses and topical antibiotics (mupirocin); extensive cases may require systemic antibiotics
Carbuncle (more common in diabetics)	Results from the coalescence of furuncles in the subcutaneous fat and involves multiple follicles; more common in the head and neck region and over the thighs; may be associated with fever, chills, and malaise; chronic infection may produce hypertrophic scars	First rule out underlying diabetes, obesity, or immunosuppression; use warm compresses to localize the lesions and help drainage; systemic antibiotic therapy is mandatory if surgical drainage is instituted

by *S. aureus*. For this reason, the following therapeutic regimen is an excellent initial therapy for most patients.

1. The correct diagnosis should be made by clinical presentation, bacterial culture, and if necessary, biopsy.
2. Good hygiene, soap and water, weight reduction, and loose-fitting clothing will help clear the initial infection and inhibit recurrence.
3. Superficial folliculitis may respond simply to soap and water. Application of moist heat helps localize the infection and promote drainage.
4. When drainage occurs, moist dressings or compresses should not be used because they may promote local spread owing to tissue maceration. The surrounding skin should be protected by applying a thin layer of mupirocin (2%) ointment. To prevent autoinoculation, all draining lesions should be covered with a sterile dressing and hands should be washed if the drainage was touched.
5. Since *S. aureus* is the most common pathogen and is often penicillin-resistant, cloxacillin or oxacillin should be the first-choice systemic antibiotics. For those allergic to penicillin, erythromycin or clindamycin should be prescribed.
6. For those patients who have recurrent lesions and either are nasal carriers or have close contact with an *S. aureus* nasal carrier, an antibiotic ointment (mupirocin) should be used in the nasal vestibule several times a day for 10 to 14 days. If this is not successful, then rifampin alone (600 mg daily for 10 days) or rifampin plus cloxacillin, minocycline, or ciprofloxacin to prevent rifampin resistance can be tried.

REFERRAL

Specialist referral may be required in the absence of rapid therapeutic response to the regimen outlined previously. This will occur in the event of an incorrect initial diagnosis or the presence of resistant organisms. The differential diagnosis is long, and many of the possible entities are relatively unusual or require complex therapeutic measures.

BIBLIOGRAPHY

Gregory DW, Schaffer W: *Pseudomonas* infection associated with hot tubs and other environments. Infect Dis Clin North Am 1987; 1:635–648.

Hedstrom SA: Treatment and prevention of recurrent staphylococcal furunculosis: Clinical and bacteriologic follow-up. Scand J Infect Dis 1985; 17:55–58.

Smith KJ, Skelton HG, Yeager J, et al: Metronidazole for eosinophilic pustular folliculitis in human immunodeficiency virus type 1–positive patients. Arch Dermatol 1995; 131:1089–1091.

CHAPTER 21

Pseudofolliculitis

A. Paul Kelly

CLINICAL APPEARANCE

Definition

Pseudofolliculitis barbae (PFB), also known as *shave bumps, barber's itch,* and *razor bumps,* is a common inflammatory disorder of the hair follicles occurring most often in the beard area of men who shave, especially black men with tightly curled hair. It may also occur on any shaved areas, in women, and in any racial group.

Typical Lesions and Symptoms

The first lesions to appear are firm, skin-colored, follicular papules. Pustules may also be present, but they are secondary lesions (see Fig. 21–1 on Color Plate 7). The lower jaw, chin, and front of the neck are most often involved, but any hairy area that is shaved closely, such as the scalp, legs, and pubic region, may develop PFB. The involved lesion may itch, causing the patient to scratch, which, in turn, creates excoriations that may result in secondary bacterial infection. Superficial traumatic razor nicks may also provide a nidus for secondary bacterial infection. The severity of PFB changes from mild (fewer than a dozen papules or pustules) to severe (more than 100 papules or pustules).

Atypical Presentations or Alternative Forms

Chronic secondary bacterial infection may lead to hair loss, scarring, lightening of the skin, focal or diffuse postinflammatory hyperpigmentation, or even keloid formation of the involved areas. The hairs in the mandibular and submandibular area often run in a haphazard direction and tend to run parallel to and hug the skin surface, thus producing linear depressed scars (grooves) that make it impossible for them to be removed by standard shaving techniques.

DESCRIPTION OF DISEASE

As the name implies, PFB is not a true bacterial infection but is a foreign body inflammatory reaction. The precipitating factor is shaving, especially close shaving in individuals with tightly curled, coarse hair. Since many blacks have a genetic predisposition for this type of hair, they have a much higher incidence than whites, Asians, or Hispanics. When present in whites, PFB is usually mild. In black men who shave, the incidence ranges from 45 to 83%.

The lesions of PFB are usually caused by the tendency of tightly curled hair to curve back to the surface of the skin; however, PFB may occur in people with straight hair in places where the hair grows at an oblique angle to the skin, such as the anterolateral neck. During shaving, the curled hair is usually cut at an oblique angle, creating a sharp tip at the distal end of the hair that enables it to penetrate the skin. Penetration by the tip is usually 1 to 2 mm from where the hair exits the follicle, but sometimes it penetrates its own follicular wall, especially when the skin is pulled tight when shaving. The hair penetrates to a depth of only 2 to 3 mm, and then the external portion of the hair coils to form a loop that in 2 to 6 weeks will function like a spring to pull the embedded tip out. Once the embedded hairs are out, clinical manifestations of PFB usually resolve spontaneously. Thus, termination of shaving and growing a beard will prevent PFB. However, in many instances, patients find it impractical, inappropriate, or impossible to grow a beard.

When the tips of hair reenter the skin, they act as a foreign body, eliciting first neutrophils, which form pustules and later granulomas and fibrosis. Most often, these pustules either are sterile or contain bacteria of the normal skin flora.

TREATMENT

Before any therapy is initiated, the patient should be given a candid explanation about the cause of PFB. It should be stressed that the only way to cure the disease is to stop shaving or permanently remove all hairs in the involved area. If the methods described previously fail or if the patient develops scarring or dyspigmentation, then he or she should be referred to a dermatologist.

Acute Management

Except for very mild cases, PFB requires medical intervention during its acute phase, when it is often painful or pruritic. Antibiotics, topical or systemic, are not beneficial unless secondary infection is present. The following therapeutic approach is recommended:

1. Shaving should be discontinued for a minimum of 1 month for mild cases, 2 to 3 months for moderate cases, and 6 to 12 months for severe cases. During this time, the beard may be trimmed with scissors or electric clippers to a minimal length of 0.5 cm.
2. Warm tap water, saline, or Burow's solution compresses are used 10 minutes three times daily to sooth the lesions, remove any crust, stop drainage secondary to inflammation or excoriations, and soften the epidermis to allow easier release of ingrown hairs.
3. With daily use of a magnifying mirror, the patient should search for ingrown hairs and release them with a sterile needle or toothpick. These hairs should not be plucked because regrowth may be fraught with irritation and penetration of the follicular wall.
4. After compressing and freeing embedded hairs, a low-potency topical corticosteroid lotion should be applied.
5. When secondary bacterial infection is present, the appropriate systemic antibiotic should be given.
6. In resistant cases, 40 to 60 mg of predisone or its equivalent every morning for 7 to 10 days may be necessary.
7. Shaving should not be resumed until all inflammatory lesions have cleared and all ingrown hairs have been released.

Shaving Methods

For those who shave, the following is recommended:

1. Remove any preexisting beard with electric clippers, leaving approximately 1 to 2 mm of stubble.
2. Wash the beard area with a nonabrasive acne soap and a rough wash cloth. In areas with ingrown hairs, gentle massaging with a soft toothbrush may be helpful.
3. Rinse the beard area with water and then compress the face with warm tap water for several minutes.
4. Use the shaving cream of your choice and massage a moderate amount of lather on the area to be shaved (do not allow the lather to dry; if it does, reapply).
5. Use a sharp blade, whichever type seems to cut the best but not too close. Shave with the grain of the hair, using short, even strokes with minimal tension. Twice over one area is usually sufficient, although in hard to shave areas, one may sometimes shave against the grain.
6. After shaving, the face should be rinsed with tap water and then compressed with cool to cold water for 5 minutes.
7. Then, using a magnifying mirror, the patient should search for and dislodge any embedded hairs with a sterile needle or toothpick.
8. The least irritating, most soothing after shave preparation of the patient's choice should then be applied. However, if excess burning or pruritus ensues, a topical corticosteroid cream or lotion (1% hydrocortisone) should be used as the after shave preparation.

Chemical Depilatories

The chemical depilatories (e.g., Magic Shave, Royal Crown) have had greater patient acceptance with the advent of "odorless" preparations. Before using a depilatory on the face, the patient should be instructed to apply a small amount to a 1- to 3-cm hair-bearing area on the forearm. If moderate or marked irritation appears in the area within 48 hours, the depilatory should not be used on the face. However, if either mild or no irritation is appreciated, then the depilatory should be used as follows:

1. Follow the instructions on the product information sheet because the prescribed use of each product may vary.

2. Patients with a beard should be instructed to trim it as short as possible without irritating or traumatizing the skin prior to using the depilatory.

3. The depilatory may be removed with a table knife, spatula, spoon, or tongue blade, after which Steps 5 to 8 of the shaving techniques previously discussed should be followed.

4. In order to prevent excessive irritation, depilatories should not be used more often than every second or third day.

Topically Applied Tretinoin

Tretinoin (Retin-A) solution, gel, or cream; 8 to 12% buffered glycolic acid; or benzoyl peroxide (Benzashave) may be used as an adjunct to shaving in patients with mild to moderate PFB. However, those with severe and chronic PFB usually have only slight improvement. These products are thought to work by alleviating hyperkeratosis and ''toughening'' the skin. Initially, tretinoin is applied every night. The patient should be told to expect some stinging, burning, and peeling. Depending on the individual's response, the dose may be changed once every second or third day. The shaving methods outlined previously should still be followed.

REFERRAL

Referral to a dermatologist may be useful for patients with chronic and recalcitrant disease that does not improve with the previously mentioned regimen.

BIBLIOGRAPHY

Alexander AM, Delph WI: Pseudofolliculitis barbae in the military: A medical, administrative, and social problem. J Natl Med Assoc 1974; 66:459, 464, 479.

Coquilla BH, Lewis CW: Management of pseudofolliculitis barbae. Military Med 1995; 160:263–269.

Kelly AP: Pseudofolliculitis barbae. Curr Concepts Skin Disord 1983; Winter, pp 10–14.

Kelly AP: Pseudofolliculitis barbae. *In* Arndt KA, LeBoit PE, Robinson JK, Wintroub BU (eds): Cutaneous Medicine and Surgery. Philadelphia: WB Saunders, 1995; pp 499–502.

Strauss JS, Kligman AM: Pseudofolliculitis of the beard. Arch Dermatol Syph 1956; 74:533–542.

CHAPTER 22

Fungal Infections

Shondra L. Smith and Matthew J. Stiller

CLINICAL APPEARANCE

Superficial fungal infections can be classified according to the infecting organism: dermatophyte infections and yeast infections (candidiasis and pityriasis versicolor). *Dermatophytosis* denotes superficial fungal infection of nonviable keratinized structures such as the stratum corneum, hair, and nails. The most common dermatophytes affecting humans include species from these three genera: *Microsporum, Trichophyton,* and *Epidermophyton*. Historically, the word *tinea* followed by the affected anatomic location has been used to refer to dermatophyte infections. These clinical types are addressed in this chapter: tinea pedis (foot), tinea cruris (groin), tinea corporis (chest, back, neck, or shoulders), tinea capitis (scalp), tinea barbae (beard), tinea unguium, (nails), and tinea manus (hand).[1]

The usual clinical presentation of tinea varies with the anatomic location and the species of dermatophyte. In general, however, dermatophytosis is manifested by a well-marginated, erythematous, annular patch with central clearing. A fine scale typically covers the plaque. Pruritus, burning, and stinging may be associated symptoms. The exception to this general description is tinea unguium, also referred to as onychomycosis, which appears as thickening, discoloration, and onycholysis of the nail bed and plate.

Atypical presentations of dermatophytosis include kerions and id reactions. Kerions result from the host's local immune response to dermatophyte infection. The lesions formed are boggy, inflamed, scaly, crusty nodules or plaques that can be painful and have purulent drainage.[2] Kerions are most often associated with tinea capitis and tinea barbae but can form at any site. An id reaction occurs in approximately 4 to 5% of dermatophytosis cases. Dermatophytid reactions are secondary inflammatory reactions that occur at sites distant from the actual fungal infection.[1] This immunologic response is not fully understood but may be associated with systemic absorption of fungal antigen. The reaction occurs shortly after initiation of systemic antifungal therapy or at the height of the dermatophytic infection and resolves once the infection is treated.

DESCRIPTION OF DISEASE

Although 39 species of dermatophytes exist, a limited number infect humans. Fungi can be categorized as geophilic (transmitted from soil to humans), zoophilic (transmitted from animal to humans), and anthropophilic (transmitted between humans), in order of increasing frequency of infection in humans. *Microsporum gypseum* is the most common geophilic species affecting humans, but infection with this organism is rare. Human infection with zoophilic species also occurs infrequently, and is most likely to occur in rural areas. Domestic pets, for example, cats and dogs, may be responsible for human infection with *Microsporum canis,* a zoophilic organism. The most likely mode of transmission of dermatophytosis is human-to-human transfer, either by direct contact or indirectly through fomites.[1]

The epidemiology of anthropophilic infections is influenced by host factors such as age, sex, race, and geographic location. The zoophile *Trichophyton tonsurans*, the predominant pathogen in tinea capitis of children, rarely infects the adult scalp. When adult infection occurs, the host is most often black or Hispanic. Adults more often experience dermatophyte infections of the feet, hands, nails, groin, and trunk. With the exception of tinea cruris and tinea barbae, no remarkable sex predilection is evident.[1,2] Certain strains of fungus are restricted to particular geographic locations, with approximately six identifiable species indigenous to the continental United States.[3] Ideal conditions for fungal growth include a warm, moist climate. Clearly, the aforementioned host factors influence the epidemiology of dermatophytosis and can alter the clinical presentation.

Chronic cutaneous fungal infection occurs in approximately 20% of the population, with greater than 90% of adult males afflicted with one or more of these conditions at some point in life.[2] Although resistance to dermatophyte infection is felt to involve both immunologic and nonimmunologic mechanisms, the increased prevalence of immunosuppressive states associated with acquired immunodeficiency syndrome (AIDS), diabetes, antineoplastic agents, corticosteroids, organ transplantation, and potent antibiotics has led to a rise in incidence of superficial fungal infections, as well as an alteration in clinical presentation. Fungal organisms are ubiquitous, and certain individuals are more susceptible to infection by these organisms. The mechanism by which the increased susceptibility occurs is not fully understood; however, certain immunologic factors decrease the chance of developing fungal infections. These include serum inhibitory factor and an α_2-macroglobin keratinase inhibitor, both of which inhibit fungal growth. However, the major immunologic defense mechanism against fungal organisms is the Type IV delayed hypersensitivity response.[1]

The natural history of fungal infection is similar for all types of disease. A suitable environment of host skin plays a crucial role in the pathogenesis of dermatophytosis. Occlusion, resulting in increased temperature and moisture, and trauma can lead to inoculation of keratinized skin with dermatophytes abundant in the environment but not previously pathogenic to that individual. The stages that follow include incubation, enlargement, a refractory period, and involution.[2] The incubation period is usually a silent state in which the dermatophyte grows in the stratum corneum, with little or no clinical signs of infection. Keratinases and proteolytic enzymes produced by dermatophytes digest the keratin, and an inflammatory response ensues. The role that such enzymes play in infection is unclear. For the fungal organisms to flourish, the rate of fungal growth must exceed the epidermal turnover rate. Once the inflammatory response is established, the rate of epidermal turnover is greatly increased, especially at the leading edge of inflammation. The centers of the lesions have fewer fungal organisms and minimal inflammation. Chronic fungal infections typically evoke a minor inflammatory response, possibly due to suppressed delayed-type hypersensitivity with resultant decreased epidermal turnover.[1] The aforementioned characteristics of the host coupled with the virulence and strain of the dermatophyte interact to create varying disease states. Each clinical dermatophytosis is discussed in more detail in the following pages.

Tinea Pedis

Tinea pedis, "athlete's foot," represents the most common dermatophyte infection. Predisposing conditions include occlusive footwear, hot and humid environments, and use of communal baths, showers, or pools. The risk of developing tinea pedis increases with age. The most common causative organisms include *Trichophyton rubrum, Trichophyton mentagrophytes,* and *Epidermophyton floccosum.* Depending on the inciting organism, tinea pedis can assume one of four common appearances. Intertriginous tinea pedis is characterized by fissuring, scaling, or maceration in the interdigital spaces, predominately the third and fourth web spaces. Typically, the interaction of dermatophytes, usually *T. mentagrophytes,* with bacteria, especially gram-negative organisms and *Staphylococcus* spp., produces prominent interdigital tinea pedis. Moccasin-type tinea pedis is characterized by minimal inflammation with prominent scaling and hyperkeratosis of the soles and lateral feet in a distribution that would be covered by a ballet slipper or moccasin. The inciting organism is usually *T. rubrum* or *T. mentagrophytes.* A third and less common variant is vesicular tinea pedis, in which small vesicles or pustules are present on the instep, midanterior plantar surface, and less frequently, the interdigital spaces. The infecting organism is usually *T. mentagrophytes* var. *interdigitale.* The relatively uncommon final form of tinea pedis is the acute ulcerative variant. Large malodorous ulcers accompany hyperkeratosis and maceration of the soles of the feet.[1,2] A secondary bacterial infection with gram-negative organisms is often present. With all four variants, microscopic potassium hydroxide examination of scrapings reveals branching septate hyphae. Biopsy specimens show hyperkeratosis, acanthosis, a sparse superficial perivascular infiltrate, and occasional epidermal neutrophils. Subcorneal or intraepithelial blisters and spongiosis are present with the vesicular variant.[3]

Tinea Cruris

Tinea cruris, ''jock itch,'' occurs almost exclusively in the groin, genitalia, and perianal and perineal skin of males. The causative organisms, in order of decreasing frequency, are *E. floccosum, T. rubrum,* and *T. mentagrophytes.* Obesity, occlusive clothing, and warm environments promote fungal growth. Transmission occurs by direct contact between infected and susceptible individuals; however, conjugal transmission rarely occurs.[3] More commonly, dermatophytes can be indirectly transmitted via scale in shared bed linens, towels, and clothing. Autoinfection is another source of fungal inoculation whereby the dermatophyte is transferred from one body part to another on the same individual. An example of this would be *T. rubrum* from tinea pedis being transferred to the groin, thus causing tinea cruris. Tinea cruris is clinically manifested by pruritus of the groin and surrounding area. Lesions are often bilateral and present as asymmetric, well-marginated, erythematous plaques with raised, scaly borders and scattered papulovesicles. Central clearing may be present. In contrast to candidiasis, in tinea cruris the scrotum and penis are usually spared. Tinea cruris may be associated with toenail or fingernail onychomycosis or tinea pedis or manus. Secondary changes that may complicate this clinical picture include lichen simplex chronicus, allergic or irritant contact dermatitis, and secondary bacterial infection.[1]

The differential diagnosis for interdigital tinea pedis includes bacterial infection, candidiasis, erythrasma, or soft corns. Moccasin-type tinea pedis has a greater differential diagnosis that includes psoriasis, hereditary or acquired keratoderma, pityriasis rubra pilaris, and Reiter's syndrome. The vesicular variety of tinea pedis may be confused with pustular psoriasis, pustulosis plantaris, and bacterial pyodermas.[1, 2] Potassium hydroxide preparation or culture should be used to confirm the diagnosis and define the offending agent.

Tinea Corporis

Tinea corporis, ''ringworm,'' occurs on the chest, back, shoulders, neck, arms, or legs. The most common etiologic agents are *T. rubrum, T. mentagrophytes,* and *M. canis.* In children, a frequent route of transmission is via pets such as cats or dogs. Although tinea corporis is uncommon in adults, they may become infected by direct human contact, autoinoculation, or transfer of fomites in clothing or other inanimate objects. Rarely, humans acquire ringworm from the soil. A variant of tinea corporis, found in the Pacific Islands, called tinea imbricata (Tokelau ringworm), is caused by *Trichophyton concentricum.* This organism is contracted relatively early in childhood and may persist for life.[3]

Tinea corporis can assume many different appearances, but the standard clinical variant is one or more discrete, sharply marginated, erythematous, annular plaques with scaling and central clearing (Fig. 22–1 on Color Plate 7). Lesions are usually limited in size and location; however, patients with diabetes or other immunosuppressive diseases may develop fulminant tinea. Variants of tinea corporis include inflammatory lesions such as kerions, nodular granulomatous perifolliculitis of the legs (unilateral lesions on the lower two thirds of women's legs secondary to trauma associated with shaving), subcutaneous abscesses, verrucous epidermophyton (verrucous lesions on the head, neck, and buttocks), mycetoma (subcutaneous masses), tinea faciale (tinea of the face associated with ill-defined borders, telangiectasia, atrophy, and photoexacerbation that may mimic lupus erythematosus), and tinea incognito (dermatophyte infection modified by corticosteroid treatment).[1]

The differential diagnosis for the typical presentation of tinea corporis includes erythema annulare centrifugum, psoriasis, nummular eczema, granuloma annulare, and erythema migrans. The differential diagnosis for inflammatory variants includes candidal, bacterial, and deep fungal infections. Granulomatous or verrucous variants may mimic blastomycosis or tuberculosis verrucosa cutis.[1, 3] Except for the absence of follicular plugging and poikiloderma, tinea faciale can resemble discoid lupus erythematosus. Careful microscopic examination and clinical suspicion are necessary to establish a diagnosis of tinea corporis.

Tinea Capitis

Infection of scalp skin, hair, and rarely, eyebrows and eyelashes is called *tinea capitis.* Children ages 4 to 14 years are the predominant population affected. *T. tonsurans* is the principal etiologic agent in the United States.[3] Infection with this organism may be self-limited and seldom extends beyond puberty. *M. canis* and *Microsporum audouinii* are other etiologic agents for tinea capitis. The four types of tinea capitis are gray-patch ringworm, black-dot ringworm, kerion, and favus. Gray-patch ringworm is predominantly a disease of children, produced by *M. audouinii* or *M. canis.* Initially, a small erythematous papule appears near a hair shaft. The papule soon regresses, and a noninflammatory, scaly area remains on the scalp, hence, the name *gray-patch ringworm.* The hair becomes brittle and may break near the scalp surface. Black-dot ringworm is noninflammatory, with breakage of hair at the follicular orifice, producing the characteristic appearance of black dots. Not all hairs are affected, and the lesions are poorly circumscribed, multiple, and scattered. Alopecia in both of the previously mentioned types may be scarring or nonscarring. Scalp kerions are boggy, purulent, painful, inflamed nodules, usually with an exudate or crust (Fig. 22–2 on Color Plate 7). Hairs do not break, but they can easily be pulled out, with resultant scarring alopecia. The final type of tinea capitis caused by *Trichophyton schoenleinii* and rare in North America and Western Europe is known as *favus.* Hallmarks of favus include cutaneous atrophy, scutula, scar formation, and scarring alopecia. Scutula are thick, yellow, adherent crusts and scales associated with favus.[2]

Diagnosis of tinea capitis should be based on a combination of gross clinical and microscopic findings, as well as culture results. Skin scrapings that include affected hair roots can be viewed microscopically, and arthrospores or hyphae can be identified. Examination of the scalp with Wood's lamp (ultraviolet A source with little or no visible output)[2] reveals bright green fluorescence of the hair shaft with *M. audouinii* and *M. canis. T. schoenleinii* fluoresces gray-green, but *T. tonsurans* does not fluoresce when examined with Wood's lamp. When cultured, each species of dermatophyte has identifiable characteristics.

The differential diagnosis of tinea capitis includes seborrheic dermatitis, atopic dermatitis, and psoriasis when signs and symptoms are mild. Trichotillomania, secondary syphilis, alopecia areata, and pseudopelade should be considered when alopecia is present. Bacterial pyodermas, folliculitis decalvans, and perifolliculitis capitis abscedens et suffodiens should be ruled out when an inflammatory component is present. The presence of scarring should prompt consideration of discoid lupus erythematosus, lichen planopilaris, pseudopelade, or radiation dermatitis in the differential diagnosis.[1, 2]

Tinea Barbae

Tinea barbae, one of the least common dermatophyte infections, affects adult males at sites of coarse hair growth such as the beard and mustache. *Trichophyton verrucosum* and *T. mentagrophytes*, the principle etiologic agents, can be introduced to humans by exposure to animals such as cattle and dogs (dairy farmers or cattle ranchers). Pruritus and a facial rash are often the presenting complaints. Follicular tinea barbae consists of erythematous pustules, with or without exudate and crusting, that surround loose facial hairs. The nonfollicular type presents as one or more scaling, circular, reddish patches, with hair broken off at the surface. Kerions may form. The differential diagnosis for tinea barbae includes *Staphylococcus aureus* folliculitis, furuncle, carbuncle, acne vulgaris, rosacea, pseudofolliculitis, and herpes simplex.[3]

Tinea Unguium

Tinea unguium is often used synonymously with the term *onychomycosis.* However, *onychomycosis* refers to infection of nails caused by any fungus, including yeasts and nondermatophytes, whereas *tinea unguium* is restricted to dermatophytosis.[1] Dermatophytes are responsible for 80 to 90% of all nail infections.[4] Tinea unguium is almost exclusively a disease of adults, with males affected more often than females. Principle etiologic agents are *T. rubrum, T. mentagrophytes* var. *interdigitale*, and *E. floccosum. T. rubrum* usually infects fingernails, but toenails can be infected by many different organisms, including *T. rubrum.*[3] Dermatophyte infection is often preceded by nail trauma or injury. Proximal subungual, distal subungual, and superficial white are types of tinea unguium. Distal subungual is the most common variety of onychomycosis. Tinea pedis often accompanies nail infection (Fig. 22–3*A* on Color Plate 7). Infection begins with invasion of the stratum corneum of the distal nail bed, then moves proximally, invading the ventral surface of the nail plate as it progresses. Proximal subungual, the least common type, begins with invasion of the proximal nail fold and travels to the nail plate. White superficial, often produced by *T. mentagrophytes*, appears as a white patch on the dorsal surface of the nail plate. Psoriasis of the nails, lichen planus, eczematoid changes of the nails, and nail trauma should be considered when nails demonstrate thickening, onycholysis (separation of the nail plate from the nail bed), and discoloration.[1, 2] The diagnosis of dermatophytosis can be established by microscopic examination or culture of the causative organism (see Fig. 22–3*B* on Color Plate 7).

Tinea Manus

Tinea manus is a form of chronic dermatophyte infection occurring on the hands. Although both hands may be affected, approximately 50% of the time only one hand is involved, typically the dominant hand.[2] *T. rubrum* is the predominant dermatophyte causing tinea manus.[1] One or more dermatophytoses usually precede the development of tinea manus (e.g., tinea pedis or onychomycosis). Recurrence of tinea manus is often associated with simultaneous presence of multiple fungal infections. Rarely, a distinctive annular, erythematous, scaly plaque with accompanying vesicles may be present on the dorsum of the hand; however, more frequently, diffuse hyperkeratosis of the palm and lateral fingers is found in tinea manus.

TREATMENT

Until the 1950s and the evolution of polyene antibiotics and *Penicillium*-derived agents, effective antifungal therapies were virtually nonexistent. The first agents successfully used to treat fungal disease included amphotericin B and nystatin; however, neither of these drugs was effective against dermatophytes. The emergence of griseofulvin, an oral agent primarily affecting dermatophytes, in 1958 was followed by tolnaftate, a topical fungicidal thiocarbamate, in 1962. The next class of agents to be added to the armamentarium was first-generation azoles, including chlormidazole, clotrimazole, and miconazole. Newer azoles include ketoconazole, oxiconazole, econazole, sulconazole, itraconazole, and fluconazole. The systemic triazoles, fluconazole and itraconazole, are particularly useful in dermatology because they can concentrate in skin and mucous membranes.[5] The allylamines, terbinafine and naftifine, are the newest group of fungicidal agents.

First-line therapy for uncomplicated tinea pedis and tinea manus includes use of one of the following topical prescription or over-the-counter preparations: clotrimazole (Lotrimin 1% cream/lotion/solution), econazole (Spectazole 1% cream), sulconazole (Exelderm 1% cream/solution), oxiconazole (Oxistat 1% cream/lotion), terbinafine (Lamisil 1% cream), naftifine (Naftin 1% gel/cream), ciclopirox (Loprox 1% cream), ketoconazole (Nizoral 2% cream/shampoo), miconazole (Monistat-Derm 2% cream), and tolnaftate (Tinactin 1% cream/solution/powder/spray). The usual treatment regimen is twice daily for 4 weeks; however, naftifine, oxiconazole, and econazole require only once-daily applications for 4 weeks; and recommended treatment with topical ketoconazole is once daily for 6 weeks. One week of twice-daily treatment with topical terbinafine is effective in interdigital tinea pedis.[5]

Adjunctive therapy for tinea pedis or manus may include Burow's wet dressings if vesiculation is present, liberal use of foot powder to prevent maceration, treatment of shoes with antifungal powders, and avoidance of occlusive footwear. Chronic tinea pedis or manus may require the use of oral agents including griseofulvin (250–500 mg ultramicrosize twice daily for up to 3 to 6 months) or itraconazole (200 mg daily for up to 3 months) with one of the aforementioned topical antifungals.[2] Secondary bacterial infections that may accompany tinea manus or pedis should be treated with appropriate antibiotics.

The topical therapies mentioned earlier can be used to treat localized tinea corporis and cruris. The topical imidazoles (miconazole, clotrimazole, ketoconazole, econazole), ciclopirox 1% cream, and terbinafine 1% cream are the most commonly used agents.[5] For widespread or inflammatory tinea cruris or corporis, consideration should be given to systemic agents such as griseofulvin, itraconazole, fluconazole, and terbinafine. Griseofulvin (ultramicrosize) 500 mg twice daily for up to 4 weeks is recommended. Alternatives to this include itraconazole 200 mg daily for 4 to 6 weeks, fluconazole in a daily or pulsed-dose regimen, or terbinafine 250 mg daily for up to 6 weeks. Topical antifungals may be used in conjunction with oral medications.[1,5]

Many cases of tinea capitis resolve within 1 year without treatment, but because of the associated signs and symptoms, treatment is advised. Topical agents are not effective with this disorder. Despite emergence of newer antifungal agents, griseofulvin remains the treatment of choice for tinea capitis. The typical adult dose of griseofulvin (ultramicrosize) for gray-patch tinea capitis is 250 mg twice daily for 1 to 2 months, whereas children receive 5 mg/kg/day until clinical and mycologic cure is achieved. Black-dot tinea capitis requires longer treatment with a higher dose. Treatment should continue for 2 weeks after Wood's lamp examination, potassium hydroxide, and culture are negative. Kerions are usually responsive to 4 to 6 weeks twice-daily dosing of 250 mg or 4 to 6 weeks of 5 mg/kg griseofulvin (ultramicrosize), for adults and children, respectively. Ketoconazole, 200 to 400 mg/day for 6 to 8 weeks, and itraconazole, 100 mg/day for 6 weeks, are alternative therapies for adult tinea capitis. With inflammatory types of tinea capitis, kerions, and favus, oral corticosteroids may decrease the risk of scar formation.[1,5]

Tinea barbae is another dermatophytosis that is unresponsive to topical antifungals. When no treatment is given, most tinea barbae infections resolve spontaneously in a few weeks. Symptomatic treatment with local compresses and débridement of crusted lesions may provide some relief. Griseofulvin 0.5 to 1 g/day (microsize) for 2 to 3 weeks following achievement of clinical cure is an effective therapy for tinea barbae.

Tinea unguium is associated with a high rate of treatment failure and recurrence, particularly in the elderly.[2] Topical preparations are of minimal benefit in nail disease. At least 6 to 9 months of treatment with griseofulvin (ultramicrosize) 500 mg twice daily for fingernails and 12 to 18 months for toenails are required in the treatment of tinea unguium. Although ketoconazole 200 mg/day for 4 to 18 months may be used for persons who are intolerant or allergic to griseofulvin or for those infected with *Candida*, neither griseofulvin nor ketoconazole should be primary agents in contemporary treatment of onychomycosis.[6] The newer triazoles (itraconazole and fluconazole) and allylamines (terbinafine) are safer and more effective. Itraconazole provides the broadest spectrum of coverage. Recommended treatment for toenail onychomycosis is itraconazole, 200 mg daily for 3 months, or pulsed-dose, 200 mg twice daily for 1 week/month for 3 to 4 months.[6, 7] Oral terbinafine, which recently became available in the United States, 250 mg daily for 6 weeks for fingernails and 12 weeks for toenails is a preferred treatment for onychomycosis. Another triazole currently under investigation for treatment of tinea unguium is fluconazole. The drug is pulse-dosed once weekly at 150 to 450 mg. The preferred treatment duration with fluconazole appears to be 6 to 9 months. Although less effective against certain *Candida* spp., oral terbinafine is fungicidal for dermatophytes, allowing for a shorter treatment course. A complete chart of oral antifungal agents and their use in the treatment of dermatophytoses can be found in Table 22–1.

PITFALLS AND PROBLEMS

A major problem associated with dermatophytoses is the difficulty in achieving and maintaining a clinical and mycologic cure. With the exception of terbinafine, the majority of currently available antifungal agents are fungistatic (inhibit growth of fungi) not fungicidal (kill fungi). The inability to actually destroy dermatophytes results in a diminished responsiveness and a high recurrence rate of fungal infection. Inadequate duration of treatment contributes to the increased incidence of fungal resistance commonly encountered; therefore, treat-

TABLE 22–1

Oral Antifungal Agents and Their Use in Treating Dermatophytoses*

Agent	Tinea Capitis	Tinea Corporis	Tinea Pedis	Tinea Unguium (Toenail)	Tinea Unguium (Fingernail)	Tinea Cruris	Tinea Manus
Griseofulvin (ultramicrosize)	250 mg bid for 1–2 months	500 mg bid for 2–4 weeks	250–500 mg bid for 3–6 months	500 mg bid for 12–18 months	500 mg bid for 6–9 months	500 mg bid for 3–4 weeks	250–500 mg bid for 3–6 months
Itraconazole	100 mg/day for 6 weeks	200 mg/day for 4–6 weeks	200 mg/day for 3 months	200 mg/day for 3 months *or* †200 mg bid for 1 week/ month for 3–4 months	200 mg/day for 6 weeks *or* †200 mg bid for 1 week/ month for 1–2 months	200 mg/day for 4–6 weeks	200 mg/day for 3 months
Ketoconazole	200–400 mg/ day for 6–8 weeks	200 mg/day for 2–3 months	200 mg/day for 4–6 months	200 mg/day for 4–18 months	200 mg/day for 4–18 months	200 mg/day for 2–3 months	
Fluconazole	50 mg/day for 20 days (kerion)	150 mg/week for up to 4 weeks	150 mg/week for up to 4 weeks	150–450 mg/ week for 6–9 months	150–450 mg/ week for 6–9 months	150 mg/week for up to 4 weeks	
Terbinafine		250 mg/day for 2–4 weeks	250 mg/day for 2–6 weeks	250 mg/day for 12 weeks	250 mg/day for 6 weeks	250 mg/day for 2–4 weeks	

Abbreviation: bid, twice daily.
*No published definitive data are available for areas that are blank.
†Pulse dosing.

ment should be continued beyond the point of clinical and mycologic cure.

Another dilemma encountered with the use of antifungal agents is the potential toxicities. The most significant side effects associated with griseofulvin are hematologic and hepatic toxicities. The cost-benefit ratio of monitoring serum chemistries and hematology while taking griseofulvin and other antifungal agents is controversial. Certainly, persons on prolonged therapy or those with known liver abnormalities should be followed more closely. Patients taking griseofulvin should be instructed not to consume alcohol because a disulfiram-like reaction may develop. Use of oral azoles may be limited by potential hepatotoxicity, effects on adrenal androgens and glucocorticosteroids (ketoconazole only), and interactions with other common therapeutic agents (e.g., hydrochlorothiazide, cimetidine, terfenadine, astemizole, loratadine, and hypoglycemic agents). Use of fluconazole and terbinafine has not been associated with any fatalities; however, hepatic toxicity may occur, and liver enzymes should be followed when a history of liver dysfunction is given. Gastrointestinal complaints such as nausea, vomiting, and anorexia are infrequently associated with the use of azole compounds.[1, 2, 5]

REFERRAL/CONSULTATION GUIDELINES

Complicated cases of tinea capitis (kerion, favus, or alopecia associated with tinea), dermatophytid reactions, ulcerative tinea pedis, nodular granulomatous perifolliculitis of the legs, dermatophyte-induced subcutaneous abscesses, verrucous epidermophyton, and mycetoma-like lesions may require the diagnostic or therapeutic assistance of a dermatologist. Dermatophytosis in the immunocompromised patient may merit consultation with a dermatologist or infectious disease specialist, as treatment can be complex. Referral to a podiatrist may be helpful in diabetic or geriatric patients with onychomycosis in whom definitive systemic therapy is contraindicated.

REFERENCES

1. Fitzpatrick TB, Eisen AZ, Wolff K, et al (eds): Dermatology in General Medicine. 4th ed. New York: McGraw-Hill, 1993; pp 2423–2442.
2. Fitzpatrick TB, Johnson RA, Polano MK, et al (eds): Color Atlas and Synopsis of Clinical Dermatology: Common and Serious Diseases. 2nd ed. New York: McGraw-Hill, 1994; pp 98–115.
3. Rippon JW (ed): Medical Mycology: The Pathogenic Fungi and the Pathogenic Actinomycetes. 3rd ed. Philadelphia: WB Saunders, 1988.
4. Roberts D: Oral therapeutic agents in fungal nail disease. J Am Acad Dermatol 1994; 31(3 Pt 2):S79–S81.
5. Rippon JW, Fromtling RA (eds): Cutaneous Antifungal Agents: Selected Compounds in Clinical Practice and Development. New York: Marcel Dekker, 1993.
6. Gupta AK, Sauder DN, Shear NH: Antifungal agents: An overview, Part II. J Am Acad Dermatol 1994; 30(6):911–932.
7. De Doncker P, Decroix J, Pierard GE, et al: Antifungal pulse therapy for onychomycosis: A pharmacokinetic and pharmacodynamic investigation of monthly cycles of 1-week pulse therapy with itraconazole. Arch Dermatol 1996; 132:34–41.

CHAPTER 23

Hand and Foot Dermatitis

Hensin Tsao and Andrew Paul Lazar

CLINICAL APPEARANCE

Definition

Hand and foot dermatitis (HFD), or hand and foot eczema, is a clinical description rather than a specific diagnosis. The thickened acral skin reacts in certain patterns to a variety of endogenous and exogenous factors; thus, a strict morphologic approach is often inadequate. Strictly speaking, hand and foot *dermatitis* implies a focus of eczematous activity limited mostly to the hands and feet. Hand and foot *involvement* describes a generalized process that includes significant disease on the hands and feet. For example, psoriasis frequently involves the palms and soles; however, it is rarely restricted to the palms and soles. The most common causes of HFD in the outpatient population are listed in Table 23–1. The appearance of HFD will change with time, and therefore, the history will often be more helpful than physical findings in determining the underlying etiology.

Usual Appearance

In the acute phase of any eczematous process, intense erythema, vesicle formation, and oozing may be present. The patients typically will complain of itching or burning. Since the stratum corneum on the palms and soles is significantly thicker than skin elsewhere, the vesicles may not fully erupt. The deep-seated fluid collections seem translucent and create a "tapioca pudding"–like appearance. As the dermatitis progresses to a subacute stage, the erythema diminishes and the skin becomes dry and scaly. Itching is still present but to a lesser degree. Finally, the changes of chronicity range from mild superficial cracks with peeling to thickened hyperkeratotic plaques. Fissuring is often seen, and painful bleeding is not uncommon. Although HFD generally refers to palmar/plantar disease, extension onto the dorsal surface of the hand and foot may be seen. Any chronic process that insults the nail matrix will alter nail plate morphology. Pits and ridges in the context of longstanding dermatitis are quite common and do not necessarily mean psoriasis.

One variant of HFD is acropustulosis. Discrete crops of pustules measuring 2 to 4 mm or confluent lakes of pus may be seen on the palms or soles. Entities that manifest with such morphology are uncommon, and management of these conditions is often complex. Another variant is fingertip eczema. This form usually localizes to the palmar tips of all fingers and most often reflects an undiagnosed irritant contact dermatitis.

TABLE 23–1

Common Causes of Hand and Foot Dermatitis

Contact dermatitis	Lichen planus
Dermatophytosis	Neurodermatitis
Atopic dermatitis	Keratoderma climactericum
Dyshidrotic eczema	Hereditary keratoderma
Psoriasis	Mycosis fungoides

DESCRIPTION OF DISEASE

Epidemiology

Most large-scale studies have focused on hand dermatitis rather than foot dermatitis. The published literature estimates the prevalence of hand dermatitis at 1.7 to 4% of the general population. Hand eczema among certain occupational groups (such as hospital personnel) tends to be higher and appears to be more common in women than in men.

Etiology/Natural History

The history may be the most important element in the evaluation of any HFD. Contact dermatitis, dermatophytosis, atopic dermatitis, and dyshidrotic eczema are the most commonly encountered etiologies.

Contact Dermatitis

By definition, *irritant contact dermatitis* is a nonallergic reaction of the skin to a noxious substance, whereas *allergic contact dermatitis* is a delayed hypersensitivity to a contact allergen. Practically speaking, it is often difficult and initially unnecessary to separate these two conditions. Accurate diagnosis may require patch-testing. The following questions are useful when contact dermatitis is suspected:

What is the patient's occupation? For instance, consider irritant detergent dermatitis in a dishwasher and latex allergy in hospital personnel.

What are the patient's hobbies? Is he or she exposed to compounds during recreation? For instance, artists may develop contact dermatitis to paint thinners.

Does the patient frequent gardens or woods? Does the patient have pets? During poison ivy season, patients are often unaware of their exposure, especially if they are highly sensitive. Furthermore, pets that roam outdoors may bring back allergens on their hair.

What cosmetics does the patient use? Fragrances are common sources of contact allergies. Fingernail polish is another offender.

Does the rash get better if the patient is away from work or home for an extended period of time? A couple of weeks is usually required to extinguish an allergic reaction.

Has the rash worsened since initiating topical medication or a new moisturizer? Neomycin is a frequent sensitizer, and albeit rare, some patients have allergies to topical steroids. Preservatives, aloe vera, and vitamin E compounds are also common allergens in moisturizers. Have the patient bring in all the products applied to his or her hands/feet.

Is the rash on the dominant hand? Preferential use of the dominant hand may cause an asymmetric dermatitis.

What kind of shoes does the patient wear? Leather processing often produces allergens in shoes.

Contact dermatitis of the hands and feet is common and yet difficult to accurately assess. Repeated inquiries and exposure diaries may be needed before a specific agent can be identified. The natural history of allergic contact dermatitis is variable. Development of a contact allergy can occur at any age. If the proper allergens are identified and avoided, most patients will improve and some will be cured. Rarely, however, some patients will continue to react despite separation from the contact agent. A reflare of allergic hand dermatitis may reflect a new allergen or an old reactant disguised in a new product.

Fungal Infections

Chronic scaling of feet should always raise the suspicion of dermatophyte infection. Furthermore, extension of tinea pedis onto the palms is not uncommon, leading to the characteristic ''two feet–one hand'' distribution. Occasionally, a zoonotic dermatophyte may induce such a inflammatory response that vesicles and bullae may form on the hands and feet, mimicking an acute contact dermatitis. Dry scales can be evaluated with a routine potassium hydroxide scraping whereas vesicles and bullae need to be vigorously scraped along the underside of the blister roof for the potassium hydroxide preparation.

Atopic Dermatitis

The major endogenous etiology for HFD is atopic disease. In a large study of patients with hand eczema, up to 22% reported an atopic history. The following constellation of findings may suggest atopic HFD:

1. Childhood history of ''sensitive'' skin or skin rashes
2. Personal or family history of asthma, allergic rhinitis, or atopic eczema at other sites
3. Other physical findings, including persistent dry, itchy skin; dermatitis in the flexural regions; hyperlinear palms; prominent infraorbital (Dennie-Morgan) lines

The atopic diathesis is quite common in the general population. However, an atopic patient can always be allergic to common allergens, and therefore, a detailed exposure history still needs to be elicited. The natural history usually starts with skin disease in childhood.

Unlike exogenous factors that can be isolated and eliminated, atopic HFD is chronic with periods of exacerbation and remission. Treatment is aimed at suppressing the symptoms rather than curing the disease.

Pompholyx or Dyshidrotic Eczema

Pompholyx accounts for 1 to 6% of all cases of HFD (Fig. 23–1 on Color Plate 8). The condition is characterized by recurrent vesiculobullous eruptions that occur on the palms, soles, and sides of the digits. A burning sensation may accompany the attack. More chronic hyperkeratosis and fissuring may eventually develop. A diagnosis of pompholyx should be rendered only when contact, dermatophyte, and atopic dermatitis have been ruled out. Since the pathogenesis of pompholyx is unknown, both the natural history and the response to treatment are variable.

Pathology

Although it is generally not necessary to perform a skin biopsy in HFD, acute dermatitis usually reflects spongiosis and vesiculation of the epidermis with superficial dermal edema. Dermal lymphocytes may eventually percolate up through the swollen epidermis. Allergic reactions may attract eosinophils. Chronic dermatitis leads to hyperkeratosis and thickening of the epidermis. Spongiosis and edema are less noticeable in chronic conditions.

TREATMENT

Preventive Measures

Instruct the patient to decrease exposure to water and potential irritants, such as detergents and heavy-duty cleaners. If exposure to chemicals is inevitable, the patient should wear heavy-duty vinyl gloves for protection. Soap-free cleansers (e.g., Cetaphil) should be used to avoid irritation. The skin should be lubricated as often as possible. In general, bland ointments (e.g., hydrated petrolatum) are the best moisturizers and are most effective if applied when the hands are still moist. If a contact allergen can be established, avoidance is the best cure.

Acute Dermatitis

If vesicles are present, astringents (Burow's solution diluted 1:20) can be applied as cold compresses for 20 to 30 minutes four times a day. Once vesicles have dried, apply potent topical steroids (e.g., halobetasol propionate [Ultravate] or clobetasol propionate [Temovate] ointment) three times a day. In severe acute contact dermatitis, systemic steroids may be required. Start prednisone at 60 mg per day with a taper schedule that lasts at least 2 to 3 weeks.

If patients complain of severe itch, use oral antihistamines (e.g., hydroxyzine hydrochloride [Atarax] 10 to 50 mg every 6 to 8 hours) as needed.

Dermatophyte infections should be treated twice daily with appropriate topical antifungals (e.g., clotrimazole [Lotrimin] 1% cream). Avoid topical steroids in documented cases of dermatophyte infection. Vesicles that have ruptured may leave open wounds. Application of topical antibiotic ointments (e.g., bacitracin or mupirocin [Bactroban]) to the erosions once daily will minimize the risk of secondary bacterial infections.

Chronic Dermatitis

In chronic dermatitis, the skin tends to be thick and dry. Proper treatment will usually bring about significant improvement within 2 weeks. Following 10- to 15-minute soaks in tepid water, patients should liberally apply hydrated petrolatum while hands or feet are still moist. Albeit brief in duration, menthol and phenol compounds (e.g., Sarna lotion) have a cooling and antipruritic effect. Although these compounds have none of the side effects of potent topical steroids (e.g., telangiectasia formation and thinning of skin), phenol should be avoided in pregnant patients. Oral antihistamines (e.g., hydroxyzine hydrochloride [Atarax] 10 to 50 mg every 6 to 8 hours) may also be helpful. Keratolytics (e.g., urea or alpha-hydroxy acids) may be helpful in diminishing the hyperkeratosis of chronic eczema.

Chronic inflammation can be reduced with super-high-potency steroids (e.g., halobetasol propionate [Ultravate] or clobetasol propionate [Temovate] ointment); two to three times a day is usually required. The patient should apply potent topical steroids after soaks and before the moisturizing ointment if they are to be used concurrently. In recalcitrant cases, topical steroids applied under occlusion may be of benefit. Dermal cotton gloves, plastic wrap (e.g., Saran Wrap), rubber gloves, or hydrocolloid membranes (e.g., DuoDerm) may be used. Depending on the patient's schedule and level of discomfort, the occlusion can be done overnight or continuously for 3 to 7 days. Topical tar products (e.g., T/Derm Tar Emollientl) may also be helpful as an anti-inflammatory agent. Hand/foot photochemotherapy with topical psoralens and ultraviolet A (PUVA) is often useful in resistant cases.

Fissures should be treated with topical antibiotics (e.g., mupirocin [Bactroban]). Flexible collodion may help to seal the fissures and diminish pain.

PITFALLS AND PROBLEMS

A worsening of the patient's dermatitis with topical steroids may signify an allergic reaction to topical steroids. Patch-testing with various topical steroids may be necessary to confirm the suspicion. Alternatively, a dermatophyte infection is often exacerbated with topical steroids. A fungal culture may be required even if the potassium hydroxide scraping is negative.

Many patients will use emollients that may be sensitizing. It is not uncommon to develop allergies to neomycin, aloe vera, and vitamin E. Bacitracin and mupirocin are relatively safe topical antibacterial ointments.

Continued exposure to an allergen will often confound all treatment plans. A prolonged respite from or a change in occupation may be required.

Both acute and chronic hand dermatitis may be worsened by *Staphylococcus aureus* colonization. Treatment with appropriate oral antibiotics may accelerate improvement.

Dyshidrotic eczema is often poorly responsive to treatment. Hyperhidrosis may be present. In many patients with dyshidrotic eczema, a nickel allergy can be demonstrated by patch-testing.

REFERRAL GUIDELINES

The treatment of chronic or recurrent HFD is often frustrating and difficult. Many therapeutic approaches may be necessary simultaneously. Dermatologic consultation should be considered in cases where patch-testing may reveal a contact allergen; in severe, recalcitrant disease unresponsive to conventional therapy; in cases where diagnosis or classification is unclear; and in chronic cases being considered for photochemotherapy.

BIBLIOGRAPHY

Abel EA, Goldberg LH, Farber EM: Treatment of palmoplantar psoriasis with topical methoxsalen plus long-wave ultraviolet light. Arch Dermatol 1980; 116:1257–1261.

Agrup G: Hand eczema and other hand dermatoses in South Sweden. Acta Derm Venereol 1969; 49:6–37.

Epstein E: Hand dermatitis: Practical management and current concepts. J Am Acad Dermatol 1984; 10:395–424.

Lammintausta K, Kalimo K, Havu VK: Occurrence of contact allergy and hand eczemas in hospital wet work. Contact Dermatitis 1982; 8:84–90.

CHAPTER 24

Herpes Simplex

Toby A. Maurer and Timothy G. Berger

CLINICAL FEATURES

Herpes simplex viruses (HSV) is one of the most prevalent infections worldwide. HSV infections can be classified as true primary infections (initial exposure to the virus), nonprimary initial episode (the initial clinical lesion from herpes simplex virus type I [HSV I] or type II [HSV II] in a person previously infected with the other virus and with partial cross-immunity), and recurrent infection. Orolabial and genital herpes are the most common forms of HSV infections (see Figs. 24–1 and 24–2 on Color Plate 8), followed by whitlow. Occasionally, erythema multiforme may be driven by HSV infections (see Fig. 24–3 on Color Plate 8). Eczema herpeticum and neonatal herpes are more rare presentations of HSV. Persons with chronic or acute immunosuppression may have prolonged and atypical clinical courses.

Orolabial Herpes

The most common form of orolabial herpes is the ''cold sore'' or ''fever blister'' and typically presents as grouped blisters on an erythematous base on the lips. Symptoms are variable. A prodrome of up to 24 hours of tingling, itching, or burning may precede the outbreak. Ultraviolet exposure, especially ultraviolet B (UVB), is a frequent trigger of recurrent orolabial HSV, and the severity of the outbreak may correlate with the intensity of the sun exposure.[1]

Recurrent erythema multiforme is most frequently due to recurrent HSV infection, most commonly HSV I orolabial disease.

In 1% or fewer patients with primary infection, herpetic gingivostomatitis develops, chiefly in children and young adults. The onset is often accompanied by high fever, regional lymphadenopathy, and malaise. The herpes lesions in the mouth are usually broken vesicles that appear as erosions or ulcers covered with a white membrane. These may become widespread on the oral mucosa, tongue, and tonsils and may produce pain, foul breath, loss of appetite, and dehydration.

Genital Herpes (Herpes Progenitalis)

Primary genital infection with HSV II has a broad clinical spectrum ranging from totally asymptomatic to severe genital ulcer disease. True primary infection in persons with no prior infection with HSV I can present as a severe systemic illness. Grouped blisters and erosions appear in the vaginal, rectal, or penile region with continued development of new blisters over 7 to 14 days. Lesions are bilaterally symmetric and often extensive, and the inguinal lymph nodes can be enlarged bilaterally. Fever and flulike symptoms may be present, but the major complaint is vaginal pain and dysuria (herpetic vulvovaginitis). The whole illness may last 3 weeks or more. Persons with prior infection with HSV I have a less severe initial infection, which may present as grouped blisters or erosions, resembling recurrent genital herpes, but perhaps lasting a few days longer. If the inoculation occurs in the rectal area, severe proctitis may occur from extensive erosions in the anal canal and on the rectal mucosa.

Typical recurrent genital herpes begins with a prodrome of burning, itching, or tingling. Usually with 24 hours, red papules appear at the site, progress blisters filled with clear fluid over 24 hours, form erosions over the next 24 to 36 hours, and heal in another 2 to 3 days. The duration of a typical outbreak of genital herpes is 7 days. Erosions or ulcerations from genital herpes are usually very tender and not indurated (as opposed to the chancre of primary syphilis). The upper buttocks is a common site for recurrent genital herpes, in both men and women.

Herpetic Whitlow

HSV I or II infection may rarely take the form of a felon or whitlow—infection of the pulp of a fingertip. There is tenderness and erythema of the lateral nail fold. Deep-seated blisters develop 24 to 48 hours after symptoms begin. Lymphangitis can occur. The blisters may be very small, requiring careful inspection to detect.

Eczema Herpeticum

Infection with HSV in patients with atopic dermatitis may lead to spread of HSV throughout the eczematous areas (Kaposi's varicelliform eruption). The same may occur in severe seborrheic dermatitis, scabies, Darier's disease, benign familial pemphigus, pemphigus (foliaceus or vulgaris), pemphigoid, Wiskott-Aldrich syndrome, or burns. Hundreds of umbilicated vesicles may be present at the onset, with fever and regional adenopathy.

Intrauterine and Neonatal HSV

Most cases of neonatal infection with HSV occur around the time of delivery. Rarely, HSV infection of the fetus can occur in utero, usually in mothers who have primary genital herpes during pregnancy. Fetal anomalies include skin lesions and scars, microcephaly, microphthalmos, encephalitis, chorioretinitis, and intracerebral calcifications. Affected neonates may die; if they survive, they virtually always suffer permanent neurologic sequelae.

Seventy percent of cases of neonatal HSV are caused by HSV II and acquired as the child passes through an infected birth canal. Neonatal HSV I infections are usually acquired postnatally through contact with a person with orolabial disease, although primary genital HSV I can also infect the neonate. The clinical spectrum of perinatally acquired HSV in the neonate ranges from localized skin infection to severe disseminated disease with encephalitis, hepatitis, pneumonia, and coagulopathy.

Immunocompromised Patients

In the setting of immune suppression, any erosive mucocutaneous lesion should be considered HSV until proved otherwise, especially lesions in the genital and orolabial regions. Atypical morphologies are also seen.

Typically, lesions appear as erosions or crusts. The early vesicular lesions may be transient or never seen. The three clinical hallmarks of HSV infection are pain, an active vesicular border, and a scalloped periphery. Untreated erosive lesions may gradually expand. In the oral mucosa, numerous erosions may be seen, involving all surfaces including the tongue. Rather than gradually expanding, mucocutaneous lesions may also appear and remain fixed and may even become papular.

DESCRIPTION OF DISEASE

Eighty-five percent of adults worldwide are seropositive for HSV I. Seroprevalence for HSV II is lower, and it appears at the age of onset of sexual activity.[2] Currently in the United States, about 23% of adults are infected with HSV II, and the seroprevalence has increased by 30% during the acquired immunodeficiency syndrome (AIDS) era.[3] Serologic data have demonstrated that many more people are infected than give a history of clinical disease. These persons may represent an important reservoir for transmission.

In the mid-1980s, the prevalence of genital herpes due to HSV I began to increase owing to changes in sexual habits, so that locally in some developed countries HSV I caused up to 70% of anogenital herpes in women. HSV I is much less likely than HSV II to recur in the genital area.[4]

Genital herpes is spread by skin-to-skin contact, usually during sexual activity. The incubation period averages 5 days. Active lesions of HSV II contain live virus and are infectious. Persons with recurrent genital herpes shed virus asymptomatically between outbreaks. Asymptomatic shedding occurs simultaneously from several sites (vagina, cervix, and rectum) and can occur through normal-appearing intact skin and mucosae. In addition, persons with HSV II infection may have lesions they do not recognize as being caused by HSV, or they may have recurrent lesions that do not cause symptoms. Barrier methods of contraception may reduce transmission.

Genital herpes infection results in recurrences six times more frequently than orolabial herpes. Twenty percent of patients have recurrent genital herpes, and 60% have clinical lesions that are culture-positive for HSV II but that are unrecognized by the patient as being due to genital herpes.

The natural history of untreated recurrent genital herpes is now well studied. Over a period of several years, the frequency of recurrences often stays the same. Over longer periods, especially in those treated with acyclovir suppression, the frequency of outbreaks decreases.

The most important predictors of neonatal infection appear to be the nature of the mother's infection at delivery (primary versus recurrent) and the presence of active lesions on the cervix, vagina, or vulvar area.[5] The risk of infection for an infant delivered vaginally when the mother has active recurrent genital herpes infection is between 2 and 5%, whereas it is 33 to 50% if the maternal infection at delivery is a primary one.[6]

Despite the frequent and severe skin infections caused by HSV in the immunosuppressed, visceral dissemination is unusual. Ocular involvement can occur from direct inoculation, and if lesions are present around the eye, ophthalmic evaluation is required as herpes keratitis is a leading cause of blindness in the United States.

TREATMENT

In most patients, recurrent orolabial herpes represent more of a nuisance than a disease. Since UVB radiation is a common trigger, all persons with recurrent orolabial herpes should use a sunblock daily on their lips and facial skin. Topical treatment with drying agents such as benzoyl peroxide or over-the-counter cold sore remedies may accelerate healing. In patients with severe individual outbreaks, or in those whose triggers for outbreaks can be identified, intermittent treatment with acyclovir 200 mg five times daily for 5 days may be indicated. Treatment should be begun 24 hours before the trigger, if possible, or at the first prodromal symptoms. Prophylaxis should be considered before skiing or tropical vacations, extensive dental procedures, or other surgical procedures in the perioral area.

The treatment of genital herpes depends on several factors including the frequency of recurrences, the severity of recurrences, the infection status of the sexual partner, and the psychologic impact of the infection on the patient. For patients with few or mildly symptomatic recurrences, treatment is often not required. Counseling regarding transmission risk is required. In patients with severe but infrequent recurrences or in those whom the psychologic complications are severe, intermittent therapy may be useful. To be effective, intermittent therapy must be initiated at the earliest sign of an outbreak. Since the patient must be given medication before the recurrence, treatment can be started whenever the first symptoms occur. Intermittent therapy only reduces the duration of the average recurrence by less than 1 day. However, it is a powerful tool in the patient who is totally overwhelmed by each outbreak. The dosage of acyclovir is 200 mg five times daily, valacyclovir 500 mg twice daily, or famciclovir 125 to 250 mg twice daily, all for 5 days.

For patients with frequent recurrences (more than 6 to 12 per year), suppressive therapy is probably more reasonable. Acyclovir 400 mg twice daily or 200 mg three times daily will suppress 85% of recurrences, and 20% of patients will be recurrence-free during suppressive therapy. In addition, chronic suppressive therapy reduces asymptomatic shedding by almost 95%. After 10 years of suppressive therapy, a large number of patients can stop treatment with a substantial reduction in frequency of recurrences. Chronic suppressive therapy is very safe. Suppression doses with famciclovir and valacyclovir are being studied.

Treatment with suppressive doses of acyclovir chronically will prevent recurrent erythema multiforme in the majority of patients. Some patients with no history of HSV as a trigger for their erythema multiforme are controlled by oral acyclovir, suggesting subclinical HSV infection is the trigger for some "idiopathic" cases of recurrent erythema multiforme.

Although the cutaneous eruption of eczema herpeticum is alarming, the disease is often self-limited in healthy individuals. In all cases, however, either intravenous or oral acyclovir therapy should be given, depending on the severity of the disease.[7]

The appropriate management of pregnancies complicated by genital herpes is complex, and there are still substantial areas of controversy. The position paper by Prober and coworkers provides guidelines for such cases.[8] Routine prenatal cultures are not recommended for women with recurrent genital herpes, as they do not predict shedding at the time of delivery.[9] Scalp electrodes should be avoided in deliveries where cervical shedding of HSV is possible, as they have been documented to increase the risk of infection of the newborn. Since the risk of neonatal herpes is much greater in women with their initial episode during pregnancy, acyclovir suppression has been used in these women to reduce outbreaks during the third trimester and thus prevent the need for cesarean section.[10] All women with active lesions at delivery are delivered by cesarean section, ideally within 4 hours of rupture of the membranes.

For the immunocompromised host, the initial dose of acyclovir is 200 mg orally five times daily. In severe infection, or in the hospitalized patient with moderate disease who has an indwelling intravenous catheter, intravenous acyclovir (5 mg/kg) can be given initially to control the disease. In patients with AIDS and those with persistent immunosuppression, consideration should be given to chronic suppressive therapy with acyclovir at a dose of 400 mg twice daily.

PITFALLS AND PROBLEMS OF DIAGNOSIS

Infections with HSV I or HSV II are diagnosed by specific and nonspecific methods. The accuracy of various tests is dependent on lesion morphology. Acute, vesicular lesions are more likely to test positive with Tzanck's smears. Crusted, eroded, or ulcerative lesions are best diagnosed by viral culture, direct fluorescent antibody (DFA), histologic methods, or polymerase chain reaction. For all these methods, it is imperative that there be a sufficient number of cells supplied. Therefore, the base of the lesion must be appropriately scraped for cells. The Tzanck smear is nonspecific, as both HSV and varicella-zoster virus infection result in the formation of multinucleated epidermal giant cells. Although rapid, this technique is very dependent on the skill of the interpreter. DFA is more accurate, will provide virus type, and results can be available in hours if a virology laboratory is nearby. Viral culture is very accurate and rapid; results are often available in 48 to 72 hours. Polymerase chain reaction is as accurate as viral culture and can be performed on dried or fixed tissue. Skin biopsies of lesions can detect viropathic changes due to HSV and with specific HSV antibodies. Serologic tests are, in general, not used in diagnosing HSV infection. A positive serologic test indicates only that the individual is infected with that virus, not that the viral infection is the cause of the current lesion. Owing to cross-reaction of HSV I and HSV II, nonspecific serologic tests can mistype HSV infection.[11]

In the immunosuppressed host, since most lesions are ulcerative and not vesicular, Tzanck's smears are of less value. Viral cultures are usually positive, but take several days. DFA testing is specific and rapid and is very useful in immunosuppressed hosts in whom therapeutic decisions need to be made.

In the immunocompromised host, chronic treatment with acyclovir or treatment of large herpetic ulcerations may be complicated by the development of acyclovir resistance. The diagnosis is suspected when high doses of acyclovir do not lead to improvement.[12] The virus isolated can be tested for acyclovir sensitivity and can be treated with intravenous foscarnet.

Herpes labialis must most frequently be differentiated from impetigo. The straw-colored serous fluid and the crusts of impetigo are distinctive; however, a mixed infection is not unusual. Herpes zoster presents with clusters of lesions along a neural dermatome.

Genital herpes, especially on the glans or corona, is easily mistaken for a syphilitic chancre or chancroid. A darkfield examination and cultures for *Haemophilus ducreyi* on selective media will aid in making the diagnosis, as will diagnostic tests for HSV (Tzanck, culture, or DFA).

Herpetic gingivostomatitis is often difficult to differentiate from aphthosis, streptococcal infections, diphtheria, coxsackievirus infections, and oral erythema multiforme. Aphthae have a tendency to occur mostly on the buccal and labial mucosae. They are usually wider and form shallow, grayish erosions, generally surrounded by a ring of hyperemia. Whereas these commonly occur on nonattached mucosa, recurrent HSV of the oral cavity primarily affects the attached gingiva.

REFERRAL/CONSULTATION GUIDELINES

The range of infections caused by HSV is most commonly seen and managed by the primary care provider. Any lesion or ulcer suspected to be caused by HSV that is not improving on maximal doses of acyclovir, famciclovir, or valacyclovir should be referred to the dermatologist for biopsy confirmation of the disease. As discussed previously, HSV in the immunocompromised host may develop acyclovir resistance and should be referred to the dermatologist or persons with experience in this area. The diagnosis of erythema multiforme usually requires biopsy confirmation. These patients may be difficult to treat, and a consultation may be considered. Intrauterine and neonatal HSV requires a multidisciplinary approach because of the morbidity and mortality of the disease. Persons with eczema herpeticum should be referred to the dermatologist regarding diagnosis and management of the underlying dermatologic condition that eventuated in widely disseminated HSV. Persons with herpetic lesions around the eyes should be seen by the ophthalmologist for management.

REFERENCES

1. Taylor JR, Schmieder GJ, Shimizu T, et al: Interrelation between ultraviolet light and recurrent herpes simplex infections in man. J Dermatol Sci 1994; 8:224.
2. Corey L: The current trend in genital herpes. Sex Transm Dis 1993; 21(2 Suppl):S38.
3. Kinghorn GR: Genital herpes: Natural history and treatment of acute episodes. J Med Virol Suppl 1993; 1:33.
4. Barton SE, Davis JM, Moss VW, et al: Asymptomatic shedding and subsequent transmission of genital herpes simplex virus. Genitourin Med 1987; 63:102.
5. Whitley RJ: Neonatal herpes simplex virus infections. J Med Virol Suppl 1993; 1:13.
6. Randolph AG, Washington AE, Prober CG: Cesarean delivery for women presenting with genital herpes lesions. JAMA 1993; 270:77.
7. Swart RNJ, Vermeer BJ, Van Der Meer JW, et al: Treatment of eczema herpeticum with acyclovir. Arch Dermatol 1983; 119:13.
8. Prober CG, Corey L, Brown ZA, et al: The management of pregnancies complicated by genital infections with herpes simplex virus. Clin Infect Dis 1992; 15:1031.
9. Brown ZA, Benedetti J, Ashley R, et al: Neonatal herpes simplex virus infection in relation to asymptomatic maternal infection at the time of labor. N Engl J Med 1991; 324:1247.
10. Arvin AM: Antiviral treatment of herpes simplex infection in neonates and pregnant women. J Am Acad Dermatol 1988; 18:200.
11. Nahass GT, Goldstein BA, Zhu WY, et al: Comparison of Tzanck smear, viral culture, and DNA diagnostic methods in detection of herpes simplex and varicella-zoster infection. JAMA 1992; 268:2541.
12. Conant MA: Prophylactic and suppressive treatment with acyclovir and the management of herpes in patients with AIDS. J Am Acad Dermatol 1988; 18:186.

CHAPTER 25

Zoster

Toby A. Maurer and Timothy G. Berger

CLINICAL FEATURES

Herpes zoster classically occurs unilaterally, often with some overflow into the neurotomes above and below. The dermatomes most frequently affected are the thoracic (55%), cranial (20%, with the trigeminal nerve being the most common single nerve involved), lumbar (15%), and sacral (5%). The cutaneous eruption is frequently preceded by several days of pain in the affected area, although the pain may appear simultaneously with or even following the skin eruption; or the eruption may be painless. Initially, the eruption presents as papules and plaques of erythema in the dermatome. Within hours, the plaques develop blisters (see Figs. 25–1 and 25–2 on Color Plate 8). Lesions continue to appear for several days. Rarely, the patient may have pain, but no skin lesions (zoster sine herpete). There is a correlation with the pain severity and the extent of the skin lesions, and elderly persons tend to have more pain. In patients under 30 years, the pain may be minimal. It is not uncommon for there to be scattered lesions outside the dermatome, usually less than 20. In the typical case, new vesicles appear for 1 to 5 days, become pustular, crust, and heal. The total duration of the eruption depends on three factors: patient age, severity of eruption, and presence of underlying immunosuppression. In younger patients, the total duration is 2 to 3 weeks, whereas in the elderly, the cutaneous lesions of zoster may require 6 weeks or longer to heal. Scarring is uncommon except in elderly and immunosuppressed patients.

The nature of the pain associated with herpes zoster is variable, but three basic types of pain have been described—the constant, monotonous, usually burning or deep aching pain; the shooting, lancinating (neuritic) pain; and triggered pain. It is usually impossible to sharply distinguish acute zoster pain from the pain that persists after the skin lesions have healed (postherpetic neuralgia).

The clinical appearance of zoster in the immunocompromised host is usually identical to typical zoster, but the lesions may be more ulcerative and necrotic and may scar more severely. Visceral dissemination and fatal outcome are extremely rare in immunosuppressed patients (about 0.3%), but cutaneous dissemination is not uncommon, occurring in 12% of cancer patients, especially those with hematologic malignancies.

Two atypical patterns of zoster have been described in patients with the acquired immunodeficiency syndrome (AIDS): ecthymatous lesions, punched-out ulcerations with a central crust; and verrucous lesions. These patterns were not reported prior to the AIDS epidemic. Atypical clinical patterns, especially the verrucous pattern, may correlate with acyclovir resistance.[1, 2]

DESCRIPTION OF DISEASE

Zoster is caused by the varicella-zoster virus. Following natural infection or immunization, the virus remains latent in the sensory dorsal root ganglion cells. The virus begins to replicate at some later time, traveling down the sensory nerve into the skin. Other than immunosuppression and age, the factors involved in reactivation are unknown.

The incidence of zoster increases with age. Below age 45 years, the annual incidence is less than 1 in 1000 persons. Over age 75 years, the rate is over four times greater. For white persons over 80 years of age, the lifetime risk of developing zoster is 10 to 30%. For unknown reasons, blacks are four times less likely to develop zoster. Immunosuppression, especially hematologic malignancy and human immunodeficiency virus (HIV) infection, dramatically increases the risk for zoster. In HIV-infected persons, the annual incidence is 30 in 1000 persons, or an annual risk of 3%.[3]

Overall, about 10% of patients have pain 1 month after the onset of the zoster. The tendency to have persistent pain is age-dependent, rarely occurring in persons under 40 years, but 50% of persons over 60 years and 75% of those over 70 years have pain beyond 1 month. Although the natural history is for gradual improvement, between 10 and 25% of those patients having pain at 1 month will still have pain at 1 year. In some patients, the pain may persist for long periods; and fortunately in a still smaller group, the pain may progressively worsen. The cause of this persistent pain is unknown.[4]

Fueyo and Lookingbill concluded that herpes zoster should not be taken as a marker of malignancy and that a screening for underlying malignancy is not indicated in patients with zoster.[5] However, since zoster is 30 times more common in HIV-infected persons, the zoster patient should be questioned about HIV risk factors, and especially in persons under 50 years in whom zoster is normally infrequent, appropriate counseling and testing should be considered. In pediatric HIV infection and in other immunosuppressed children, zoster may rapidly follow primary varicella.

Although it is not cost-effective to search for underlying malignancy in patients with zoster, patients with malignancy (especially Hodgkin's disease and leukemia) are five times more likely to develop zoster than are their age-matched counterparts. Patients with deficient immune systems, such as those immunosuppressed for organ transplantation, by carcinomatosis, by connective tissue disease, and by the agents used to treat these conditions (especially corticosteroids), also have a higher incidence of zoster. Mortality of zoster in bone marrow transplantation is 5%. Prophylactic antiviral agents are used in this high-risk group.[6] In AIDS patients, ocular and neurologic complications of herpes zoster are increased. Immunosuppressed patients often have recurrences of zoster, up to 25% in patients with AIDS.

Diagnosis

The same techniques used for the diagnosis of varicella are used to diagnose herpes zoster. The clinical appearance is often adequate to suspect the diagnosis, and the in-office Tzanck smear can rapidly confirm the clinical suspicion. Beyond Tzanck, direct fluorescent antibody is preferred to viral culture, since it is rapid, types the virus, and has a higher yield than culture. In atypical lesions, biopsy may be necessary to demonstrate the typical herpesvirus cytopathic effects.

Differential Diagnosis

The distinctive clinical picture permits a diagnosis with little difficulty. The unilateral painful eruption of grouped vesicles along a neurotome, with hyperesthesia and regional lymph node enlargement, is typical. Occasionally, segmental cutaneous paresthesias or pain may precede the eruption by 4 or 5 days. In such patients, prodromal symptoms are easily confused with the pain of angina pectoris, duodenal ulcer, biliary or renal colic, appendicitis, pleurodynia, or early glaucoma. The diagnosis becomes obvious once the cutaneous eruption appears. Herpes simplex infections may occasionally have a similar clinical presentation. Direct fluorescent antibody or viral culture will distinguish them.

TREATMENT

Antiviral therapy has become the cornerstone in the management of herpes zoster. The main benefit of therapy is the reduction in the duration of zoster-associated pain. Therefore, treatment in immunocompetent patients is restricted to those at highest risk for persistent pain, those over 50 years of age. Exceptions are patients with very painful or severe zoster, ophthalmic zoster, Ramsay Hunt syndrome, and probably patients with motor nerve involvement. In the most severe cases, especially in the case of ophthalmic zoster, and in disseminated zoster, initial intravenous therapy may be considered. Therapy should be started as soon as the diagnosis is confirmed, preferably within the first 3 to 4 days. In immunocompetent persons, the efficacy of starting treatment beyond this time is unknown. Treatment leads to more rapid resolution of the skin lesions and, most importantly, substantially decreases the duration of zoster-associated pain. Initially, acyclovir at a dose of 800 mg five times daily was used. The newer antivirals, valacyclovir (1000 mg) and famciclovir (500 mg), may be given only three times daily. These agents are as effective or superior to acyclovir, probably due to better absorption and higher blood levels. They are as safe as acyclovir. If not contraindicated, they are preferred. For acyclovir, as well as the new antivirals, the recommended length of treatment is 7 days. The newer antivirals are recommended for 7 days also. Valacyclovir and famciclovir must be dose-adjusted in the setting of renal impairment.[7] In an elderly patient, if the renal status is unknown, the newer agents may be started at twice-daily dosing (almost as effective) pending laboratory renal evaluation, or acyclovir can be used. For patients with renal failure (creatinine clearance less than 25 ml/min), acyclovir is preferred.[8]

In the setting of immunosuppression, an antiviral agent should always be used owing to the increased risk of dissemination and zoster-associated complications. The doses are identical to those used in immunocompetent hosts. In immunosuppressed patients with ophthalmic zoster or Ramsay Hunt syndrome, and in patients failing oral therapy, intravenous acyclovir should be used at a dose of 10 mg/kg three times daily, adjusted for renal function.[9]

The importance of early and adequate antiviral therapy to reduce the duration of pain must be stressed. Topically, capsaicin applied every few hours may reduce pain, but the application itself may cause burning, and the benefits are modest. Local anesthetics such as 10% lidocaine in gel form or 5% lidocaine-prilocaine may acutely reduce pain, but long-term results are not available.

Topical aspirin dissolved in ether or chloroform (750 mg of aspirin in 20 to 30 ml of liquid) in the form of a poultice or paste is also effective.

Nerve blocks are effective for the reduction of acute herpetic pain. For patients with severe or incapacitating acute pain, this option should be offered, as most patients get relief for at least 8 hours and some for much longer periods. The benefit of nerve blocks in the prevention of persistent zoster-associated pain seems limited, however.

Tricyclic antidepressants such as amitriptyline and desipramine are the first-line systemic treatments beyond simple analgesics such as aspirin and acetaminophen. They are given at a dose of 25 to 75 mg in a single nightly dose. Anticonvulsants such as carbamazepine and valproate, neuroleptics such as chlorprothixene and phenothiazines, and H_2 blockers such as cimetidine have all been advocated but have been not been studied critically. Many of these agents are difficult for the elderly to take owing to frequent side effects. Opiate analgesia is effective and may be the next reasonable step if tricyclics alone are ineffective.[4, 10]

Middle-aged and elderly people are urged to restrict their physical activities or even stay home in bed for a few days. Bedrest may be of paramount importance in prevention of neuralgia. Younger patients may usually continue with their customary activities. Local applications of heat, as with an electric heating pad or a hot water bottle, are recommended. Simple local application of gentle pressure, with the hand or an abdominal binder, often gives great relief. Topical anesthetics such as discussed previously may be useful.

The value of systemic corticosteroids in preventing postherpetic neuralgia is controversial.[11] Systemic steroids do reduce acute pain during the first week.[12] Most recent studies have failed to show reduction in the duration of zoster-associated pain.[13, 14] Systemic steroids should not be used in immunosuppressed hosts, as they may increase the risk of dissemination. Steroids do not increase complications in immunocompetent hosts, however. Until there are definitive studies, no recommendation can be made. Steroids may be most useful in patients with severe pain, ophthalmic zoster where immunologic complications are greater, and in patients in whom there is no relative contraindication (e.g., fragile diabetes, severe hypertension).

PITFALLS AND PROBLEMS

Disseminated Herpes Zoster

Herpes zoster generalisatus is a generalized varicelliform eruption accompanying the segmental eruption. It has been defined as more than 20 lesions outside the affected dermatome. It occurs chiefly in old or debilitated persons, especially in the setting of lymphoreticular malignancy or AIDS. Fever, prostration, headache, and signs of meningeal irritation or viral meningitis may be present. Zoster encephalomyelitis may rarely follow and is often fatal.

Ophthalmic Zoster

In herpes zoster ophthalmicus, the ophthalmic division of the fifth cranial nerve is involved. If the external division of the nasociliary branch participates, with vesicles on the side and tip of the nose (Hutchinson's sign), the eyeball is involved 76% of the time, as compared with 34% when this branch is not involved. Vesicles on the lid margin are virtually always associated with ocular involvement. Ocular involvement is most commonly uveitis (92%) and keratitis (50%). Less common but severe complications include glaucoma, optic neuritis, encephalitis, hemiplegia, and acute retinal necrosis. Unlike the cutaneous lesions, ocular lesions of zoster and their complications tend to recur, sometimes as long as 10 years after the zoster.[15]

Other Complications of Zoster

Motor nerve neuropathy occurs in about 3% of patients with zoster, and is three times more common if zoster is associated with underlying malignancy. Seventy-five percent of cases slowly recover, leaving 25% with some residual motor deficit. If the sacral dermatome S3, or less often S2 or S4, is involved, urinary hesitancy or actual urinary retention may occur. The prognosis is good for complete recovery. Similarly pseudo-obstruction, colonic spasm, dilatation, obstipation, constipation, and reduced anal sphincter tone can occur with thoracic (T6–T12), lumbar, or sacral zoster. Recovery is complete.

Ramsay Hunt syndrome results from involvement of the facial and auditory nerves by varicella zoster virus. Herpetic inflammation of the geniculate ganglion is felt to be the cause of this syndrome. The presenting features include zoster of the external ear or tympanic membrane; herpes auricularis with ipsilateral facial paralysis; or herpes auricularis, facial paralysis, and auditory symptoms. Auditory symptoms include mild to severe tinnitus, deafness, vertigo, nausea and vomiting, and nystagmus.

REFERRAL/CONSULTATION GUIDELINES

Zoster and its management can be handled by the primary care provider. In the case of disseminated zoster or zoster in the immunocompromised host, a consultation may be beneficial. Zoster-associated pain, especially of long duration, is very difficult to manage. As in all pain syndromes, pain control should be achieved as quickly as possible. Adequate medication should be provided to control the pain. Patients with persistent moderate to severe pain may benefit from referral to a pain clinic.

The patient with ophthalmic zoster should be seen by an ophthalmologist.

REFERENCES

1. Alessi E, Cusini M, Zerboni R, et al: Unusual varicella-zoster virus infection in patients with AIDS. Arch Dermatol 1988; 124:1011.
2. Glesby MJ, Moore RD, Chaisson RE: Clinical spectrum of herpes zoster in adults infected with human immunodeficiency virus. Clin Infect Dis 1995; 21:370.
3. Straus SE, Ostrove JM, Inchauspe G, et al: Varicella-zoster virus infections. Ann Intern Med 1988; 108:221.
4. Lee JJ, Gauci CA: Postherpetic neuralgia: Current concepts and management. Br J Hosp Med 1994; 52:565.
5. Fueyo MA, Lookingbill DP: Herpes zoster and occult malignancy. J Am Acad Dermatol 1984; 11:480.
6. Rusthoven JJ, Ahlgren P, Elhakim T, et al: Varicella-zoster infection in adult cancer patients. Arch Intern Med 1988; 148:1561.
7. Tyring S, Barbarash RA, Nahlik JE, et al: Famciclovir for the treatment of acute herpes zoster: Effects on acute disease and postherpetic neuralgia. Ann Intern Med 1995; 123:89.
8. Balfour HH Jr: Current management of varicella zoster virus infections. J Med Virol Suppl 1993; 1:74.
9. Balfour HH Jr, Bean B, Laskin OL, et al: Acyclovir halts progression of zoster in immunocompromised patients. N Engl J Med 1983; 308:1448.
10. Rowbotham MC: Treatment of postherpetic neuralgia. Semin Dermatol 1992; 11:218.
11. Post BT, Philbrick JT: Do corticosteroids prevent post-herpetic neuralgia? J Am Acad Dermatol 1988; 18:605.
12. Eaglstein WH, Katz R, Brown JA: The effects of early corticosteroid therapy on the skin eruption and pain of herpes zoster. JAMA 1970; 211:1681.
13. Esmann V, Geil JP, Kroon S, et al: Prednisolone does not prevent post-herpetic neuralgia. Lancet 1987; 1:126.
14. Keczkes K, Basheer AM: Do corticosteroids prevent post-herpetic neuralgia? Br J Dermatol 1980; 102:551.
15. Harding SP: Management of ophthalmic zoster. J Med Virol Suppl 1993; 1:97.

CHAPTER 26

Hidradenitis Suppurativa

Suzanne Grevelink

CLINICAL APPEARANCE

Hidradenitis suppurativa is a chronic cicatrizing disease involving primarily the apocrine gland–bearing areas. Other names for the disease used occasionally in the literature include *apocrinitis, hidradenitis axillaris,* and *abscess of the apocrine sweat glands.* Hidradenitis suppurativa may be seen in association with acne conglobata and dissecting cellulitis of the scalp, a grouping known as the *follicular occlusion triad.* An increased incidence of pilonidal sinus has also been seen with this triad.

Hidradenitis suppurativa most commonly involves the axillary, inguinal, and perianal areas (see Figs. 26–1 and 26–2 on Color Plate 9). Other areas of involvement include the upper thighs and inframammary areas, and rarely, the disease may also affect the abdomen, chest, eyelid, and scalp. The disease usually presents at or after puberty as recurrent episodes of comedones in the inguinal or axillary areas that may be diagnosed initially as a folliculitis. The patient later develops pruritus or mild tenderness followed by the appearance of 0.5- to 1.5-cm, tender, inflammatory, subcutaneous nodules in the affected areas. These nodules rapidly enlarge and may perforate the overlying skin, yielding a seropurulent drainage. Multiple recurrent episodes of similar abscesses lead to sinus tracts and fibrotic scars of the band or bridge type. Although the condition has been reported to resolve spontaneously, hidradenitis more typically runs a gradually progressive, chronic course.

DESCRIPTION OF DISEASE

Hidradenitis suppurativa generally begins after puberty and affects females more commonly than males with a preponderance of approximately 66%. Females have a greater tendency to develop axillary involvement, whereas males are more likely to develop perianal disease. The incidence is unknown but has been estimated at 1 in 300 individuals. Hidradenitis may occur more readily in warmer climates, but it is present throughout the world. Blacks may be affected more often than whites. Genetic studies have revealed a high incidence of patients with a positive family history of hidradenitis, suggesting an autosomal dominant inheritance. Apparent risk factors for the development of hidradenitis suppurativa include a family tendency toward acne, obesity, and smoking.

Hurley[1] delineated a clinical classification of hidradenitis suppurativa consisting of three stages. Stage I disease comprises "isolated abscesses, single or multiple, without scarring or sinus tracts." Stage II disease occurs when the patient develops "recurrent abscesses with tract formation and cicatrization" and "widely separated lesions." Stage III disease involves the formation of "diffuse or near-diffuse involvement, or multiple interconnected tracts and abscesses across an entire area." This staging system facilitates selection of a treatment approach.

Hidradenitis suppurativa may be complicated by a restriction of mobility of an affected limb or by fistula formation to the urethra, bladder, rectum, or perineum.

Apocrine sweating may be decreased or absent in affected areas. Patients are also at risk for ulceration and acute infection. A variety of organisms may be cultured from the seropurulent drainage including *Staphylococcus aureus,* streptococci (especially *Streptococcus milleri*), *Escherichia coli,* and less commonly, *Bacillus proteus, Pseudomonas aeruginosa,* and *Bacteroides* spp. Longstanding cases of hidradenitis suppurativa may occasionally be complicated by squamous cell carcinoma, a phenomenon reported most commonly with perianal disease.

Obstruction, dilatation, and subsequent inflammatory changes of the apocrine gland have traditionally been considered to be the initating events in hidradenitis suppurativa. However, this hypothesis has been challenged by data revealing an absence of apocrine glands in mammary, inguinal, upper thigh, and buttock areas where hidradenitits may present. In addition, apocrine gland enlargement and inflammation are not prominent features on histopathology. Instead, the histopathology of hidradenitis is most notable for multiple sinuses of follicular origin and epithelium-lined cysts. The primary event may be occlusion followed by cystic alteration of the hair follicle, with perhaps secondary or incidental involvement of the apocrine gland. Bacterial infection appears to play an important role in extension of the disease, with formation of sinus tracts and scarring.

Hormonal factors appear to play an integral role in the initiation and subsequent continuation and exacerbation of hidradenitis. The disease begins after puberty when the development of secondary sexual characteristics as well as apocrine gland function has just been completed. Hidradenitis appears to be more active during pregnancy and the second half of the menstrual cycle, and the use of oral contraceptives with a low estrogen to progesterone ratio or high androgenicity may exacerbate the disease. Experimental studies have shown that androgens increase keratin production, and systemic androgen administration in animals leads to keratinaceous follicular occlusion. In addition, antiandrogen therapy has been reported to have efficacy in the treatment of hidradenitis.

As mentioned previously, the initial changes seen histopathologically include keratinaceous occlusion of the follicular orifice and cystic dilatation. Apocrine glands, if involved, may also show occlusion of the ductal orifice with dilatation of the secretory tubules, a histologic pattern considered pathognomic for hidradenitis. Polymorphonuclear leukocytes and bacteria may infiltrate the follicle, glands, and later, the surrounding dermis and subcutaneous tissue. Later changes include the destruction of the apocrine and eccrine glands as well as the entire pilosebaceous unit. Pseudoepitheliomatous hyperplasia and tract formation with fibrosis and scarring are prominent features of late disease.

TREATMENT

Treatment of hidradenitis suppurativa is generally based on the clinical stage as outlined previously under ''Description of Disease.'' Stage I disease may be cured or at least minimized with aggressive dermatologic and medical management and prophylactic measures. Newly formed abscesses should be injected with intralesional triamcinolone acetonide (TAC) at a dose of 5 to 10 mg/ml. If an abscess is fluctuant and may rupture, incision and drainage should be performed followed by injection of TAC into the base and sides of the abscess. Patients should be given a 10- to 14-day course of tetracycline (1 to 1.5 g/day) or one of the tetracycline derivatives (doxycycline or minocycline at 100 to 200 mg/day). Alternative antibiotic choices include ciprofloxacin, cephalosporins, or clindamycin. Bacterial culture and antibiotic sensitivity testing should guide this antibiotic therapy.

Local maintenance care should include avoidance of tight-fitting clothing such as blue jeans, pantyhose, and undergarments, which may induce friction in affected areas thereby exacerbating disease. Affected areas should be cleansed daily with a germicidal soap such as chlorhexidine gluconate. Topical antibiotics such as 2% clindamycin or erythromycin may be helpful in prophylaxis. In addition, 6.25% aluminum chloride hexahydrate in absolute ethanol (Xerac AC) may be effective as both an antiperspirant and a deodorant because it has strong antibacterial properties. Regular antiperspirants may be used once inflammation has subsided, provided the liquid or spray types are used rather than the roll-on or stick types, which may induce excessive friction during application.

The treatment of choice for recurrent hidradenitis with fibrosis, scarring, and sinus tract formation (Stages II and III disease) is surgical management. Options for surgical management include unroofing and destruction of sinus tracks (''exteriorization surgery''), excision with primary closure, and excision with a flap or a split-thickness skin graft. Unfortunately, studies have revealed high rates of recurrence after excision with primary closure (54%), excision with flap closure (19%) and excision with split-thickness skin grafting (13%). Wide en bloc excision of all affected areas is probably the most successful surgical procedure and is the treatment of choice for Stage III disease. The resultant defects may be allowed to heal secondarily or may be closed with a flap or graft. It is important to note that skin grafts are frequently unsuccessful in the perineal and perianal areas. These areas are more effectively treated with localized excisions, by unroofing of the sinus tracts, and curettage.

Other therapeutic options include corticosteroids, oral contraceptives, antiandrogen therapy, retinoids, cyclosporine, and carbon dioxide laser. Oral prednisone at a dose of 60 to 80 mg/day has been used in treatment of the acute inflammation of recurrent hidradenitis. An oral contraceptive containing 50 mg of ethinylestradiol has shown efficacy as monotherapy in some cases. Antiandrogen therapy with spironolactone, cyproterone acetate, or leuprolide, a synthetic gonadotropin-releasing hormone, may be helpful in controlling disease, but reports of efficacy are conflicting. Retinoid therapy is also unpredictable. Isotretinoin (1 mg/kg/day), acetretin (0.5 mg/kg/day), and etretinate (0.5 mg/kg/day) have all been tried in the treatment of hidradenitis with variable degrees of success. Cyclosporine may be helpful in the prevention of recurrent disease, but its usage is associated with multiple side effects. Finally, a recent report described the use of a carbon dioxide laser to vaporize affected tissue followed by second intention healing. The authors stated that the carbon dioxide laser provided an efficient treatment method for for early lesions of hidradenitis. The use of the carbon dioxide laser as well as the use of other alternative therapies described previously requires further study to accurately determine their potential therapeutic value in the treatment of hidradenitis.

PITFALLS AND PROBLEMS

Early hidradenitis may be difficult to distinguish from a variety of dermatologic disorders. Infectious disorders that may mimic hidradenitis include furuncles, carbuncles, erysipelas, tuberculosis, actinomycosis, granuloma inguinale, lymphogranuloma venereum, cat-scratch disease, and tularemia. Early isolated lesions may also resemble inflamed or infected epidermal inclusion cysts or Bartholin's cysts. Perianal hidradenitis must be distinguished from perianal Crohn's disease, pilonidal sinus, and sigmoidal diverticulitis. Finally, hidradenitis suppurativa should not be confused with neutrophilic eccrine hidradenitis. The latter eruption consists of erythematous papules, plaques, and nodules, especially on the upper trunk, and is associated with the use of a chemotherapeutic agent such as cytarabine or, less commonly, methotrexate, cyclophosphamide, and 5-fluorouracil. The characteristic recurrent abscess formation, sinus tract formation, scarring, and distribution of lesions should help to establish the diagnosis of hidradenitis suppurativa.

Optimal treatment of hidradenitis includes an awareness of several important issues. First, patients should be referred for surgical consultation early in the disease course, as many clinicians now advocate early surgical intervention for control of hidradenitis. Second, lesions of hidradenitis not responding to the initial antibiotic chosen should be cultured to guide further antibiotic usage. A skin biopsy should be performed on any longstanding ulcerated lesions to rule out squamous cell carcinoma. Thorough conservative management coupled with excellent surgical intervention should help to minimize many of the debilitating complications of hidradenitis including fistulas and constricting scars.

REFERRAL AND CONSULTATION GUIDELINES

Surgical consultation should be obtained early in the disease course, and repeatedly on a regular basis while the disease is active. Early surgical intervention may be helpful in prevention of morbidity due to complications associated with this disease.

REFERENCE

1. Hurley HJ: Axillary hyperhidrosis, apocrine bromhidrosis, hidradenitis suppurativa, and familial benign pemphigus. Surgical approach. *In* Roenigk RA, Roenigk HH Jr (ed): Dermatologic Surgery. Principle and Practice. New York: Marcel Dekker, 1989; p 735.

BIBLIOGRAPHY

Banerjee AK: Surgical treatment of hidradenitis suppurativa. Br J Surg 1992; 79(9):863–866.

Dicken CH, Powell ST, Spear KL: Evaluation of isotretinoin treatment of hidradenitis suppurativa. J Am Acad Dermatol 1984; 11:500–502.

Hogan DJ, Light MJ: Successful treatment of hidradenitis suppurativa with acetretin. J Am Acad Dermatol 1988; 19:355–356.

Mendonca H, Rebelo C, Fernandes A, et al: Squamous cell carcinoma arising in hidradenitis suppurativa. J Dermatol Surg Oncol 1991; 17(10):830–832.

Rubin RJ, Chinn BT: Perianal hidradenitis suppurativa. Surg Clin North Am 1994; 74(6):1317–1325.

CHAPTER 27

Human Immunodeficiency Virus–Related Cutaneous Disease

Neil S. Sadick

CLINICAL DISEASE SPECTRUM

Cutaneous disease occurs in up to 92% of human immunodeficiency virus (HIV)–infected individuals at some time in the course of their illness. The cutaneous manifestations of infection with HIV may be directly attributable to infection by this retrovirus or may be the result of complicating secondary events that occur as a consequence of immune dysfunction caused by the underlying infection.[1] The atypical presentation of common dermatoses, as well as the occurrence of rare or previously undescribed skin diseases in patients infected with HIV, provides the physician with a great diagnostic challenge. It is in this setting that this chapter outlines important diagnostic and therapeutic approaches to cutaneous diseases seen in the HIV patient.

Cutaneous manifestations of retroviral disorders may be classified according to underlying pathophysiologic mechanisms (Table 27–1).

DESCRIPTIONS OF DISEASE STATES

Infectious Manifestations

The inability of HIV-infected patients to mount a normal immunologic response has led to a wide clinical spectrum of cutaneous opportunistic infections and rare atypical presentations of more common infectious dermatoses. The utilization of biopsies with special stains and appropriate cultures plays an important role in this setting.

Viral Infections

ACUTE EXANTHEM OF HIV INFECTION

Prior to seroconversion, patients infected with HIV may develop fever and clinical signs of an upper respiratory or serum sickness–like illness.[2] These symptoms may be associated with either a truncal maculopapular exanthematous eruption or an urticaria-type eruption, the latter occurring more commonly in the pediatric HIV population. The eruption is most often nonpruritic, af-

TABLE 27–1

Classification of Cutaneous Manifestations of Retroviral Disorders

Infections
Vascular
Papulosquamous
Hypersensitivity dermatoses
Miscellaneous

fecting the trunk, face, neck, and upper extremities, and rarely, the palms and soles. Less frequently, the eruption may manifest an ulcerative component. This constellation of signs and symptoms occurs in 75 to 80% of patients who develop HIV infection.

HERPES SIMPLEX VIRUS INFECTION

Reactivation of the herpesvirus is common in HIV infection and may be the source of significant morbidity secondary to secondary bacterial superinfection. Herpes simplex virus (HSV) type I may be associated with widespread disseminated lesions consistent with Kaposi's varicelliform eruption. Other unusual presentations include diffuse mucous membrane ulcerations, herpetic whitlow, and persistent hemorrhagic ulcerative lesions. HSV type II disease may present with multiple recurrences that mimic hemorrhoids. Lesions may present as chronic crusted erosions and ulcers. Deeply destructive perirectal ulcers may become secondarily infected and result in gram-negative sepsis.

CYTOMEGALOVIRUS INFECTION

Although retinitis and gastroenteritis are the most common manifestations, the skin may also be a target of infection, presenting with ulcerations of the orofacial and perineal regions. These ulcerations are often painful, deep, and confluent with elevated borders. Other less commonly reported presentations include petechiae, purpura, and vesiculobullous and morbilliform eruptions, as well as recalcitrant diaper dermatitis in the pediatric HIV population. Skin biopsy is often helpful in this setting, as it may show infected fibroblasts or endothelial cells.

VARICELLA-ZOSTER VIRUS

Herpes zoster infection is often the first manifestation of compromised immune function in progressive HIV infection. Multidermatomal vesicular lesions and disseminated cutaneous disease may occur in this setting (see Fig. 27–1 on Color Plate 9). Patients may also suffer from prolonged severe postherpetic neuralgia. Two unusual clinical patterns of varicella-zoster virus have been described. Ecthymatous destructive phagadenic ulcers occurring most commonly on the buttocks and lower extremities may be seen. In addition, verrucous hyperkeratotic persistent lesions resembling giant warts or keratoacanthomas may also be noted. These associated strains are often thymidine kinase–deficient and may be associated with acyclovir resistance. Biopsy material from verrucous or ecthymatous lesions may be necessary because swab cultures and fluorescent antibody testing are often negative in this setting.

EPSTEIN-BARR VIRUS

Oral hairy leukoplakia, although occurring most commonly in HIV-infected patients, has also been reported in organ transplant recipient patients as well as sporadic case reports in HIV-seronegative individuals. Lesions present as hyperplastic, verrucous, grayish-white plaques on the dorsal and marginal sides of the tongue. Of diagnostic importance, the lesions are potassium hydroxide/culture-negative and do not respond to antifungal therapy.

HUMAN PAPILLOMAVIRUS

There is an increased incidence of warts in HIV-infected adults and children. The most common presentations are classic verrucous papules of condylomata acuminata in the penis and perianal zones. Special patterns intrinsic to the HIV setting include pigmented hemorrhagic facial warts and extensive flat verrucous papules consistent with verrucae plana. Such lesions are similar to those noted in the epidermodysplasia verruciformis in which human papillomavirus type 5 may be detected.

MOLLUSCUM CONTAGIOSUM

Umbilicated papules most commonly presenting on the face, particularly the beard area and neck, are often noted in the HIV setting (see Fig. 27–2 on Color Plate 9). Giant molluscum lesions up to 10 mm and miliary molluscum papules presenting with hundreds of lesions are unique for the HIV setting. There is a predilection for periorificial and flexural intertriginous locations. It is important to curette a lesion in order to make a specific microscopic or pathologic diagnosis because deep fungal infections such as cryptococcosis, coccidioidomycosis, and histoplasmosis may present with similar clinical lesions.

Arthropod Infections

SARCOPTES SCABIEI

Scabetic infestation is a common cause of pruritus in the HIV setting. Classic crusted pruritic lesions may occur in the flexural and intertriginous locations, or generalized scaling hyperkeratotic lesions may occur. Absence of classic distribution, hyperkeratotic Norwegian crusted scabies-type presentation, minimal inflammatory response to mites, intense pruritus, and frequent posttherapy recurrences are features noted in the HIV-infected population.

DEMODECOMICOSIS

Demodex mites may cause a pruritic papular eruption of the scalp and face. Diagnosis is made by demonstration of multiple *Demodex* mites on wet smear.

Superficial Fungal Infections

CANDIDA ALBICANS

Infection of the oral mucosa with white curdlike plaques is often the initial presenting manifestation of HIV infection.[3] Erythematous plaques and papillary atrophy of the tongue as well as angular cheilitis with associated fissuring may also be present. In the later stages of disease, diffuse plaque formation with altered or lost sense of taste may occur. Vulvovaginal infection with associated discharge and cutaneous erythema and symptomatic soreness occurs in close to 100% of female patients infected with HIV.

PITYROSPORUM INFECTION

Extensive seborrheic dermatitis has been associated with *Pityrosporum ovale* colonization; this association is felt to be more significant in the HIV-infected population. Extensive tinea versicolor secondary to *Pityrosporum orbiculare* infection may also be manifest. In addition to classic hyperpigmented and hypopigmented patches, extensive disease involving the face and scalp and unusual plaquetype lesions may occur. A pruritic papulopustular folliculitis on the trunk and proximal extremities has also been described.

DERMATOPHYTE INFECTION

Unusual presentations in the HIV-infected population include scaling patches on the face indicative of tinea faciale. These lesions may mimic seborrheic dermatitis. Severe dermatophyte infections of the palms and soles may present with thickened hyperkeratotic plaques resembling keratoderma blennorrhagicum. A characteristic superficial whitening of the nail plate (proximal superficial white onychomycosis) may be present secondary to infection with *Trichophyton rubrum*. Tinea capitis may be associated with diffuse rapid hair loss, and infection with the superficial fungus *Scopulariopsis brevicaulis* may lead to patchy hair loss. Generalized papulosquamous scaling patches involving large percentages of the torso may present in patients with significant CD4 depletion.

Deep Fungal Infections

CRYPTOCOCCUS NEOFORMANS

Blood borne dissemination of *Cryptococcus neoformans* occurs in 5 to 10% of patients with disseminated disease. Four characteristic presentations occur in the HIV-infected population: (1) numerous disseminated umbilicated papules resembling molluscum contagiosum; (2) disseminated ulcerative lesions resembling HSV; (3) single or multiple reddish-purple papules, nodules, or plaques resembling cellulitis; and (4) discrete papular lesions with central keratotic horn occurring on the sides of the palms and soles.

COCCIDIOIDES IMMITIS

Disseminated *Coccidioides immitis* infection may present as papulopustular or noduloplaque type complexes. Facial lesions, which occur commonly, may resemble molluscum contagiosum. These lesions may result in draining sinus tracts and ulcers, leading to severe cribriform scarring. Appropriate diagnostic culture and biopsy techniques with special stains are indicated in this setting.

HISTOPLASMA CAPSULATUM

Histoplasmosis presents with cutaneous findings in 10% of disseminated cases of HIV-infected individuals. Common presentations in this setting include (1) generalized maculopapular exanthematous eruptions, (2) necrotic-ulcerative plaque lesions, (3) keratin-plugged papules resembling molluscum contagiosum, (4) follicular acneiform and rosacea-like lesions, and (5) panniculitis-like lesions. The face followed by the extremities and trunk are the most common areas of involvement.

PENICILLINOSIS

Penicillium marneffei, a dimorphic fungus endemic to southeast Asia, may produce reactivation from a latent pulmonary focus and spread hematogenously causing a clinical picture of fever, anemia, weight loss, cough, lymphadenopathy, and hepatomegaly. Cutaneous involvement manifests as papules on the palate and molluscum-like papules and nodules on the face, pinnae, upper trunk, and arms. Diagnosis is made by isolating *P. marneffei* from lesional skin biopsy specimens, blood, or bone marrow cultures. A touch preparation from a lesional skin biopsy shows yeast forms resembling *Histoplasma capsulatum* but with central septae.

Bacterial Infections

Unusual manifestations of bacterial infection in the HIV setting include intractable abscesses, lymphedema, and ulcerative ecthyma-type lesions.

STAPHYLOCOCCUS AUREUS

Early in the course of disease, crusted plaques of impetigo may occur, particularly in the pediatric HIV population. Crusted lesions on the neck or beard area are characteristic. Abscess-type lesions over catheter insertion and needle tract sites may also occur. Tender red plaques of cellulitis may occur. Finally, thickened lichenified plaques resembling prurigo nodularis may occur on the trunk and upper arms.

BACILLARY ANGIOMATOSIS

Lesions caused by the *Rochalimaea* spp. are characterized by asymptomatic, cutaneous vascular nodules resembling Kaposi's sarcoma, occasionally associated with systemic dissemination.[4] The lesions are violaceous to red papules and nodules, which vary from one to several hundred in number and may occur at any site except the palms, soles, and oral mucous membranes. The organism can be found on skin biopsy utilizing the Warthin-Starry stain.

SYPHILIS

Atypical and aggressive clinical manifestations have been described in HIV-infected individuals. In addition to aberrant antibody responses, frequent relapses and rapid progression to tertiary disease are characteristic in the HIV setting. Two points are of importance as related to treponemal skin disease in the HIV-infected population: (1) There is an increased incidence of painful chancres owing to secondary bacterial infection, and (2) there is an increased incidence of "lues maligna," a rare form of secondary disease characterized by papulopustular lesions on the torso and extremities with associated histologic necrotizing vasculitis.

Mycobacterial Infection

Although the incidence of tuberculosis in the United States has risen since the mid-1980s, particularly in the HIV-infected population, disseminated skin lesions are rare because of the short natural history of disease in this patient population. However, cutaneous infection with atypical mycobacteria presenting as abscesses and noduloulcerative complexes on the torso and extremities has frequently been reported with *Mycobacterium haemophilum, Mycobacterium fortuitum,* and *Mycobacterium avium–intracellulare* (see Fig. 27–3 on Color Plate 9). In addition, *M. avium–intracellulare* has been detected within skin lesions of Kaposi's sarcoma.

Vascular Disorders

Retroviruses may elicit cutaneous angiogenic and antigenic factors. In this setting, various vascular manifestations of HIV infection of the skin may occur. Telangiectasia occur with increased incidence on the chest and earlobes. Subungual splinter hemorrhages may be noted. Nonpalpable purpura secondary to both immune and thrombotic thrombocytopenia may occur.

Palpable purpura as a manifestation of leukocytoclastic vasculitis may present in this setting and may be related to HIV as an immunologic antigen.

Finally, hyperalgesic pseudothrombophlebitis, a newly described HIV entity, may manifest as painful, swelling plaques of the lower extremities.

Papulosquamous Disorders

Seborrheic Dermatitis

One of the most common manifestations of HIV disease, this occurs in up to 80% of HIV-infected patients. In addition to the classic butterfly rash, intense erythema, thickened plaques on the scalp, and associated alopecia may occur. Severe cases may eventuate in exfoliative erythroderma.

Psoriasis

Psoriasis occurs in 5 to 10% of patients infected with HIV. Two variants are noted in the HIV population: (1) classic psoriasis with a positive family history and classic, silvery-scaled hyperkeratotic plaques on the scalp, buttocks, torso, and extensor extremities. An increased incidence of the pustular variant and associated arthritis in up to 35% of patients may occur in this variant and in (2) the so-called acquired immunodeficiency syndrome (AIDS) psoriasiform dermatoses, where a more generalized scaling eruption progressing from an early "dry skin syndrome" has also been described (see Fig. 27–4 on Color Plate 10). These two variants are summarized in Table 27–2.

Xerosis Generalisata

A generalized dry skin syndrome is noted in up to 80% of HIV-infected individuals, particularly in the late stages of disease associated with downward-spiraling immune competence.

TABLE 27–2

AIDS-Related Psoriasis Syndromes

Classic Psoriasis	AIDS Psoriasiform Dermatoses
Family history positive	No family history
Munro's microabscesses	Perivascular inflammation, keratinocyte necrosis
Common arthropathy	Rare arthritis
Monomorphous morphology	Continuum of seborrheic dermatitis, ichthyosis, keratoderma
Bacterial etiology rare, i.e., guttate psoriasis	Viral etiology common, i.e., retrovirus
Responds to classic therapeutic intervention, i.e., topical steroids, phototherapy, calcipotriene, tar preparations	Responds to immune modulation following antiretroviral drugs, i.e., zidovudine (AZT), didanosine (DDI)

Abbreviation: AIDS, acquired immunodeficiency syndrome.

Acquired Ichthyosis

Acquired lower extremity rhomboidal scaling has been noted with increased frequency in the HIV-infected population, particularly in black individuals and in drug addicts. Malnutrition with associated fatty acid deficiency and immunologic aberrations have been hypothesized as possible etiologic factors.

Keratoderma Blennorrhagicum

Thickening of the palms and soles with or without associated pustular lesions occurs with increased frequency in the HIV setting. The true incidence of Reiter's syndrome in this setting is unclear, and many of these cases may be a result of dermatophyte infection or may represent an overlapping spectrum of HIV psoriatic disease.

Exfoliative Erythroderma

All of the HIV-associated epidermal hyperproliferative states previously described may eventuate in their most severe forms as generalized erythroderma with associated skin exfoliation.

Neoplastic Disorders

Kaposi's Sarcoma

Epidemic Kaposi's sarcoma is the most common malignant manifestation of AIDS. The lesions present as violaceous macules or plaquetype lesions that are often widespread and tend to follow the cleavage lines of the skin (see Fig. 27–5 on Color Plate 10). Mucous membrane involvement, particularly of the hard palate, and associated lymphadenopathy are noted with increased frequency in the HIV setting. The role of the herpesvirus group in the vascular process is now being actively investigated.

Other HIV-Related Malignancies

An increased incidence of aggressive non-Hodgkin's lymphoma commonly of the B-cell type and peripheral nonepidermatotropic T-cell lymphoma have also been described. These lesions commonly present as violaceous, plum-colored plaques and nodules. Cloacogenic carcinoma, presenting as anal ulcerations, occurs with increased frequency in homosexual HIV-infected individuals. Squamous cell carcinoma of the oral mucous membranes and anal canal may present as nonhealing ulcerative or infiltrative nodular lesions. The latter may arise in preexisting lesions of bowenoid papulosis. Finally, an increased incidence of basal cell carcinomas presenting as pearly ulcerated tumors commonly on the face have been noted. Associated increased recurrences and an increased incidence of metastatic disease have been reported.

Hypersensitivity Dermatoses

Hypersensitivity dermatoses in HIV infection may be related to abnormalities in delayed hypersensitivity or cytokine function or altered antigen processing.

Eosinophilic Folliculitis

This disorder is most specific of the HIV hypersensitivity dermatoses in that it presents with papular and pustular lesions, often on an erythematous base, most commonly localized to the face, neck, proximal extremities, and upper torso. The lesions are pruritic and sterile. They may be accompanied by peripheral leukocytosis and eosinophilia and are characterized histologically by neurophilic and eosinophilic infiltration of the hair follicles.

Pruritic Papular Eruption of AIDS

This disorder presents with pruritic papules in a distribution similar to that of eosinophilic folliculitis; however,

TABLE 27–3

Therapeutic Options in HIV-Related Cutaneous Disease

Type of Disorder	Therapeutic Alternatives
Infectious Manifestations	
VIRAL INFECTIONS	
Acute exanthem of HIV infection	1. Self-limited—diagnostic recognition 2. Appropriate serologic testing of importance
Herpes simplex infection	1. Acyclovir (Zovirax): PO 200 mg 5 times per day for 5 days; IV 5 mg/kg every 8 hours for 5 days ***Alternatives*** 2. Foscarnet for acyclovir-resistant strains (thymidine kinase–deficient): IV 40–60 mg/kg every 8 hours for a minimum of 10 days 3. Vidarabine for acyclovir-resistant strains: IV 15 mg/kg/day for 7 days
Cytomegalovirus	1. Ganciclovir (DHPG): induction IV 5 mg/kg every 8–12 hours for 3 weeks *Maintenance:* IV 6 mg/kg/day 5 times per week or 5 mg/kg/day 2. Foscarnet: IV 60 mg/kg every 8 hours or 20 mg/kg bolus over 30 minutes followed by 230 mg/kg/day for 2–3 weeks *Maintenance:* IV 90–120 mg/kg/day
Varicella-zoster virus	1. Acyclovir: PO 800 mg (5 times per day for 7 days; IV 10 mg/kg every 8 hours for 7 days) 2. Famciclovir (Famvir): PO 500 mg tid for 7 days 3. Valacyclovir (Valtrex): PO 1000 mg tid for 7 days ***Alternatives*** 4. Foscarnet for acyclovir-resistant strains: IV 40–60 mg/kg every 8 hours for a minimum of 10 days
Epstein-Barr virus Oral hairy leukoplakia	1. Zidovudine (AZT): 100 mg every 4 hours while awake or 200 mg tid for 1 day 2. Acyclovir: PO 400–800 mg 5 times per day until healed 3. Ganciclovir: induction 5 mg/kg every 8–12 hours for 3 weeks, then 6 mg/kg/day 5 times per day for 1 week until clearing 4. Foscarnet: 40–60 mg/kg every 8 hours until clearing 5. Retinoic acid topical solution 0.025% (Retin-A) 6. Podophyllin topical 25% suspension
Human papillomavirus	1. Cryosurgery 2. 10–20% salicylic or lactic acid preparations (Occlusal-HP, DuoFilm, Mediplast) ***Alternatives*** 3. IFN-α2b, IFN-αn3: 1 million IU/0.1 ml per wart 3 times per week for 3 weeks
Molluscum contagiosum	1. Cryosurgery 2. Curettage/electrosurgery 3. 40–100% trichloroacetic acid solution ***Alternatives*** 4. Cantharidin (Cantharone): occlude for 4–12 hours, weekly application
Arthropod Infections	
Sarcoptes scabiei	1. Lindane 1% lotion (Kwell): 8-hour application, second application in 1 week 2. Permethrin 5% cream (Elimite): 10-hour application, second application in 1 week ***Alternatives*** 3. Precipitated sulfur 6% in petrolatum: nightly application for 3 nights, wash off in 24 hours 4. Ivermectin: single oral dose of 200 mg/kg
Demodecomicosis	1. Permethrin lotion 1–5%: weekly applications overnight 2. Lindane 1% lotion (Kwell): 1 overnight application, repeat as necessary weekly 3. Crotamiton lotion or cream (Eurax): overnight application, repeat as necessary weekly ***Alternatives*** 4. 3–6% salicylic acid ointment 5. 6–12% lactic acid lotion (Lac-Hydrin) 6. 10–20% urea lotion (Carmol, Ultra Mide)

TABLE 27-3

Therapeutic Options in HIV-Related Cutaneous Disease *Continued*

Type of Disorder	Therapeutic Alternatives
SUPERFICIAL FUNGAL INFECTIONS	
Candida albicans	1. Ketoconazole (Nizoral): PO 200 mg/kg until clearing 2. Fluconazole (Diflucan): PO 200 mg/day, day 1, then 100 mg/day until clearing 3. Itraconazole (Sporanox): PO 2 100-mg tabs/day until clearing 4. Nystatin suspension: oral suspension 500,000 U/5 ml bid until clearing ***Topical Agents*** IMIDAZOLES 1. Sulconazole 1% (Exelderm) bid until clearing 2. Clotrimazole 1% (Lotrimin): bid until clearing 3. Econazole 1% (Spectazole): bid until clearing 4. Miconazole 2% (Monistat): bid until clearing 5. Ketoconazole 2%: bid until clearing 6. Terconazole 2% (Terazol): bid until clearing ALLYLAMINES 1. Naftifine hydrochloride 1% (Naftin): bid until clearing
Pityrosporum infection	1. Ketoconazole: PO 200 mg/day for 3–7 days 2. Selenium sulfide 2.5% lotion (Selsun/Exsel); 20-minute application once a day for 2 weeks, then once a month in order to prevent recurrences ***Alternatives*** 3. Topical imidazole creams 4. Topical allylamine creams: bid applications until clearing (see *Candida albicans* therapy)
Dermatophytes	***Systemic Agents*** 1. Griseofulvin (Gris-PEG): PO 250 mg bid until clearing 2. Ketoconazole: PO 200 mg qid until clearing 3. Fluconazole: PO 200 mg/day, day 1, then 100 mg/day until clearing 4. Itraconazole: PO 2 200-mg tabs/day until clearing ***Topical Agents*** 1. Topical allylamine creams Terbinafine hydrochloride 1% (Lamisil): bid application until clearing Other allylamines (see *Candida albicans* therapy) 2. Topical imidazole creams (see *Candida albicans* therapy)
DEEP FUNGAL INFECTIONS	
Cryptococcus neoformans	1. Amphotericin B (Fungizone) 0.1 mg/ml (1 mg/10 ml): IV infusion over 2–6 hours 2. Flucytosine (Ancobon): PO 50–150 mg/kg/day in divided dosages at 6-hour intervals 3. Fluconazole: PO 800 mg on day 1, followed by 200 mg/day
Coccidioides immitis	1. IV amphotericin B: 0.1 mg/ml (1 mg/10 ml) IV infusion over 2–6 hours 2. Fluconazole: PO 400 mg/day on day 1, followed by 200 mg/day
Histoplasma capsulatum	1. IV amphotericin B: 0.1 mg/ml (1 mg/10 ml) IV infusion over 2–6 hours ***Alternatives*** 2. Ketoconazole: PO 200–400 mg/day 3. Itraconazole: PO 2 100-mg–200-mg tabs/day 4. Fluconazole: 200–400 mg/day on day 1, then 100–200 mg/day
Penicillium marneffei	1. IV amphotericin B: 0.1 mg/ml (1 mg/10 ml) IV infusion over 2–6 hours 2. 5-Flucytosine: PO 50–150 mg/kg/day in divided dosages at 6-hour intervals ***Alternatives*** 3. Ketoconazole: PO 200–400 mg/day 4. Itraconazole: PO 2 100-mg–200-mg tabs/day
Bacterial Infections	
Staphylococcus aureus	1. Penicillinase-resistant penicillins: e.g., dicloxacillin PO 1–2 g/day for 7–14 days ***Alternatives*** 2. Cephalosporins, e.g., cephalexin (Keflex): PO 1–2 g/day for 7–14 days *or* Cefadroxil (Duricef) PO 1000–2000 mg/day for 7–14 days 3. Ampicillin–clavulanic acid derivatives: Amoxicillin/clavulanate potassium (Augmentin) PO 750–1500 mg/day for 7–14 days *or* 4. Macrolides Erythromycin (ERYC) PO 1–2 g/day for 7–14 days Clarithromycin (Biaxin): PO 500 mg bid for 7–14 days Azithromycin (Zithromax): PO 500 mg/day on day 1, followed by 250 mg once daily on days 2–5 for a total dose of 1–5 g

Table continued on following page

TABLE 27-3

Therapeutic Options in HIV-Related Cutaneous Disease *Continued*

Type of Disorder	Therapeutic Alternatives
Bacillary angiomatosis	1. Erythromycin: PO 500 mg qid for 3–6 weeks 2. Doxycycline: PO 100 mg bid for 3–6 weeks ***Alternatives*** 3. Ceftazidime: IV 2 g tid for 2–3 weeks
Syphilis	CDC Treatment Guidelines for primary, secondary, and early latent syphilis in HIV-infected patients: Penicillin G benzathine 2.4 million U IM for 1 dose ***Alternatives*** Penicillin G benzathine 2.4 million U for 3 doses 1 week apart *or* For penicillin-allergic patients Doxycycline: PO 100 mg bid for 14 days *or* Erythromycin: PO 500 mg qid for 14 days
MYCOBACTERIAL INFECTIONS	
Mycobacterium tuberculosis	Active disease—9-month regimen: First 2 months: isoniazid 5 mg/kg/day plus rifampin 10 mg/kg/day plus pyrazinamide 15–25 mg/kg/day If isoniazid resistance is likely, add ethambutol 15–25 mg/kg/day, then switch to isoniazid plus rifampin daily as above or twice-weekly at isoniazid 15 mg/kg/day plus rifampin 10 mg/kg/day
Atypical mycobacterium	Multidrug regimens include ethambutol plus three to four of the following drugs (based on sensitivities): clarithromycin 500–1000 mg bid or azithromycin 500–1000 mg every day, Rifampin, 10 mg/kg/day, ciprofloxacin 750 mg bid, or ofloxacin 400 mg bid, clofazimine 100 mg every day, amikacin 7.5 mg/kg IV every day
Vascular Disorders Telangiectasis Subungual splinter hemorrhages Thrombocytopenic purpura Palpable purpura (leukocytoclastic vasculitis) Hyperalgesic pseudothrombophlebitis	***Antiretroviral Therapy*** 1. Zidovudine: PO 100 mg every 4 hours while awake or 200 mg tid ***Alternatives*** 2. Didanosine (DDI): PO 250–375 mg bid day 3. Zalcitabine (DDC): PO 0.75 mg tid alone or in combination with zidovudine (oral, 200 mg tid)
Papulosquamous Disorders Seborrheic dermatitis Psoriasis Xerosis generalisata Acquired ichthyosis Keratoderma blennorrhagicum Exfoliative erythroderma	***Oral Agents*** 1. Zidovudine: PO 100 mg every 4 hours while awake or 200 mg tid 2. Etretinate (Tegison): PO 0.5–1 mg/kg once daily ***Phototherapy*** 3. Ultraviolet B phototherapy: modified Goeckerman's regimen 4. PUVA—5-methoxypsoralen 0.5–1 mg/kg/day plus ultraviolet A (questionable role of immunosuppression) ***Topical Agents*** 1. Corticosteroids (Classes I–VII) 2. Vitamin D analogs: calcipotriene (Dovonex) 3. Topical tar derivatives (Estar gel, Doak Tar solution, Balnetar) 4. Topical anthralin derivatives (Anthra-Derm) 5. Keratolytic agents (3–6% salicylic acid ointment, 6–12% lactic acid lotion, 10–20% urea lotion) 6. Shampoos: ketoconazole, selenium sulfide, 1–2% pyrithione zinc (DHS-Zinc, Head & Shoulders, Zincon), tar shampoos (Pentrax, T/Gel, Zetar, DHS Tar, Ionil T)
Neoplastic Disorders Kaposi's sarcoma	***Systemic Therapy*** 1. Radiotherapy 2. Cryosurgery 3. Surgical excision 4. IFN-α2a 36 million IU sub q *or* IFN-α2b, 30 million IU sub q Therapy is continued until no residual tumor is present ***Local Intralesional Therapy*** 1. Vinblastine sulfate (Velban): 1 mg vinblastine dissolved in 10 ml sodium chloride (0.3–0.5 ml injected per lesion intralesionally) 2. Bleomycin sulfate (Blenoxane): 1 vial (15 U) dissolved in 5 ml sterile water (0.3–0.5 ml injected per lesion intralesionally) 3. IFN-α2b (1 million IU/0.1 ml per lesion) 4. Sodium tetradecyl sulfate 1–3%: 0.5 ml injected intralesionally

TABLE 27-3

Therapeutic Options in HIV-Related Cutaneous Disease *Continued*

Type of Disorder	Therapeutic Alternatives
Non-Hodgkin's lymphoma Nonepidermitropic T-cell lymphoma Cloacogenic carcinoma Squamous cell carcinoma	1. Surgical excision 2. Radiotherapy 3. Chemotherapy (COPP [cyclophosphamide {Cytoxan}, vincristine {Oncovin}, procarbazine, prednisone], regimen commonly employed for non-Hodgkin's lymphoma)
Basal cell carcinoma	1. Surgical excision 2. Cryosurgery 3. Electrosurgery 4. Intralesional IFN-α2b (1 million IU/0.1 ml per lesion) IFN-αn3 (225×10^3 IU/0.1 ml per lesion)
Hypersensitivity Dermatoses	
Eosinophilic folliculitis Papular eruption of AIDS	1. Ultraviolet B phototherapy (modified Goeckerman's regimen) ***Alternatives*** SYSTEMIC 1. Itraconazole: PO 200 mg/day until clearing 2. Dapsone: 50–300 mg/day (taper to lowest maintenance dose) 3. Astemizole (Hismanal): PO 10 mg/day TOPICAL 1. Potent topical corticosteroids: betamethasone diproprionate 0.05% (Diprolene), clobetasol propionate 0.05% (Temovate), halobetasol propionate 0.05% (Ultravate) 2. Pramoxine hydrochloride (Pramosone) (1.0–2.5% lotion or cream)
Drug hypersensitivity dermatoses	Removal of drug antigen
Miscellaneous Associations	
Autoimmune phenomena Vitiligo	1. Potent topical corticosteroids: betamethasone diproprionate 0.05% clobetasol propionate 0.05%, halobetasol propionate 0.05% 2. PUVA (Oxsoralen-Ultra) 0.5–1 mg/kg plus ultraviolet A light
Sicca syndrome	Mucous membrane lubricants (Clerz 2)
HAIR ABNORMALITIES	***Antiretroviral Therapy***
Telogen effluvium Graying of hair Acquired trichomegaly	1. Zidovudine: PO 100 mg every 4 hours while awake or 200 mg tid ***Alternatives*** 2. Didanosine: PO 250–375 mg bid 3. Zalcitabine: PO 0.75 mg tid alone or in combination with zidovudine (PO 200 mg tid) Rapid diagnosis and treatment of opportunistic infection
PHOTOSENSITIVITY DISORDERS	
Porphyria cutanea tarda	1. Broad-spectrum ultraviolet B/ultraviolet A sun screens 2. Avoidance of inciting drugs 3. Phlebotomy
Granuloma annulare	***Systemic Therapy*** 1. Antimalarials: hydroxychloroquine (Plaquenil) PO 200 mg bid for 1 day, quinacrine (Atabrine) PO 100 mg/day ***Local Therapy*** 1. Intralesional corticosteroids: triamcinolone diacetonide (5 mg/ml) 0.2–0.3 ml per lesion 2. Potent topical corticosteroids with/without occlusion, e.g., betamethasone diproprionate 0.05%, clobetasol propionate 0.05%, halobetasol propionate 0.05%
Erythema elevatum diutinum	Sulfones: PO 50–300 mg/day

Abbreviations: HIV, human immunodeficiency virus; PO, by mouth; IV, intravenous; tid, three times a day; bid, twice a day; qid, four times a day; CDC, Centers for Disease Control and Prevention; IM, intramuscular; sub q, subcutaneous; IFN, interferon; AIDS, acquired immunodeficiency syndrome.

there is no associated eosinophilia, and histopathology reveals a nonspecific perivascular inflammation.

Drug Hypersensitivity Dermatoses

An increased incidence of drug hypersensitivity reactions has been noted in the HIV population. The spectrum of cutaneous disease runs from the more common generalized morbilliform eruptions to the more severe Stevens-Johnson syndrome and toxic epidermal necrolysis. Trimethoprim-sulfamethoxazole (Bactrim, Septra) and ampicillin–clavulanic acid (Augmentin) are the most common drug antigens responsible for these reactions.

Miscellaneous Associations

Other disorders noted with increased frequency that may serve as cutaneous markers of underlying retroviral infection include:

1. Autoimmune phenomena. An increased incidence of both vitiligo and the sicca syndrome has been reported.
2. Hair abnormalities. Diffuse thinning of scalp and body hair (telogen effluvium) may occur as well as premature hair graying and elongation of the eyelashes (''acquired trichomegaly'').
3. Photosensitive disorders. An increased propensity for photosensitivity as well as porphyria cutanea tarda manifesting as bullae in sun-exposed areas and facial temporal hirsutism have been reported. Retrovirus-induced impairment of porphyrin metabolism has been hypothesized to be the cause.
4. Granuloma annulare. Both localized and generalized forms of granuloma annulare have been described. In HIV infection, lesions present as dermal papules and plaques. Atypical forms mimicking AIDS papular hypersensitivity dermatoses have been reported.
5. Erythema elevatum diutinum. Infiltrative inflammatory plaques, 3 to 5 cm, on the acral extremities, showing characteristic inflammatory neutrophilic changes, may occur. Distinction from granulomatous infectious processes is important.

TREATMENT

Many treatment options are available for the wide spectrum of disorders presented in this review. Although noninclusive, Table 27–3 presents some of the treatment options found in both the dermatologic literature and the author's experience.

PITFALLS AND PROBLEMS

Patients who are infected with HIV may suffer from profound immunocompromise, so that the response to infectious agents may be abnormal and the classic appearance of cutaneous disease states may not be observed.[5] For example, nonhealing ulcers may be caused by a number of infectious agents, varying from infections with deep fungi to atypical *Mycobacteria.* Neoplastic processes also need to be excluded. Appropriate biopsies and cultures must be performed to render an accurate diagnosis.

Nondescript papules may be found in disseminated histoplasmosis, cryptococcosis, and acid-fast infection as well as in botryomycosis and pneumocystosis. Diffuse erythematous plaques resembling cellulitis may be found in bacterial infections, as well as in disorders caused by systemic fungi, *Nocardia*, and atypical mycobacteria.

Opportunistic infections in patients with immunocompromise may have clinical features similar to more common, less serious diseases, leading to diagnostic errors. For example, cutaneous histoplasmosis may resemble psoriasis and cryptococcosis. *Penicillium* infection may mimic molluscum contagiosum. Thus, in managing HIV-infected patients, the clinician should always be alert that a skin lesion could be a manifestation of an infectious process and appropriate biopsies with special stains and cultures should be performed.

REFERRAL AND CONSULTATION GUIDELINES

When the physician is unable to recognize or come to a reasonable differential diagnostic approach to a given skin lesion or cutaneous eruption, or if conventional therapy has failed for a suspected clinical cutaneous problem, referral is indicated.

REFERENCES

1. Sadick NS, Pahwa S: Cutaneous diseases associated with human immunodeficiency virus infection. Curr Opin Infect Dis 1992; 5:673–682.
2. Cowley NC, Staughton RCD: Human immunodeficiency virus–related skin disease. Curr Opin Infect Dis 1991; 4:659–666.
3. Smith KJ, Skelton RCD, Yaeger J, et al: Cutaneous findings in HIV-1 positive patients: A 42-month prospective study. J Am Acad Dermatol 1994; 31:746–754.
4. Dover JS, Johnson RA: Cutaneous manifestations of human immunodeficiency virus infection. Arch Dermatol 1991; Part I, 127:1382–1391; Part II, 127:1549–1558.
5. Cockerell CJ: Cutaneous clue to HIV infections: Diagnosis and treatment. Semin Dermatol 1994; 13:275–285.

CHAPTER 28

Impetigo

Lawrence F. Eichenfield and Sheila Fallon Friedlander

CLINICAL APPEARANCE

Definition

Impetigo is a common superficial bacterial infection of the skin caused by group A beta-hemolytic streptococcus (GABHS) or *Staphylococcus aureus,* alone or in combination. It most commonly occurs in infants and young children and is highly infectious. Impetigo primarily occurs on intact skin, but it can develop in sites of skin trauma such as insect bites, scratched varicella, or eczema lesions. Impetigo may be seen in isolated cases or in epidemics, especially in conditions of crowding and poor hygiene. There is an increased prevalence in summer and autumn.

Typical Lesions and Symptoms

Impetigo is classified as bullous or nonbullous. Nonbullous impetigo is much more common. Although group A streptococcus was once the cause of most nonbullous cases of impetigo, it now appears that *S. aureus* is the predominant pathogen in both forms.

Nonbullous Impetigo

Nonbullous impetigo presents with thin, erythematous vesicles or pustules that rupture easily. The purulent material often dries with a honey-colored crust (see Fig. 28–1 on Color Plate 10). Soft débridement of the crust reveals shallow, pink-red erosions that soon recrust. Lesions may be present anywhere, although exposed surfaces including the face, neck, and extremities are most common. Satellite lesions often appear at the periphery of the initial lesion. Perinasal and perioral lesions are very common, and these often occur after upper respiratory tract infections. Autoinoculation contributes to the spread of lesions. Lesions generally heal without scarring or atrophy owing to the superficial location of the infection.

Bullous Impetigo

Bullous impetigo appears as small vesicles that evolve into annular bullae (see Fig. 28–2 on Color Plate 10). Lesions may be up to 1 cm or more in diameter. The lesions are initially clear in color, become more purulent, and may display a "fluid level." They have a shallow, moist, erythematous base on rupture, which dries to form a lacquered or varnished appearance. Lesions may dry with annular crust.

Atypical Presentations or Alternative Forms

Impetigo is generally asymptomatic and localized. It is usually nonpainful, only occasionally pruritic, and generally does not have constitutional symptoms. Regional adenopathy is usually present, and leukocytosis may be found in approximately half of patients. Generalized skin involvement may be seen with varicella, with large denuded areas extending from varicella lesions. This condition is often termed *bullous varicella.* Extensive impetigo may also be seen in immunosuppressed patients and in those with secondarily infected bug bites or dermatitis. Neonates with bullous impetigo may have lesions localized to the inguinal area and lower trunk or generalized lesions.

DESCRIPTION OF DISEASE

Impetigo is more common in children than in adults and is the most common bacterial skin infection in infants and young children, especially of preschool age. It is estimated that impetigo accounts for 10% of skin disorders in pediatric clinics.[1] There is no sex predilection.

Impetigo is caused by group A beta-hemolytic streptococcus (GABHS) and *S. aureus* bacteria. Lesions begin after exposure to bacteria, with a latency of 10 to 20 days. Streptococcal infections generally occur in previously traumatized skin, but *S. aureus* is capable of infecting intact epithelium. Streptococcal impetigo may induce lesions after transfer of bacteria from infected skin to normal skin.

Staphylococcal organisms will often colonize nasal passages, with subsequent spread to normal skin and development of impetigo. The axillae, perineum, and toe webs may also be colonized. Impetigo may spread rapidly and is highly infectious to individuals with intimate contact with open sores. Spontaneous resolution may occur in weeks, although treatment is warranted to minimize spread and risks of secondary complications.

Classic bullous impetigo is caused by *S. aureus* capable of producing an exfoliative toxin, most commonly phage group II. Nonbullous impetigo was thought to be due only to GABHS, with cultures showing *S. aureus* thought to be secondary contaminant. It is now clear that *S. aureus* is a primary pathogen of nonbullous and bullous impetigo and appears to be the predominant causative agent of impetigo.[2, 3]

Diagnosis may be confirmed by bacterial culture, with evaluation of sensitivity profile. Gram's stained smears reveal gram-positive cocci. Antistreptolysin O titers are generally not elevated, but anti-DNAse B and antihyaluronidase are increased significantly.[4]

TREATMENT

Standard Treatment

Standard treatment of impetigo is based on elimination of the bacterial pathogen. Systemic or topical antibiotics with coverage against *S. aureus* and GABHS are indicated.

1. First-line oral agents are semisynthetic penicillinase-resistant penicillins such as cloxacillin or dicloxacillin. However, oral suspensions of these agents are generally not well tolerated by young children owing to unpleasant taste, and cephalosporins such as cephalexin may be used. A 10-day course is standard.

2. Gentle débridement of crusts and debris with warm water soaks is appropriate.

3. Local antibacterial preparations, such as bacitracin or mupirocin ointment, may be useful in treating impetigo and in limiting person-to-person spread. It has been documented that 2% mupirocin ointment applied three times a day for 10 days is as safe and effective as oral erythromycin for treatment of localized impetigo.[5]

4. Recurrent disease occasionally results from chronic colonization in the nares or groin with *S. aureus*. Topical mupirocin applied twice daily to the nares for 5 days has been shown to eliminate the carrier state in more than 90% of patients for 6 months or more.[6]

Age Considerations

Dosages of antibiotics for infants and children should be based on weight.

ALTERNATIVE THERAPEUTIC OPTIONS

1. The prevalence of penicillin resistance of *S. aureus* bacteria has increased greatly, rendering penicillin an inadequate medication. (Penicillin should not be used owing to a high percentage of resistance in *S. aureus* spp.)[3]

2. Erythromycin resistance is variable by geographic location. Staphylococcus resistance to erythromycin is fairly common and appears to be increasing, although there is significant regional variation.[7, 8]

3. Other systemic antibiotics including amoxicillin plus clavulanic acid, cefaclor, and the newer macrolides azithromycin and clarithromycin may be used.

PITFALLS AND PROBLEMS

Impetigo may complicate atopic dermatitis (eczema) in children, adolescents, and adults (see Fig. 28–3 on Color Plate 10). Bacterial colonization with *S. aureus* is very common in patients with atopic dermatitis, seen in greater than 90% of skin sites with active eczematous lesions and in greater than 70% of nondermatitic skin.[9] *S. aureus*–colonized skin may look "impetigo-like," with honey-colored crusting, or may appear like typical dermatitis with erythema and scaling without vesicles, pustules, or crust. Similar colonization and infection may occur with other dermatoses, including ichthyosiform conditions, Darier's disease, and irritant contact dermatitis. It is thought that colonization of the skin with forms of *S. aureus* capable of elaborating toxins may lead to refractory and persistent erythema in some children with atopic dermatitis. This may be the result of such *S. aureus* toxins functioning as "superantigens" that are capable of stimulating excessive inflammatory reactions via cytokine stimulation.

Secondary complications from impetigo are uncommon but of great medical significance. Acute glomerulonephritis is caused by nephritogenic strains of streptococcus (M-T serotypes 2, 49, 55, 57, 60). There is no evidence that treatment of impetigo prevents nephritis, although prompt treatment of these strains is appropriate to minimize the risk to others. Cellulitis, bacteremia, septic arthritis, and osteomyelitis are rare complications of impetigo. Toxin-producing staphylococcal and streptococcal bacteria may colonize the skin or penetrate the epidermal barrier through superficial impetigo infection, with subsequent local toxin production (seen in bullous impetigo) or systemic toxin spread, causing staphylococcal scalded skin syndrome, toxic shock syndrome, or necrotizing fasciitis.

REFERRAL/CONSULTATION GUIDELINES

Failure of response to appropriate antistaphylococcal/antistreptococcal antibiotics warrants reappraisal of the diagnosis. Although the diagnosis of impetigo is generally straightforward, a variety of conditions may resemble impetigo in its different stages. These include early varicella vesicles, herpes simplex virus vesicles and crusts, chronic dermatitis (seborrheic, atopic, contact, and phototoxic), and vesiculobullous bug bite hypersensitivity reactions. Older impetigo lesions may mimic fungal infection, as active erythema, scale, and crust may develop at the border of the lesions with central clearing. Impetigo secondarily complicating primary skin disease may require treatment of the underlying disease process.

REFERENCES

1. Darmstadt GL, Lane AT: Impetigo: An overview. Pediatr Dermatol 1994; 11(4):293–303.
2. Barton LL, Friedman AD: Impetigo: A reassessment of etiology and therapy. Pediatr Dermatol 1987; 4(3):185–188.
3. Demidovich CW, Wittler RR, Ruff ME, et al: Impetigo. Current etiology and comparison of penicillin, erythromycin, and cephalexin therapies. Am J Dis Child 1990; 144:1313–1315.
4. Habif TP (ed): Bacterial Infections, Clinical Dermatology. St. Louis: Mosby–Year Book, 1996; p 241.
5. Barton LL, Freidman AD, Sharkey AM, et al: Impetigo contagiosa III. Comparative efficacy of oral erythromycin, and topical mupirocin. Pediatr Dermatol 1989; 6:134–138.
6. Doebbeling BN, Reagan DR, Pfaller MA, et al: Long-term efficacy of intranasal mupirocin ointment. A prospective cohort study of *Staphylococcus aureus* carriage. Arch Intern Med 1994; 154:1505–1508.
7. Misko ML, Terracina JR, Diven DG: The frequency of erythromycin-resistant *Staphylococcus aureus* in impetiginized dermatoses. Pediatr Dermatol 1995; 12(1):12–15.
8. Seppala J, Nissinen A, Jarvinen H, et al: Resistance to erythromycin in group A streptococci. N Engl J Med 1992; 326:292–297.
9. Hoeger PH, Lenz W, Boutonnier A, et al: Staphylococcal skin colonization in children with atopic dermatitis: Prevalence, persistence, and transmission of toxigenic and non-toxigenic strains. J Infect Dis 1992; 165:1064–1068.

CHAPTER 29

Inflamed Epidermal Cysts

Daniel B. Dubin

CLINICAL APPEARANCE

Definition

Epidermal cysts are lined by keratinocytes that proliferate, terminally differentiate, and directionally deposit keratin-rich material into the cyst core, which is topologically equivalent to the external cutaneous surface. However, unlike surface epidermis that innocuously sheds its outer layer of dead keratinocytes, the cyst sac traps and accumulates keratinaceous material. Either with or without secondary infection, cyst rupture into the dermis triggers an exuberant foreign body inflammatory reaction that prompts afflicted patients to seek treatment.

Usual Appearance

Epidermal inclusion cysts (EICs) account for about 80% of all cutaneous cysts. Inflamed EICs most commonly present over the head, neck, upper trunk, and genitalia as tender, erythematous, firm to fluctuant dermal nodules, often bearing a small overlying punctum. Infected cysts tend to be larger, more erythematous, and more painful than those that are sterile.

Less Common Forms

Trichilemmal (pilar) cysts account for approximately 5 to 15% of skin cysts and occur predominantly over the scalp. Uncommonly, these cysts can rupture and become inflamed. Traumatic disruption of trichilemmal cysts can trigger an epidermal proliferative response that grossly appears as a progressively enlarging lobular mass that may ulcerate and resemble a squamous cell carcinoma.

Trauma-induced cysts over non–hair-bearing areas such as the palms and soles may also rupture and become inflamed. Pilonidal as well as embryonic dermoid, branchial cleft, preauricular, and thyroglossal duct cysts can all present as inflamed and infected keratinized cysts.

Dermoid cysts appear at embryologic fusion lines, such as the nasal root, lateral eyebrow, scalp, submental area, anterior neck, chest wall, and anogenital areas. Many have sinus tracts from which hairs may protrude.

Branchial cleft cysts most often present in the upper neck over the anterior border of the sternocleidomastoid muscle. Thyroglossal duct cysts appear as midline neck masses, usually over the hyoid bone, but they may be as inferior as the suprasternal notch. Infected thyroglossal duct cysts may drain directly to the skin, into the pharynx, or through a patent foramen cecum onto the base of the tongue, thus eliciting a foul taste.

Preauricular cysts and sinuses arise from imperfect fusion of the first and second branchial arches and may be associated with other developmental abnormalities. Pilonidal cysts present over the superior natal cleft. Steatocystoma multiplex manifests as small rubbery dermal nodules over the upper trunk and proximal extremities that occasionally become inflamed.

Ruptured urachal (umbilicus), omphalomesenteric (umbilicus), bronchial (chest wall), Bartholin's (vulvar), and ganglion cysts (over joints) can mimic inflamed epidermal cysts.

DESCRIPTION OF DISEASE

Epidemiology

Typical EICs usually appear in young and middle-aged adults. Pilar (trichilemmal) cysts are more common in women of middle age and may be inherited in an autosomal dominant fashion. Gardner's syndrome and basal cell nevus syndrome are autosomal dominant disorders that predispose to the development of epidermal cysts, particularly over the extremities. Embryologic and pilonidal cysts often present in childhood or early adulthood. The cysts of steatocystoma multiplex typically appear in young adults and are often inherited in an autosomal dominant pattern. Preauricular cysts may occur as an autosomal dominant trait.

Natural History

Inflamed sterile epidermal cysts are usually less than 1 cm, painful erythematous nodules that resolve in 1 to 3 weeks without treatment; however, without either complete removal or destruction of the cyst wall, they may recur. By contrast, infected epidermal cysts often require antibiotics and surgical attention. Rupture of trichilemmal cysts induces a proliferative but benign and self-limited response; excision is often desired for cosmetic concerns. Chronically infected pilonidal and embryologic cysts often merit surgical intervention.

Pathology

Typical epidermal cysts are lined by squamous epithelium whose keratinization is akin to that of the interfollicular and distal follicular epidermis. However, the keratinization of pilar (trichilemmal) cysts mimics that of the follicular external root sheath (lower portion of the follicle); therefore, the contents of pilar cysts are often not as cheesy and fetid as that of typical epidermal cysts. The histopathology of proliferating trichilemmal cysts mimics that of squamous cell carcinoma. Steatocystoma multiplex cysts are lined by squamous epithelium but are filled mostly with oily sebum, not keratinaceous debris. Dermoid cyst walls may contain appendageal structures such as follicles and sweat glands. Branchial cleft cysts often have associated lymphoid tissue. Thyroglossal duct cysts may include rests of thyroid tissue. The histopathology of all inflamed cysts will demonstrate various degrees of inflammatory foreign body reaction and scarring. Rarely, frank squamous cell carcinoma may arise from the wall of a chronically inflamed cyst.

Etiology/Pathogenesis

Occlusion of pilosebaceous units, traumatic implantation of keratinocytes into the dermis, and trapping of either differentiated or pluripotential epithelium along embryonal fusion planes or morphogenetic tracts result in the formation of dermal cysts lined by keratinizing stratified squamous epithelium. Occluded follicles account for the majority of epidermal cysts. Acne vulgaris can predispose to follicular occlusion, disruption, and infection—all of which contribute to the pathogenesis of inflamed epidermal cysts. Pilonidal cysts may be congenital or may arise as a consequence of chronic trauma to appendageal structures in the sacrococcygeal area. The etiology of cysts that arise in conjunction with Gardner's syndrome, basal cell nevus syndrome, and steatocystoma multiplex is not known. Any of these cysts can become secondarily infected via communication with the external environment or traumatic manipulation. One study of infected EICs demonstrated 44% aerobic, 30% anaerobic, and 26% mixed infections. Overall, *Staphylococcus aureus* was the most common etiologic pathogen. Group A streptococci, *Escherichia coli, Peptostreptococci,* and *Bacteroides* spp. were other commonly isolated pathogens.

TREATMENT

Inflamed Epidermal Cysts

Treatment of uninfected, yet inflamed, epidermal cysts requires no specific therapy. However, injection of 2.5 to 5.0 mg/ml of triamcinolone acetonide (diluted in either 1% lidocaine or normal saline solution) into the inflamed surrounding dermis in an amount sufficient to slightly distend the lesion can hasten resolution. Injection of large amounts of triamcinolone can result in residual, usually temporary, atrophic scarring. The cyst can be electively excised once the inflammation has resolved; however, it is reasonable to wait for recurrence before recommending surgery, as many inflamed cysts do not recur.

Proliferating Trichilemmal Cysts

Proliferating trichilemmal cysts require excision with a margin of normal tissue to prevent recurrence.

Infected Typical Epidermal or Trichilemmal Cysts

Management of infected cysts entails drainage of purulent material. Especially over the face, where scarring is of particular cosmetic concern, one should attempt to withdraw the infected cyst contents through a 16- or 14-gauge needle. If drainage through a large-bore needle proves inadequate, the area should be locally anesthetized, incised with a no. 11 blade, and drained. This incision should be oriented along natural relaxed tension lines to minimize subsequent scarring. The tips of a small hemostat are useful for disrupting loculations and allowing for optimal drainage of the infected contents, which should be sent for Gram's stain and bacteriologic culture.

Some surgeons recommend packing the evacuated cyst with iodophor-impregnated gauze that is gradually removed over the 2- to 3-week healing period to ensure continued drainage. Others contend that this wick serves as a foreign body that impedes wound healing, exacerbates scarring, and may serve as a nidus for secondary infection. Proper incision and drainage followed by warm soaks three or four times daily often provide adequate treatment. However, infected cysts associated with significant cellulitis or constitutional symptoms, occurring in immunocompromised patients, or not responding to drainage and warm soaks require systemic antibiotics.

Amoxicillin-clavulanate, ampicillin-sulbactam, cefoxitin, or clindamycin plus either a fluoroquinolone or gentamicin will provide adequate empirical coverage against most of the anaerobic and aerobic organisms typically cultured from infected cysts. Infected perirectal cysts warrant empirical coverage against *Pseudomonas* spp. with either gentamicin or a fluoroquinolone. Gram's stain, culture, and clinical response permit specific honing of the antibiotic regimen, which should be continued for 10 to 14 days. Most surgeons recommend waiting 4 to 6 weeks before attempting to excise an infected cyst in order to reduce the risk of wound infection, dehiscence, and scarring. However, one recent small study claims that immediate surgical excision and irrigation result in faster resolution, less pain, and a more acceptable scar.

Infected Embryologic and Pilonidal Cysts

Generally, treatment of these cysts requires systemic antibiotics and consultation with a skilled surgeon. Chronically infected dermoid cysts often extend deep to periosteum and require complete excision to prevent recurrence. Infected frontal, temporoparietal, and occipital scalp dermoid cysts may have intracranial extensions that require neurosurgical intervention. Infected pilonidal cysts often communicate with numerous deep sinus tracts that must be completely cleaned, externalized, or removed in order to effect a cure. Because of their anatomic location, branchial cleft and thyroglossal duct cysts are optimally managed by excision with the patient under general anesthesia. It is important to ascertain by ultrasound or radionuclide scan that the thyroglossal duct cyst does not represent the patient's only source of thyroid tissue before excision. Preauricular cysts and sinuses may blend with the periosteum of the external auditory canal and, thus, require complete visualization before excision.

BIBLIOGRAPHY

Atherton DJ: Naevi and other developmental defects. *In* Champion RH, Burton JL, Ebling FJG (eds): Rook/Wilkinson/Ebling Textbook of Dermatology. 5th ed. Oxford: Blackwell Scientific, 1992; pp 509–516.

Bennett RG: Cystic lesions. *In* Fundamentals of Cutaneous Surgery. St. Louis: CV Mosby, 1988; pp 734–749.

Brook I: Microbiology of infected epidermal cysts. Arch Dermatol 1989;125:1658–1661.

Kitamura K, Takahashi T, Yamaguchi T, et al: Primary resection of infectious epidermal cyst. J Am Coll Surg 1994;179:607.

CHAPTER 30

Leg Ulcers

Theodora Mauro

CLINICAL APPEARANCE

Definition

An ulcer is a cutaneous wound that destroys all of the epidermis and at least part of the dermis. All ulcers discussed in this chapter are chronic ulcers, that is, ulcers that persist for longer than 6 weeks. Most leg ulcers occur in elderly populations, especially ulcers due to venous insufficiency, arterial insufficiency, or neuropathy, the three most common causes of leg ulceration in industrialized countries. Signs and symptoms vary according to the etiology of the ulcer (see later in this chapter).

Typical Lesions and Symptoms

Venous Insufficiency

Venous stasis ulcers cause approximately 70 to 80% of the chronic leg ulcers in industrialized countries. Ulcers due to venous insufficiency are most commonly located over the ankle malleoli, tend to be painful, and are often associated with leg edema (see Fig. 30–1 on Color Plate 11). A history of venous thromboses can often be elicited. These ulcers have shallow, irregular borders and are often surrounded by skin changes characteristics of venous insufficiency: venous varicosities, deposition of hemosiderin, and induration and fibrosis of the dermis (lipodermatosclerosis).[1] Unless there is coexistent arterial insufficiency, arterial pulses are palpable.

Arterial Insufficiency

These ulcers make up 5 to 10% of ulcers in industrialized societies. Patients with ischemic heart disease, cerebral vascular disease, hypertension, or diabetes are at increased risk to develop this type of ulcer. Unlike ulcers due to venous insufficiency, ulcers due to arterial insufficiency tend to be located in distal locations, such as the toes. These ulcers have a ''punched-out'' appearance and are often quite painful. As opposed to venous insufficiency ulcers, whose pain is relieved by leg elevations, pain due to arterial insufficiency is relieved by placing the leg lower than the heart. Foot pulses are usually absent. These ulcers are best treated by a vascular surgeon.

Neuropathic

These ulcers are found in patients, most commonly diabetics, with diminished sensation in their feet. Resulting from repetitive, often minor trauma, the ulcers are found over the heels, toes, or plantar areas of these patients. Typically, the ulcer extends beyond the area of epidermis that is damaged and may extend into joint spaces or underlying bone. Ulcer infection occurs commonly and is often polymicrobial.

Infections

Although ulcers due to infection constitute only a small minority of ulcers in the United States, their effects can be devastating. Thus, prompt recognition and treatment of these ulcers are essential.

ECTHYMA GANGRENOSUM

This lesion originates as a vesicopustule that becomes hemorrhagic and rapidly develops into a punched-out ulcer with necrotic edges. The ulcer can enlarge rapidly, is usually caused by *Pseudomonas* (although other gram-negative organisms such as *Klebsiella* can also be responsible), and is often associated with septicemia. Ecthyma gangrenosum is usually seen in immunocompromised or debilitated patients.

GROUP A STREPTOCOCCI

This infection, popularized in the lay press as ''flesh-eating bacteria,'' has reemerged recently after decades when its incidence was rare. Unlike ecthyma gangrenosum, this infection can occur in healthy individuals. Thought to be precipitated by minor trauma, this suppurative ulcer may progress within hours to myositis, necrotizing fasciitis, and multiorgan system failure.[2] Prompt treatment with both antibiotics and tissue débridement is necessary.

Other Types of Leg Ulcers

VASCULITIC ULCERS

Leg ulcers can be caused by vasculitis of either large or small vessels. Vasculitic leg ulcers are caused most commonly by rheumatoid arthritis[3] but are also seen in systemic lupus erythematosus, scleroderma, and the other entities listed in Table 30–1. Depending on the size of the blood vessel involved, these ulcers present as digital infarcts, well-defined punched-out ulcers, geographic ulcers, or peripheral gangrene. The ulcers tend to be extremely painful.

PYODERMA GANGRENOSUM

Pyoderma gangrenosum presents as a purple nodule that enlarges over days, with necrosis and ulceration at the center. An overhanging border of the ulcer is characteristic, as is a violaceous hue to the rim of the ulcer. This condition is associated with a variety of conditions, most commonly inflammatory bowel disease, hematologic malignancies, and chronic active hepatitis. The lesion occurs at sites of trauma (pathergy), so débridement of the ulcer is not advised until the patient has begun immunosuppressive therapy.

Uncommon causes of leg ulcers are listed in Table 30–1.

DESCRIPTION OF DISEASE

Pathogenesis

The most common types of leg ulcers are not caused by pathology of the skin per se, but rather by alterations in the vessels or nerves that supply the skin.

Thus, venous insufficiency is associated with incom-

TABLE 30–1

Causes of Leg Ulcers

Vascular	Embolic	Infectious
Venous insufficiency	Subacute bacterial endocarditis	Bacterial
Arterial insufficiency	Meningococcemia	Group A streptococcus
Raynaud's disease	**Neurologic**	Pseudomonas
Malignant atrophic papulosis (Degos' disease)	Peripheral neuropathy	Klebsiella
Buerger's disease	Tabes dorsalis	Mycobacteria
Antiphospholipid syndrome	**Metabolic**	Anthrax
Vasculitic	Diabetes mellitus	Fungal
Rheumatoid arthritis	Prolidase deficiency	''Madura foot'' (actinomycetes, eumycetes)
Systemic lupus erythematosus	Calciphylaxis	Sporotrichosis
Scleroderma	Gout	Blastomycosis
Dermatomyositis	**Miscellaneous**	Histoplasmosis
Periarteritis nodosa	Sickle cell anemia	Other
Livedoid vasculitis	Cryoglobulinemia	Tertiary syphilis
	Thalassemia	Yaws
	Pyoderma gangrenosum	Leishmaniasis
	Sarcoidosis	Neoplastic
	Epidermolysis bullosa	Squamous cell carcinoma
	Lichen planus	Basal cell carcinoma
	Necrobioses lipoidica diabeticorum	Kaposi's sarcoma
		Cutaneous lymphoma
		Metastatic tumors

petent venous valves of the superficial or deep venous system, leading to venous hypertension, edema, leakage of fibrin, and formation of perivascular fibrin cuffs, which are thought to cause the ulcers by acting either as a barrier to oxygen diffusion or as a sink for growth factors needed for tissue repair.

In contrast, ulcers resulting from arterial insufficiency are associated with pathologic changes of arteriosclerosis: occlusion of arteries by deposition of lipids within arterial vessel walls. Patients suffering from arterial insufficiency in other organ systems are more likely to acquire these ulcers, as are patients who smoke cigarettes or who suffer from hypertension or diabetes.

Ulcers caused by vasculitis will often demonstrate vasculitis of the small or large vessels supplying the skin. Because occlusion of a medium or large artery causes necrosis of the entire cutaneous area that it supplies, ulcers due to these etiologies are often large (see Fig. 30–2 on Color Plate 11) with jagged edges (''geographic purpura'').

Laboratory Tests

Since most patients suffer from ulcers due to arterial or venous insufficiency, noninvasive vascular studies are often valuable in aiding diagnosis. An ankle-brachial index (ABI), which compares the systolic pressure in arm and ankle, can diagnose arterial insufficiency. Values less than 0.7 correlate with impaired arterial flow, although these values may be falsely elevated in diabetics. Studies that assess venous value competence include photoplethysmography, air plethysmography, light rheography, and duplex ultrasound imaging.

Other laboratory tests should be ordered as warranted by the physical examination. Hematologic causes (see Table 30–1) can be detected with the appropriate screens, as can ulcers caused by some vasculitic processes such as systemic lupus erythematosus or rheumatoid arthritis. The edge of a longstanding ulcer should be biopsied to rule out neoplastic causes. A punch or wedge biopsy can be helpful in diagnosing lesions caused by vasculitis or infection.

Finally, x-rays or bone scans of the bones underlying chronic ulcers should be examined to rule out osteomyelitis.

TREATMENT

General Considerations

Patients suffering from systemic diseases such as diabetic mellitus or malnutrition will heal their wounds poorly, regardless of ulcer etiology. These underlying conditions, some medications, and other systemic diseases that impair wound healing (Table 30–2) should be treated or modified in addition to any therapy for a specific type of ulcer. In addition, any infection of the ulcer should be treated with appropriate antibiotics. Advantages and disadvantages of various topical dressings are listed in Table 30–3.

Dressings

Because wounds heal more quickly in a moist environment, traditional therapies such as wet-to-dry dressings have been supplanted by occlusive wound dressings, such as hydrocolloids.[4] These dressings enhance granulation tissue, promote débridement, and improve rates of epithelialization.[5]

Application Before Dressing

Although dressings may be applied to ulcers with fibrinous bases, ulcers with necrotic material should be debrided, either by sharp débridement, using a scalpel or curette, or chemical débridement placed under the dressing (see Table 30–3). Before the dressings are applied, the wound should be flushed with normal saline solution. The wound edges should be dry. If wound edges are macerated, absorptive, nonadherent dressings such as alginates or foam are the best choice.

Choice of Dressing

Several factors are important in choosing an appropriate wound dressing (see Table 30–3). Hydrocolloids and hydrogels are similar in their uses: both are suitable for shallow ulcerations with mild to moderate drainage. For deeper ulcers, or ulcers with greater exudate, calcium alginates or foam dressings are more appropriate.

TABLE 30–2

Conditions That Impair Healing

Diabetes mellitus	Medications
Nutritional deficiencies	Glucocorticoids
Protein	Cytotoxic drugs
Vitamin C	Nonsteroidal anti-inflammatory drugs
Zinc	
Iron	
Malignancies	

TABLE 30-3
Wound Dressings

Types	Uses	Comments
Hydrocolloids (DuoDerm, Tegasorb, Comfeel)	Uninfected wounds with mild/moderate fibrin and moderate drainage	Initially, change frequently (3–4 days) to prevent wound fluid leakage and maceration
Hydrogels (Vigilon)	Painful ulcers; moderate drainage	More expensive than hydrocolloids; nonadherent
Calcium Alginates (Sorbsan, Kaltostat)	Ulcers with moderate/heavy drainage	Can be shaped into wound cavity; good for deep ulcers
Foam Dressings (Allevyn, Hydrasorb)	Ulcers with heavy drainage; ulcers that require padding or protection	May remove healing epithelium if drainage dries and adheres dressing to wound
Wound Cleaners		
Collagenase (Santyl)	Ulcers with fibrin	Inactivated by metal salts, hexachlorophene, or acidic solutions
Cadexomer Iodine (Iodosorb)	Ulcers with moderate amounts of necrotic material	Will damage living tissue; stop use when necrotic debris is removed

Application of Dressing

Hydrocolloids and foam dressings should be cut so the dressings cover an area about 1 inch around the ulcer. Hydrogels and alginates can be cut to fit directly in the wound. Hydrocolloids generally adhere to the wound edges; the other dressings do not and must be secured. Alginates require an absorptive dressing to be placed over them.

Venous Insufficiency

Relief of venous hypertension and leg edema is the cornerstone of treating this condition. Although bedrest and leg elevation will theoretically alleviate venous hypertension, in practice some form of leg compression is usually required. Leg compression can be achieved by one of several methods. The venerable Unna boot, developed in 1896, is a semipermeable zinc oxide paste bandage that is usually applied weekly. Compressive wraps or support stockings are more convenient methods of applying pressure to the leg. Finally, compression pumps can be used in patients who cannot tolerate compressive dressings. If lymphedema is absent, 30 to 40 mmHg compression should be applied. Since many patients with venous insufficiency have coexistent impairment of arterial blood flow, care must be taken not to apply compression greater than the ankle diastolic pressure (which can be measured using the ABI). Most wound care dressings can be used under these compressive wraps, although if there is a large amount of wound exudate, the dressings and compressive wraps may need to be changed more frequently than once each week. Stanozolol, pentoxifylline, and aspirin have also been reported to aid healing in these types of ulcers. Application of cultured keratinocyte autografts or allografts can speed healing of recalcitrant ulcers.

Neuropathic Ulcers

Relief of external pressure and treatment of infection are the most effective measures to treat neuropathic ulcers. The ulcers heal most effectively when all weight-bearing activities on the affected area are avoided, using crutches, a wheelchair, or total-contact casting. After the ulcer heals, the patient must be carefully managed to prevent a recurrence. Custom-fitted shoes and the service of a podiatrist are valuable in this regard. The physician should make a special effort to educate the patient to immediately report even small breaks in the skin.

Vasculitic Ulcers

Systemic suppression of the rheumatologic disease causing the ulcers is required to treat these lesions. The mainstay of treatment remains corticosteroids, although other agents such as azathioprine, methotrexate, cyclophosphamide, dapsone, and cyclosporine have been used, usually as steroid-sparing agents. Treatment of vasculitic ulcers can be difficult, as the medications that suppress the underlying conditions can themselves retard wound healing. Application of hydrogel wound dressings often aids healing and decreases pain.

Other Types of Ulcers

Ulcers due to infectious etiologies must be treated with appropriate antibiotics. In addition, ulcers caused by group A streptococci must be thoroughly débrided immediately after the diagnosis is made.

Pyoderma gangrenosum is usually treated with corticosteroids. These can be injected intralesionally, given as oral prednisone (usual dose 60 to 100 mg a day for adults), or in very severe cases, given as intravenous pulse therapy. Dapsone, azathioprine, or cyclosporine can be used as steroid-sparing agents or as the sole therapeutic agent (especially cyclosporine).

Ulcers in patients with antiphospholipid (formerly known as lupus anticoagulant) antibody may require anticoagulation with warfarin or heparin.

PITFALLS AND PROBLEMS

It is important to remember that a nonhealing ulcer may have more than one cause. For example, venous insufficiency may be complicated by compromised arterial blood flow in 10% of patients. Neuropathic ulcers are often worsened by an accompanying soft tissue infection or underlying osteomyelitis. A patient with venous insufficiency may also develop vasculitis. Thus, additional investigation may be warranted if the ulcer does not improve after 1 to 2 months of treatment. If vascular studies have not been performed, arterial blood supply should be assessed. The ulcer edge should be biopsied to rule out a neoplastic process or to diagnose vasculitis, panniculitis, or pyoderma gangrenosum. If clinically appropriate, radiographic studies to rule out osteomyelitis or hematologic tests to diagnose rheumatologic disease should be performed. All ulcers are colonized with bacteria, so culture of tissue biopsied from the ulcer edge may yield a more accurate picture of possible bacterial fungal, or mycobacterial infection.

Because maceration of the periulcer skin can occur in ulcers with a great deal of drainage, care must be taken to change wound dressings at appropriate intervals. In addition, growth of anaerobic bacteria in the wound fluid may cause an unpleasant odor. This colonization can be controlled with topical metronidazole. Finally, these dressings should not be applied to frankly infected wounds.

REFERRAL GUIDELINES

A patient with an ulcer suspected to be ecthyma gangrenosum or necrotizing fasciitis should be examined by a dermatologist, surgeon, or infectious disease specialist immediately. Patients with significant arterial disease should be referred to a vascular surgeon.

An ulcer suspected to be caused by neoplastic or vasculitic processes should be referred if a biopsy is warranted, as should an ulcer suspected of being pyoderma gangrenosum.

REFERENCES

1. Phillips TJ, Dover JS: Leg ulcers. J Am Acad Dermatol 1991; 25:965–987.
2. Wolf JE, Rabinovitz LG: Streptococcal toxic shock–like syndrome. Arch Dermatol 1995; 131(1):73–77.
3. McRorie ER, Jobanputra P, Ruckley CV, Nuki G: Leg ulceration in rheumatoid arthritis. Br J Rheumatol 1994; 33(11):1078–1084.
4. Helfman T, Ovington L, Falanga V: Occlusive dressings and wound healing. Clin Dermatol 1994; 12(1):121–127.
5. Kirsner RS, Eaglstein WH: The wound healing process. Dermatol Clin 1993; 11(4):629–640.

CHAPTER 31

Lice

James E. Rasmussen

CLINICAL APPEARANCE

Definition

Infestation of blood-sucking insects of the order Anoplura produces three distinct clinical presentations depending on the type of organism: pediculosis capitis, pubis, and corporis. *Pediculus humanus* var. *capitis* (head louse) and *Pediculus humanus* var. *corporis* (body louse) are 2 to 4 mm long. *Phthirus pubis* (pubic louse) (Fig. 31–1) is more rounded with a well-developed first pair of legs, giving rise to the common term *crabs*.

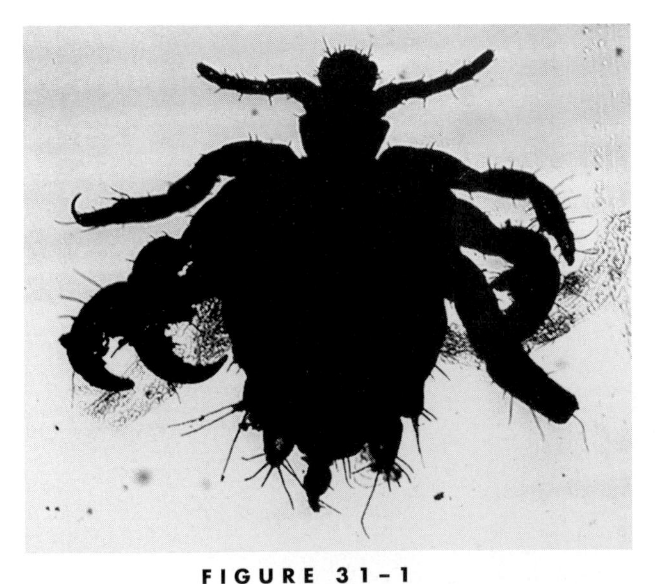

FIGURE 31–1
A pubic louse.

Usual Appearance

Itching is the symptom of all forms of infestation with lice. Only in severe and longstanding cases are other physical signs and symptoms usually noticed. With heavy infestations and significant scratching, hemorrhagic papules and secondary infection may suggest a primary pyoderma in the scalp or groin or over the chest or back. In the scalp, considerable hair matting results from poor hygiene and frequent rubbing.

Head Lice[1]

A typical patient with head lice usually has few, if any, easily observable signs of infestation with the disease. The patient may complain of itching around the ears and over the sides of the neck, but these changes occur so gradually that patients frequently give them little attention. Longstanding cases produce hemorrhagic papules, matting of the scalp hair, pyoderma, and lymphadenopathy.

Nits represent eggs cemented to the side of hairs (Fig. 31–2). They are most commonly seen around the fringes of the lateral and posterior scalp. They cannot be removed easily.

Pubic Lice

Infestation with pubic lice is usually noted by the individual because of the constant crawling of the insects. Other than the physical presence of the insects and their eggs, there is usually very little secondary infection, except in the most severe cases. In prepubertal children, pubic lice may colonize eyelashes, eyebrows, and the

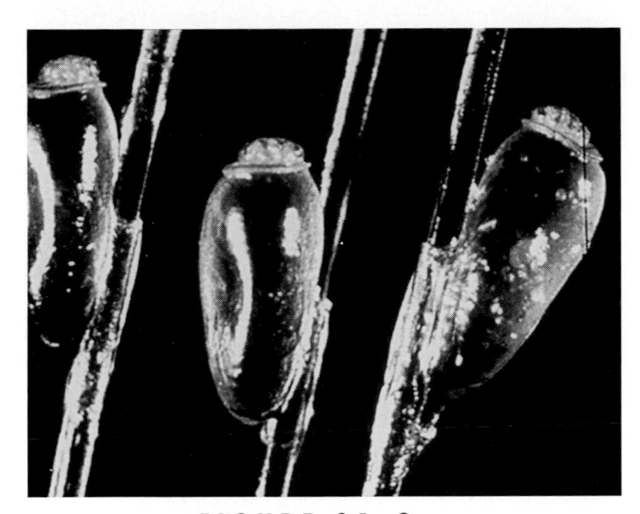

FIGURE 31-2
Nits.

fringes of the scalp. Rarely, transient blue macules (maculae cerulae) may appear on the abdomen or chest. These probably represent hemorrhage secondary to lice bites.

Body Lice

Patients infected with body lice are frequently homeless and indigent. These cases often go undetected for long periods of time, so that scratching, secondary infection, and scarring are common. Body lice frequently live and lay their eggs in the seams of clothing and on body hair.

DESCRIPTION OF DISEASE

Age/Population/Demographics

Head Lice

Head lice can be found worldwide in individuals of any age but are much more common in children from 4 to 12 years old. This probably represents exposure and transmission in social settings such as school. Head lice infection is distinctly uncommon among blacks.

Pubic Lice

Since infestation with pubic lice is usually transmitted through sexual exposure, it is uncommon to see affected individuals who are younger than 10 years old. Teenagers and younger adults are the most commonly affected with pubic lice. Although the disease is often transmitted sexually, it can also be more casually spread by fomites.

Body Lice

Although patients of any age are susceptible, infestation with body lice is commonly seen in older individuals. Vagabonds, street people, and indigent people in communal living situations are at greatest risk.

Natural History of Disease

All forms of lice will probably persist indefinitely unless treated. The individual's general state of hygiene may determine the severity of infection with body and head lice. Head lice are much more common in tropical and near-tropical parts of the world, probably because the environment is more friendly for transmission. For practical purposes, no significant diseases are transmitted in the United States by any of these blood-sucking insects, although this is potentially possible.

Pathology

Since these organisms do not live in the human skin, they are rarely found in pathologic specimens. Reactions to their bites are nonspecific and are not useful in diagnosing the disease.

Etiology/Pathogenesis

All three of these diseases are spread from human to human by direct physical contact and through fomites. Body and pubic lice probably depend more on direct physical contact, whereas head lice can be transmitted through the use of towels, caps, combs, and other articles of clothing. Itching becomes more noticeable as more organisms and, consequently, the number of bites increase.

Diagnosis

Nits in the scalp or pubic area are the usual diagnostic sign. The organisms are quite shy and are usually not seen unless infestation is heavy. Because of the scarcity of pubic hair, it is easier to see lice in this area than it is on the scalp. Nits are egg cases of lice that have been cemented at an oblique angle to the shaft of the hair. The body louse lays its eggs primarily in clothing near the seam lines or occasionally on body hair as well. It is important to thoroughly examine this area in order to make this diagnosis. Some patients may change from more frequently worn clothes into their "Sunday best" for a visit to the doctor, and the organisms may be missed.

TREATMENT[2–5]

Goals of treatment include killing the adults and the incubating eggs with biochemical and physical modalities. In addition, all contaminated articles of clothing, bedding, and personal hygiene products need to be disinfected. For head lice, the primary focus should be on brushes, combs, hats, scarves, and coats. Most of these personal hair care items can be treated with rubbing alcohol or placed in the home dishwasher. Towels, sheets, pillowcases, and bedding should be laundered in hot water. For items that are difficult to clean or disinfect, freezing works well. This might be used for hats, parkas, and other such items. It is not necessary to fumigate the house to rid the patient of head lice.

For pubic lice, emphasis should be placed on underwear and body clothes as well as bedding articles. These should be laundered thoroughly in hot water.

Patients with body lice will need to disinfect a substantial portion of their surroundings, and since many of these people are indigent, it is hard to identify exactly where they sleep and to what they are exposed. Bedding, sleeping bags, and all clothing articles must be washed or dry-cleaned. This is not easy, given the financial state of the usual person involved with body lice.

Therapeutic Agents

Scalp and Pubic Lice

A multitude of agents are used for the treatment of head, pubic, and body lice. In the United States, only two groups of compounds are currently commonly used: lindane and pyrethrins/permethrin.[2, 3] Lindane 1% in the form of a shampoo has long been considered the treatment of choice. It has an outstanding record of efficacy but has recently come under criticism because of its potential for neurotoxicity with prolonged, frequent use, misuse, or ingestion. It is generally applied as a shampoo, lathered on for 5 or 10 minutes, and rinsed off. Some feel that the lathering and rinsing should be done in the sink rather than in the shower, so that the residual does not run over the rest of the body. However, I do not follow this practice.

Permethrins are synthetic pyrethrins (originally extracted from a specific type of chrysanthemum). Pyrethrins are frequently used with the synergistic agent piperonyl butoxide. These are available as over-the-counter (OTC) products such as RID and A-200. They come in a variety of lotions and shampoos, which are applied to the scalp for 5 or 10 minutes and then rinsed out. Permethrin (Nix) is a synthetic pyrethroid available as an OTC 1% creme rinse. The scalp is lathered with a commercial soap and rinsed. The creme rinse is applied for 5 to 10 minutes and then rinsed out. Permethrin is reported to be more effective against nits than other products.

In general, I follow the initial application with vigorous nit combing. Nit combs are included in most commercial prescription and OTC products (Fig. 31–3). It is difficult to show that the use of nit combs increases the effectiveness of these agents, but it probably does no harm and certainly does make the patient and parent feel like they are contributing to the removal of the disease. However, if the goal of a nit-free scalp is emphasized in too hard a fashion, some patients develop psychologic problems because of the less than 100% efficacy of these combs. For a brief period in the United States, a product was marketed to aid in nit removal (Step 2). To my knowledge, this product is no longer available, however.

In other parts of the world, malathion is commonly used. This product was marketed briefly in the United States under the brand name Prioderm as a 0.5% lotion. It must be left in contact with the scalp hair for 8 to 12 hours. It has both ovacidal and pediculcidal activity, but once again, I recommend a repeat application after an

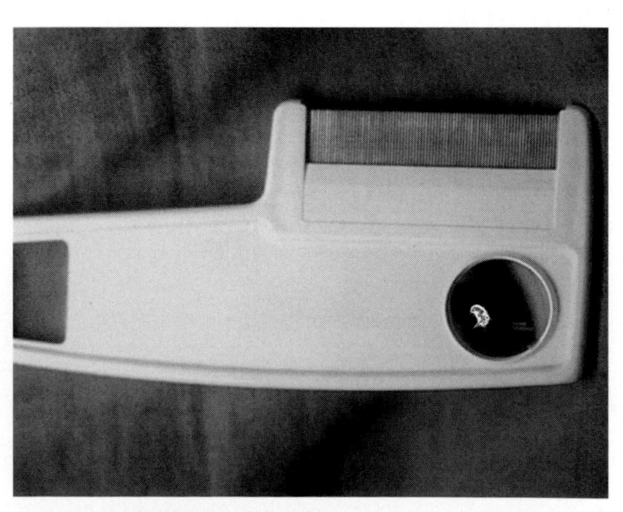

FIGURE 31–3
A nit comb demonstrating closely spaced teeth.

interval of 1 week. It is apparently a very safe compound, and adverse effects have rarely been reported. It does, however, have a somewhat objectionable odor.

In some countries, a mixture of disulfuram, benzyl benzoate, and dichlorodiphenyltrichloroethane (DDT) (Tenutex) has been used. These components have also been used individually. Tenutex is left on the hair for several hours and then washed out with common shampoo.

In some Scandinavian countries, tincture of quassia is also used for the treatment of pediculosis capitis. Quassia is a plant extract that is prepared in 86% alcohol. The scalp hair is rinsed with the tincture, followed by drying. The tincture is left in contact with the scalp for 18 hours and then rinsed out. Apart from the odor and slight stinging from the alcohol, no side effects have been reported with this compound.

In England, carbaryl has been used. Carbaryl is napthy-1-yl methyl carbamate. It is applied as a 0.2% emulsified lotion or as a shampoo. The lotion is applied to the scalp for 24 hours before being washed off with a bland shampoo. Shampoo preparations are applied for 3 to 5 minutes and then rinsed off with warm tap water.

Crotamiton (Eurax) is used as a 10% lotion or cream. It is applied for 24 hours and then shampooed out. This product is sold in many parts of the world but is not very effective.

The treatment for head lice and pubic lice is similar, only different areas are treated. Lindane is not reported to be as effective in the treatment of pubic lice as it is in head lice. To my knowledge, no product is specifically marketed for the treatment of pubic lice.

Eyelash Lice

Eyelash lice are occasionally found and usually represent pubic lice in a prepubertal patient, although they have occasionally been reported in patients with head lice. The most effective treatment for eyelash lice is petrolatum (Vaseline) applied vigorously 3 to 4 times a day. Other options are yellow oxide of mercury, physostigmine (Eserine), and fluorescence, each applied 3 to 4 times a day for 2 to 3 days.

Body Lice

All the agents effective against head and pubic lice are also effective against body lice. It is important to appreciate that body lice are much more likely to infest the patient's general surroundings, including their clothing and bedding, than head and pubic lice. In addition, these patients are frequently indigent, so that much care must be given to laundering and disinfecting their environment. It is not necessary to apply insecticides to the clothing, since simple laundering in hot water is quite effective. In areas where laundry facilities are scarce, dusting of the patient's clothing and bedding may be necessary, especially in large-scale treatment programs.

The effectiveness of all these preparations depends on how they are used and who has done the investigation. It is my experience that none of these agents is remarkably effective when given as a single treatment. Consequently, I suggest that all patients use the OTC agents (permethrin/pyrethrins) because of lower cost, greater availability, and increased public awareness of lindane's potential for side effects. Therapy should be administered according to product directions as single treatments interrupted by 1-week intervals.

Permethrin 1% has been noted to have greater effectiveness in killing organisms in eggs, but I have still not found that one application is uniformly successful. Information on its use in body lice is lacking.

Attention must be given to treatment of all exposed persons, whether symptomatic or not. My general rule of therapy involves treatment of all symptomatic patients followed by a second treatment given after an interval of 1 week. Asymptomatic patients are treated only once.

Resistance to Therapy

Several studies have discussed problems of resistance specifically to lindane but also to other ingredients. Most of these have occurred in countries where pharmaceutical standards are not as rigorous as in the United States, and the use of multiple insecticides on a frequent routine basis is much more common. A study from France showed definite resistance of head lice to 0.3% D-phenothrin. Only 40% of patients responded to this agent versus 95% with 0.5% malathion.[6] In my experience, resistance to any of the previously mentioned pediculocides has never been a factor influencing therapy.

Toxicity

Although lindane has been described as a more toxic compound, I have never seen a reaction to it following proper use. From a study comprising tens of thousands of patients,[4] there were no differences in reactions to lindane versus pyrethrins. Because of the notoriety given lindane, however, I think it prudent to use other agents.

None of these compounds has been proved safe for use during pregnancy.

Alternate Therapeutic Options

Oral therapy of head lice has been successful using combinations of cotrimoxazole and sulfamethoxazole for 3 to 5 days.[5] Treatment has no effect on the nits, so it will need to be repeated. This therapy is little used in the United States and, of course, should not be given to patients who are allergic to sulfa drugs.

None of these products should be used in a prophylactic sense.

PITFALLS AND PROBLEMS

The difficulty in making the diagnosis of pediculosis is that the number of adult organisms is usually few. Consequently, diligent search must be made on the scalp, pubic area, or clothing for presence of nits. Hair casts, hair spray, trichorrhexis nodosa from vigorous scratching, and other causes of pseudonits must also be given careful consideration. If doubt exists, then the hair should be plucked or cut from the scalp and examined under a microscope for the characteristic morphology of the egg case. It is rarely necessary to shave the scalp hair, and this should be considered only in cases where matting of the hair is beyond a manual reduction.

When pediculosis occur on the eyelashes, it usually represents pubic lice and not head or body lice. Symptoms here are referable to crusting and blepheritis in addition to itching. Most of the therapeutic modalities available for the treatment of head, body, and pubic lice are not suitable for use around the eyes. On the eyelashes, the treatment of choice should be manual removal (which is quite difficult, particularly in an uncooperative child) versus petroleum jelly applied liberally with a swab 2 or 3 times a day for 2 to 3 days. Fluorescein, physostygmine, and yellow oxide of mercury are mentioned as useful, but I have no experience with any of these.

REFERRAL/CONSULTATION GUIDELINES

This group of diseases can be effectively treated by general practitioners, pediatricians, or dermatologists. In fact, any physician who has patient contact should be familiar with the diagnosis and therapy.

REFERENCES

1. Rasmussen JE: Pediculosis and the pediatrician. Pediatr Dermatol 1984; 2:74–79.
2. Taplin D, Meiking TL, Castillero PM, et al: Permethrin 1% creme rinse for the treatment of *Pediculus humanus* var *capitis* infestation. Pediatr Dermatol 1986; 3:344–348.
3. Carson DS, Tribble PW, Weart CW: Pyrethrins combined with piperonyl butoxide (RID) vs 1% permethrin (NIX) for the treatment of head lice. Am J Dis Child 1988; 142:768–769.
4. Andrews EB, Joseph MC, Magenheim MJ, et al: Postmarketing surveillance study of permethrin creme rinse. Am J Public Health 1992; 82:857–861.
5. Shashindran CH, Gandhi IS, Krishnasamy S, et al: Oral therapy of pediculosis capitis with cotrimoxazole. Br J Dermatol 1978; 98:699–700.
6. Chosidow O, Chastang C, Brue C, et al: Controlled study of malathion and D-phenothrin lotions for *Pediculus humanus* var *capitis*–infested school children. Lancet 1994; 344:1724–1727.

CHAPTER 32

Lichen Simplex Chronicus (Neurodermatitis)

Jack L. Arbiser

CLINICAL APPEARANCE

Definition

Lichen simplex chronicus (neurodermatitis) is a chronic idiopathic condition characterized by localized and severe pruritus (see Fig. 32–1 on Color Plate 11). Usually, the lesion is a raised erythematous plaque with exaggerated skin lines that often demonstrates evidence of excoriation. This condition can occur at all ages, but it is most prominent in the elderly.

Typical Lesions and Symptoms

The patient with lichen simplex chronicus has single or multiple erythematous plaques that may be several centimeters in diameter. These lesions may be accompanied by postinflammatory hyperpigmentation or hypopigmentation in darker-skinned patients. Sites often involved include the ankles, anogenital area, and nuchal scalp. Some patients have multiple lesions on the trunk and extremities. Facial involvement is uncommon, and lesions are not seen in anatomic areas that the patient is unable to scratch. This suggests that itching serves to propagate further development of the lesions. Superinfection, especially with staphylococcal and streptococcal spp. may occur.

The hallmark of lichen simplex chronicus is pruritus, and the presence of clinically suggestive lesions in the absence of pruritus should make the physician consider alternative diagnoses.

DESCRIPTION OF DISEASE

The etiology of lichen simplex chronicus is poorly understood. Continued itch is necessary for initiation and propagation of this disorder, but not all patients with chronic pruritus with repeated rubbing and scratching demonstrate lesions consistent with lichen simplex chronicus. This makes it clear that other factors are necessary for the development of this disorder. This disorder also appears to have a behavioral component, but a consistent behavioral profile or response to psychotropic agents has not been observed.

The histopathologic findings of lichen simplex chronicus demonstrate epidermal hyperplasia, with scale, crust, and neutrophils seen in excoriated lesions at the surface, and lymphocytes, mast cells, and eosinophils. Thickening of dermal nerve bundles is sometimes observed in the lesions.

Nerves in lichen simplex chronicus have been demonstrated to contain the neurotransmitter calcitonin gene-related peptide (CGRP).[1] The role of CGRP in lichen simplex chronicus is not known, but it may present a therapeutic target in the treatment of lichen simplex chronicus.

TREATMENT

Therapeutic Expectations

Control of the behavioral component of lichen simplex chronicus may be necessary for the control of cutaneous symptoms.[2] Clinical relief followed by relapse is the usual course. Atypical-appearing lesions or lesions that do not respond to treatment require biopsy to rule out conditions that may clinically resemble lichen simplex chronicus.

First-Line Therapy

Twice-daily application of potent topical glucocorticoids (e.g., fluocinonide, betamethasone diproprionate) usually induces lesions to subside. Ointments work better than creams. Use of overnight occlusion over the corticosteroid often provides additional benefit in that it prevents further excoriation of the lesion and increases the anti-inflammatory effect. Resolution of lesions may require 2 to 4 weeks and is often followed by postinflammatory hyperpigmentation.

Alternative Therapies

1. Intralesional corticosteroid injection (e.g., triamcinolone acetonide 2.5 mg/ml) induces remission of 1 to 3 months' duration.
2. Topical doxepin is often useful in the treatment of pruritus, especially in atopic dermatitis.[3] Topical and systemic doxepin, as well as sedating H_1 oral antihistamines, may have a beneficial effect in this condition.
3. The substance P–depleting agent capsaicin (Zostrix) may also prove to have benefit.
4. Behavioral therapy administered by a qualified psychiatrist may be of benefit in severe cases.
5. Cryotherapy with liquid nitrogen has several advantages. It causes rapid destruction of nerve fibers that may drive the itch-scratch-itch propagation of lichen simplex chronicus. As well, it is relatively easy to freeze a large number of lesions in a single session.
6. Thalidomide, a sedative notorious for its teratogenicity, has been shown to have benefit in the treatment of lichen simplex chronicus, but a significant number of patients developed neuropathy.[4]

DIFFERENTIAL DIAGNOSIS

Whereas lichen simplex chronicus is usually readily diagnosed, a number of conditions may mimic its appearance. Atypical distribution, rapid growth, and failure to respond to proven therapies should alert the clinician to other diagnostic possibilities. Conditions that may mimic lichen simplex chronicus include contact dermatitis, lichen planus, atopic dermatitis, T-cell dyscrasias, psoriasis, dermatophytosis, and scabies. Skin biopsy is helpful in reaching a definitive diagnosis.

PITFALLS

Common pitfalls include untreated accompanying bacterial infection, misdiagnosis, and complications of chronic topical steroid therapy. When lichen simplex chronicus involves genitalia or flexural skin, cutaneous atrophy and striae from application of potent topical steroids are most likely. For these reasons, these agents should be used sparingly in these areas.

REFERRAL AND CONSULTATION

Poor response to initial therapy and presence of genital lesions are strong reasons for referral.

REFERENCES

1. Gupta MA, Gupta AK, Haberman HF: The self-inflicted dermatoses: A critical review. Gen Hosp Psychiatry 1987; 9:45–52.
2. Vaalasti A, Suomalainen H, Rechart L: Calcitonin gene-related peptide immunoreactivity in prurigo nodularis: A comparative study with neurodermatitis circumscripta. Br J Dermatol 1989; 120:619–623.
3. Drake LA, Millikan LE: The antipruritic effect of 5% doxepin cream in patients with eczematous dermatitis. Doxepin Study Group. Arch Dermatol 1995; 131:1403–1408.
4. Johne H, Zachariae H: Thalidomide treatment of prurigo nodularis. Ugeskr Laeger 1993; 155:3028–3030.

CHAPTER 33

Melasma

Pearl E. Grimes

CLINICAL APPEARANCE

Melasma is a common acquired disorder of hyperpigmentation characterized by often symmetric, irregular, light tan to brown macules affecting sun-exposed areas of skin (see Fig. 33–1 on Color Plate 11). The most common areas of involvement include the cheeks, forehead, upper lip, chin, and nose. Three clinical patterns of hyperpigmentation—centrofacial, malar, and mandibular—are recognized in patients with melasma.

DESCRIPTION

The true incidence of melasma is unknown. Women constitute the majority of cases. The disease affects all racial groups but is most prevalent in darker-complexioned individuals (skin types IV through VI), especially women of Hispanic descent who live in areas with intense ultraviolet radiation exposure.

The precise cause has not been delineated. However, multiple etiologies have been implicated in the pathogenesis of melasma and include genetic factors, oral contraceptives, pregnancy, intense solar radiation exposure, use of certain cosmetics, estrogen-progesterone therapies, thyroid dysfunction, and antiseizure medications.[1]

Histologic examination of lesions reveals three patterns—epidermal, dermal, and mixed—of increased pigment deposition. The mixed pattern is characterized by deposition of both dermal and epidermal pigment.

TREATMENT

Therapeutic Expectations

Because of the recurrent or persistent hyperactivity of melanocytes in melasma, the disorder is a therapeutically challenging and frustrating one. Intermittent long-term topical therapy is often necessary to control moderate to severe disease. A variety of medical and surgical approaches have been used to "lighten" the hyperpigmented areas of skin typical of this disease. Phenolic and nonphenolic bleaching agents and chemical peels are most often recommended.[1, 2] Laser therapy is not useful.

First-Line Therapies

Phenolic Bleaching Agents

HYDROQUINONE. Hydroquinone is used extensively worldwide for treatment of melasma. Hydroquinone is a hydroxyphenolic chemical that inhibits the conversion of dopa to melanin by inhibiting the tyrosinase enzyme. It induces hypopigmentation, in contrast to monobenzylether of hydroquinone (Benoquin), which induces permanent depigmentation. Monobenzylether of hydroquinone should only be prescribed as a depigmenting agent for severe vitiligo. Concentrations of hydroquinone vary from 2% (over-the-counter) to 3 to 4% (by prescription). The 2% formulations (e.g., Esoterica, Ambi) can be recommended for patients with mild disease. However, the higher concentrations, 3% (Melanex) or 4% (Eldoquin Forte, Solaquin, Eldopaque), are usually considered for more severe disease. Products are applied twice daily for up to 3 months, with subsequent tapering of the frequency of use once the desired effects are achieved.

Higher concentrations of hydroquinone are often extemporaneously compounded for treatment of more severe disease. The efficacy of hydroquinone may be improved when combined with keratolytic agents such as salicylic acid, glycolic acid (Neostrata), and tretinoin. The Kligman formula combines hydroquininone 5%, tretinoin 0.1% in a steroid vehicle. In addition, lower concentrations of tretinoin (i.e., 0.01% and 0.025%) offer significant efficacy when combined or used in conjunction with hydroquinone. Compared with tretinoin 0.1%, the lower concentrations are less irritating. Side effects associated with hydroquinone use include acute and chronic complications. The most common acute reactions are irritant or allergic contact dermatitis. Hydroquinone also causes hypopigmentation of the surrounding lesional skin and, rarely, depigmentation. These changes are temporary and resolve on cessation of hydroquinone therapy. Chronic complications of hydroquinone therapy are hydroquinone-induced ochronosis, a chronic disfiguring condition generally resulting from the prolonged use of high concentrations of hydroquinone.[3] Although ochronosis is common in Africa, there have been no more than 18 cases reported in the American scientific literature. Most occurred in response to short-term or long-term use of 2% hydroquinone. Therefore, ochronosis in the United States appears to be an idiosyncratic reaction to hydroquinone.

N-ACETYL-4-S-CYSTEAMINYLPHENOL. The efficacy of a new depigmenting agent, *N*-acetyl-4-S-cysteaminylphenol, has been reported.[1] Marked improvement was noted in 75% of the 12 subjects treated. Side effects were minimal. This drug, however, is not approved by the U.S. Food and Drug Administration.[3]

Nonphenolic Bleaching Agents

AZELAIC ACID. Azelaic acid is a dicarboxylic acid that has demonstrated beneficial therapeutic effects in the treatment of acne vulgaris and hyperpigmenting disorders such as melasma and lentigo maligna. It inhibits tyrosinase and has cytotoxic and antiproliferative effects against hyperactive melanocytes.[1] Multiple clinical trials have reported the efficacy of azelaic acid for treatment of melasma. Azelaic acid 20% (Azelex, Allergan Pharmaceuticals) has recently been approved for use in the United States as an antiacne agent. It should be applied to affected areas twice daily and appears to be well tolerated. However, adverse reactions include erythema, pruritus, burning, and scaling.

TRETINOIN 0.1%. Tretinoin 0.1% has shown beneficial effects in the treatment of melasma and postinflammatory hyperpigmentation. It is applied once daily at bedtime. When used as a monotherapy for treatment of melasma, efficacious results often necessitate prolonged use for 6 to 9 months. Factors limiting the prolonged use of tretinoin 0.1% include severe erythema and desquamation. Postinflammatory hyperpigmentation often ensues in response to tretinoin-induced irritant reactions. These side effects are particularly severe in darker-skinned ethnic groups.

KOJIC ACID. Kojic acid is a newer product gaining popularity in the treatment of melasma. As with hydroquinone and azelaic acid, it inhibits the tyrosinase enzyme, hence blocking the conversion of tyrosine to melanin. A recent study documented efficacy comparable with hydroquinone, when both products were combined with 2% glycolic acid.[4] Over-the-counter formulations frequently combine kojic acid 2% or 4% with keratolytic agents such as glycolic acid or salicylic acid. Kojic acid formulations may be applied twice daily. Side effects are burning and desquamation.

Chemical Peels

A variety of chemical peels have been used to treat the pigmentary imperfections of melasma.[5] These include trichloroacetic acid, resorcinol, buffered and unbuffered phenol, and alpha-hydroxy acids (glycolic acid). Chemical peels should be used with caution in darker-skinned ethnic groups because of the tendency to induce areas of hyperpigmentation or hypopigmentation. Chemical peels are indicated in patients with moderate to severe disease who have failed to respond to topical bleaching agents. Of the aforementioned peels, glycolic acid peels appear to be associated with fewer acute and chronic complications. Concentrations of 35%, 50%, and 70% glycolic acid are used to treat hyperpigmentation. If no response occurs with the lower concentrations, patients are progressively titrated to the higher concentrations in a series of peels repeated weekly, biweekly, or monthly. After surface oils are removed with prepeel cleansers, glycolic acid is applied with a gauze sponge or sable brush for 3 to 5 minutes, then neutralized. Appropriate neutralization of the applied acid avoids burning or scarring. Most peeling protocols recommend the use of lower concentrations of glycolic acid between chemical peels and the concomitant use of topical bleaching agents applied twice daily (e.g., Neostrata).

Alternative/Adjunctive Therapies

Alternative Therapies

Although a few studies have demonstrated some success with laser therapy for hyperpigmentation, its efficacy and place in the treatment of melasma have yet to be established.

Adjunctive Therapies

The routine daily use of broad-spectrum sunscreens providing ultraviolet B and ultraviolet A protection is an essential part of the management of melasma. Opaque sunblocking agents must be used to truly prevent the increased pigmentation induced by ultraviolet light exposure.

PITFALLS AND PROBLEMS

Melasma may sometimes be confused with erythema dyschromicum perstans or lichen planus actinicus. Therefore, in extremely difficult, recalcitrant cases, a skin biopsy may be indicated.[2]

REFERENCES

1. Grimes PE: Melasma: Etiologic and therapeutic considerations. Arch Dermatol 1995; 131:1453–1457.
2. Grimes PE: Diseases of hyperpigmentation. *In* Sams WM, Lynch PJ (eds): Principles and Practice of Dermatology. 2nd ed. New York: Churchill Livingstone, 1996; pp 825–841,
3. Findley GH, Morriso JGL, Simon IW: Exogenous ochronosis and pigmented colloid millium from hydroquinone bleaching creams. Br J Dermatol 1995; 93:613–622.
4. Garcia A, Fulton JE: The combination of glycolic acid and hydroquinone or kojic acid for the treatment of melasma and related conditions. Dermatol Surg 1996; 22:443–447.
5. Brody H: Chemical Peels. St. Louis: Mosby–Year Book, 1992; pp 53–73.

CHAPTER 34

Moles and Melanoma

Jason K. Rivers

CLINICAL APPEARANCE

Definition

Mole

A *mole* (also called *melanocytic nevus)* is a benign, localized proliferation of melanocytes in the skin. The clinical appearance of a mole depends, in part, on the location of the melanocytes within the cutis. Melanocytes either are confined to the dermoepidermal junction (junctional nevus), extend farther into the dermis (compound nevus), or are localized to the dermis (intradermal nevus). Moles are occasionally present at birth, but most are acquired lesions that first appear in childhood.

Melanoma

Melanoma refers to a malignant proliferation of melanocytes that most often arises from pigment cells located in the skin (as opposed to mucosal or ocular sites of origin). Melanoma is characterized by a pigmented lesion that undergoes a change (in size, shape, color, or symptoms) usually over a span of weeks to months. Rare in childhood, the age-specific incidence increases steadily over the lifetime of predisposed individuals.

Typical Lesions

Mole (see Fig. 34–1 on Color Plate 11)

A mole is a well-defined oval to round pigmented macule or papule with uniform color ranging from light to dark brown, although it may be flesh colored. The surface of a nevus may be smooth or mamillated, and the margin is distinct.

Common moles can be identified anywhere on the skin surface, although they predominate on sun-exposed sites (i.e., it is unusual to find moles on the breasts or buttocks). For the most part, moles are asymptomatic. Occasionally, moles may itch or bleed when traumatized. These findings do not persist, and the general morphology of the mole remains unchanged.

Melanoma (see Figs. 34–2 on Color Plate 11 and 34–3 on Color Plate 12)

The typical textbook melanoma is characterized by the mnemonic *ABCD: a*symmetry, *b*order irregularities, *c*olor variegation, and *d*iameter. Unlike moles, melanoma is usually asymmetric (i.e., it cannot be evenly bisected). The border of the lesion is irregular, but the edge usually remains distinct, at least in part. Melanomas display an admixture of colors, including black, blue, and even pink. An area of pigment loss in some part of the lesion (regression) is an important distinguishing feature for some early melanomas. Once fully developed, benign melanocytic nevi seldom change in diameter. If a lesion doubles in size over a period of a few months, malignant degeneration should be considered. Although melanoma can be identified at any size, lesions measuring larger than 6 mm in diameter should be assessed carefully for other atypical clinical features in order to rule out a malignant process.

Change in size also includes a change in surface elevation: a part of the tumor will become raised from the skin. It is important to make the diagnosis of melanoma before this event, as the development of a nodular component is a sign of an advanced lesion. These nodules are usually black or blue-black but are sometimes red (amelanotic).

The development of an intermittent, nonsevere itch is a useful sign in the diagnosis of melanoma. Tenderness or pain is a late sign and is of no help in making the diagnosis in the majority of patients.

Atypical Presentation or Alternative Forms

CONGENITAL MOLES. Congenital moles (see Figs. 34–4 and 34–5 on Color Plate 12) have been arbitrarily classified into three categories based on the size of the lesion: small (<1.5 cm); medium (≥1.5 cm and ≤19.9 cm); and large (≥20 cm). Small and medium-sized lesions are well demarcated from the surrounding skin, may be macular or raised, range in color from light brown to almost black, and may have increased hair growth within them. They are generally solitary lesions but can occur as "satellites" when they develop in association with a large congenital mole. Large congenital nevi can have a more varied appearance, often developing a coarse surface texture and displaying subcutaneous nodules that represent tumors derived from neuroectodermal structures.

ATYPICAL NEVUS. The atypical nevus (see Figs. 34–6 through 34–8 on Color Plate 12) (previously called *dysplastic nevus)* is a benign acquired lesion that is both a potential precursor to melanoma and a marker for people with an increased risk to develop this neoplasm. Atypical nevi are usually greater than 5 mm in diameter (although they can be smaller), have an irregular border, and show a variegation of color with hues of tan, brown, and red. Sometimes, small areas tend to become hypopigmented, suggesting clinical regression. However, white is never seen in an atypical nevus as it is in regressing melanoma. Atypical nevi often display a "shoulder": a macular tan area of pigmentation at the perimeter of the lesion that fades imperceptibly into the surrounding normal skin. Compound/dermal moles are often dome-shaped papules that are elevated throughout the lesion. By contrast, atypical nevi, if palpable, generally have greater breadth than height—atypical nevi are usually raised in the center, flattening out toward the edge. This gives rise to the so-called target nevus. Generally, atypical nevi are heterogeneous lesions, with each individual atypical nevus differing from its neighbor.

HALO NEVUS. A halo nevus (see Fig. 34–9 on Color Plate 13) is a benign lesion that most often develops in childhood or adolescence. These red to brown macules or papules are centered on a circular area of depigmentation and result from an immunologic response to presumably altered antigens on the melanocytes of one or more nevi. At times, when the regression of the mole is complete, only a circular area of depigmented skin and hair may remain as the telltale sign of a preexisting pigmented lesion.

SPITZ' NEVUS. Spitz' nevus (see Fig. 34–10 on Color Plate 13), formerly called *Spitz' juvenile melanoma,* is a rapidly growing, benign pigmented lesion predominantly seen in children. Although the histologic features may at times suggest melanoma, there is no evidence that these lesions can become malignant. Most Spitz' nevi are dome-shaped, pink to red papules measuring less than 5 mm in diameter. Less than 50% present as some shade of brown to black. The fact that these lesions occur primarily in children is an important diagnostic clue because melanoma is rarely encountered in children. Nonetheless, these nevi should be excised for histologic assessment.

BLUE NEVUS. A blue nevus (see Fig. 34–11 on Color Plate 13) can be confused with melanoma but should not be difficult to diagnose. The lesion is almost always round or oval, with a uniform bluish pigmentation evenly distributed throughout the lesion. These nevi are characteristically small, measuring less than 5 mm in diameter. In larger lesions, hairs will be present within the nodule if it occurs on hair-bearing skin. By contrast, melanomas will lose hair as they destroy hair follicles when they invade into the reticular dermis. A large nodule of melanoma will, therefore, hardly ever contain hair. A history of a longstanding stable lesion is commonly obtained from these patients.

MELANOMA VARIANTS. Melanoma variants (see Figs. 34–12 and 34–13 on Color Plate 13) do exist. Although the majority of melanomas are quite characteristic in appearance, some tumors may develop initially as dome-shaped papules or nodules, subungual pigmented streaks, or even reddish plaques devoid of observable pigment. A history of change in a pigmented lesion that occurs over a 2- to 6-month period is suggestive of malignancy.

DESCRIPTION OF DISEASE

It has been estimated that 1 to 2% of the population is born with a small (<1.5 cm diameter) congenital mole, and these lesions may be somewhat more common in darkly pigmented populations.[1] Large (>20 cm) or bathing trunk–type nevi are rare and develop in 1:20,000 to

1:500,000 live births. Most occur sporadically, and these lesions are often centered over the posterior aspect of the trunk, although they can appear in any location.

For the most part, congenital moles are benign lesions and remain so throughout the life of the individual. Although malignant transformation has been documented in all types of congenital melanocytic nevi regardless of size, it is important to emphasize that this is a rare event for small to medium-sized lesions, especially before the teenage years. By contrast, the lifetime risk for melanoma developing in a large congenital nevus is substantial (approximately 6%), and many of the reported cases have occurred before the age of 10 years.

Common acquired and atypical moles usually appear in childhood and, in some populations, continue to increase in number into the third or fourth decade of life before slowly disappearing with age. Loss of moles through an immunologic mechanism (halo nevus formation) is common in children and young adults.

Studies have shown a relationship between the number of moles and increasing ambient ultraviolet light.[2] Mole numbers are correlated with a number of phenotypic risk factors including light skin color, freckling, light eye color, greater tendency to burn, and lesser tendency to tan. Finally, immunosuppression seems to play an additional role in the development of moles: increased numbers of nevi have been reported in children after renal transplantation or chemotherapy for malignancy.

Melanoma is the most rapidly increasing cancer in white populations. It is rare in children (under 14 years of age), accounting for less than 1% of all melanoma cases. Risk factors for the development of melanoma in childhood include giant congenital moles, the atypical mole syndrome, xeroderma pigmentosum, and immunodeficiency states. In the adult population, additional factors include sun-sensitive skin type, numerous common moles, atypical moles, immunosuppression, a family history of melanoma, and a history of nonmelanocytic skin cancer. In many populations, both sexes have a similar predilection to the disease, and the average age at diagnosis is around 50 years.

At least 25 to 50% of melanomas arise de novo (i.e., not associated with a precursor lesion) and may appear as a new, flat, darkly pigmented lesion that undergoes a noticeable change over a 2- to 6-month period. Melanoma proliferates locally for a time and then develops the ability to metastasize to distant sites through lymphatics and blood.

For patients with localized primary cutaneous melanoma, the most important prognostic factor is tumor thickness, measured in millimeters from the granular cell layer of the skin to the base of the lesion. Melanoma in situ does not metastasize, since the malignant cells are confined to the epidermis. Patients with lesions less than 1.0 mm in thickness (''thin'' or ''early'' melanoma) have a predicted 10-year survival that approximates 90%, whereas half of all patients with tumors larger than 4 mm will succumb to their disease within 5 years. Often, melanoma first spreads to the regional draining lymph nodes before appearing at other sites such as the lung, liver, and brain.

It has been estimated that 80% of melanomas are caused by sun exposure. Although the mechanism remains unclear, many investigators have concluded that acute, intense exposure to sunlight that causes sunburn is strongly linked to the development of melanoma. For the remaining 20% of melanomas that are estimated to develop in black, African, and Asian populations and are not clearly related to sunlight exposure, the pathogenesis remains elusive.

Occupational and environmental factors related to melanoma have been explored, but nothing conclusive has materialized. There is a link to high socioeconomic status, which provides the individual with the opportunity to experience significant recreational sun exposure. There is no strong evidence of a relationship between diet, alcohol, vitamin A, or betacarotene in the pathogenesis of melanoma.

Approximately 10% of melanomas develop in the familial setting, and an autosomal dominant gene with incomplete penetrance seems to be operative in this setting.

TREATMENT

Therapeutic Expectations

Acquired Moles

Acquired melanocytic nevi, including atypical nevi, are benign, stable lesions and therefore require no treatment unless they become irritated (e.g., from clothing or shaving) or undergo a significant change in size, shape, or color in a relatively short time. Moles are often removed for cosmetic reasons.

Congenital Moles

Controversy surrounds the management of congenital moles. Treatment recommendations are often suggested based on lesion size. Most investigators advise that large congenital nevi be removed whenever possible. However, it is important to note that complete excision of these lesions may be impossible, and the risk for malignant degeneration is not totally eliminated because the tumor may originate from an extracutaneous site (e.g., muscle or the central nervous system).

As the majority of small congenital nevi never undergo malignant change, many authors have suggested a conservative approach to their management (e.g., observation with or without photodocumentation). Lesion removal is advocated only if the mole undergoes a significant change in clinical features (see earlier in this chapter) or is of significant cosmetic concern.

Melanoma

The prognosis of melanoma is directly related to the thickness of the primary lesion at the time of excision. Therefore, the key to maximizing cure is to remove the malignancy when it is at an early stage of development. Once metastases appear, the hope for cure falls precipitously.

First-Line Therapy

Acquired Moles

Total surgical excision is the preferred method of removing these lesions, either by means of an elliptical excision or by deep saucerization into the subcutaneous tissue. A 2-mm margin beyond the clinical border is adequate for almost all moles.

Congenital Moles

Biopsy of a portion of a small or intermediate-sized lesion is rarely of any value, and complete excision is recommended when it has been decided to remove these lesions. For large congenital nevi, multiple surgical procedures are often required to excise the lesion, and the attendant morbidity is not insignificant. Split-thickness skin grafts or the use of tissue expanders is often incorporated into the closure of the surgical wound.

Melanoma

A biopsy should be performed when a lesion is suspected to be a melanoma. Total excision biopsy with narrow margins is recommended. When the lesion is large or located in an area where tissue sparing is required, a punch or incision biopsy is acceptable. This should be taken from the darkest or thickest portion of the lesion.

LOCALIZED CUTANEOUS MELANOMA

In situ melanoma should be excised with a margin of at least 0.5 cm of normal-appearing skin. The results of prospective randomized studies have led to the current recommendation that melanoma 1.0 mm or less in thickness can be safely excised with a 1-cm margin.[3] A 2-cm margin is adequate for lesions between 1 and 4 mm in thickness and does not appear to compromise disease-free or long-term survival. For the subset of patients with melanoma between 1 and 2 mm in thickness, a 1-cm margin would be acceptable in anatomic locations where a 2-cm margin would jeopardize the function of a vital structure (e.g., the area around the eye). The optimal surgical margin has not been determined for melanomas larger than 4 mm, but the accepted standard is 3 cm and has been advocated as a way to reduce the risk of local recurrence.

Controversy remains about the role of elective lymph node dissection for melanoma of intermediate thickness (tumors between 1.5 and 4 mm). It would appear that the number of centers advocating this procedure is in decline,[4] but the results of two ongoing prospective randomized trials should help to resolve the debate.

REGIONAL LYMPH NODE METASTASES

A regional lymph node dissection is always recommended when there is clinical evidence of regional lymph node involvement by tumor. This may prevent further dissemination of disease and will reduce the morbidity associated with nodal ulceration that may develop with time. Adjuvant chemotherapy does not appear to alter the prognosis after therapeutic lymph node dissection.

METASTATIC DISEASE

Metastatic disease can be managed surgically if there are limited accessible lesions (e.g., skin, subcutaneous tissue, lung, brain, or gastrointestinal tract). Isolated hyperthermic limb perfusion, using melphalan alone or in combination with other drugs, can significantly extend the disease-free interval but has little impact on overall survival. Chemotherapy using dacarbazine alone or in combination with other agents can achieve response rates up to 50%, but the duration of response is generally limited. There is no survival advantage of combination chemotherapy over single-agent therapy.

Age Considerations

Acquired Moles

There is no urgency to remove these lesions in childhood, as malignant transformation is rare during this time period. However, in patients at high risk for melanoma (e.g., immunosuppressed or familial melanoma setting), the author believes that atypical lesions of the scalp should be excised because they are difficult to monitor over time. Treatment is deferred to an age when the child can understand and cooperate with the procedure (usually a ''psychologic window'' between 8 and 12 years of age).

Congenital Moles

If one is inclined to remove small or intermediate-sized nevi, it is important to emphasize that malignant degeneration is extremely rare before the age of 10 years, and therefore, there is no urgency to have these lesions excised within the first weeks to years of life. Again, the anatomic location of the lesion does have some bearing on the author's approach to these lesions. In general, the prophylactic removal of small congenital moles of the scalp is advised. Nevi of the face may be psychologically distressing to the patient and are removed for cosmetic reasons.

By contrast, large congenital melanocytic nevi present a significant risk for malignant degeneration early in life, and therefore, it has been the recommendation of many authorities that these lesions be surgically removed as early as a year of life.

Melanoma

Although uncommon, melanoma does occur in childhood. The therapeutic principles advocated for adults should be applied to children because the biology of the disease appears to be similar.

Alternative Therapeutic Options

Acquired Moles

1. Destructive techniques such as cryotherapy, fulguration, or laser surgery.
2. Topically applied retinoids (e.g., vitamin A acid 0.05%).

Congenital Moles

1. Destructive techniques such as cryotherapy, laser surgery, or dermabrasion.

Melanoma

1. Radiation therapy for biopsy-confirmed in situ lentigo maligna melanoma of the head and neck in elderly patients.
2. Biologic response modifiers (interleukin-2, interferons) show modest activity against melanoma in the setting of adjuvants to high-risk primary and metastatic disease.
3. Tumor vaccines and gene therapy are experimental at present.

PITFALLS AND PROBLEMS

1. Removal or destruction of a pigmented lesion without a confirmatory biopsy may result in missing the diagnosis of melanoma.
2. Benign acquired moles that are incompletely excised may recur, and on reexcision, atypical histologic features may appear pronounced. Whether this observation has any biologic significance is unclear at present.
3. In the case of large congenital moles, the malignant change may occur deep to the skin or even directly from the leptomeninges itself. In this setting, early detection of malignancy may be impossible, and the clinician is only alerted to the fact when other signs or symptoms develop (e.g., pain, headache, or seizures).
4. Some melanomas occur on sites rarely exposed to the sun, and this emphasizes the importance of performing a complete skin examination including the scalp and soles. The latter location is especially important in darkly pigmented populations, since the soles and nail beds are sites of predilection in these individuals.
5. Although rare, melanoma does develop in children. Any pigmented lesion suspicious for malignancy should be excised and submitted for histologic assessment, regardless of the patient's age.
6. Melanoma may at times be red (amelanotic). In this situation, the diagnosis of melanoma becomes difficult or impossible to establish on clinical grounds alone. The patient's history of a change to a previously stable lesion then becomes critical in guiding the physician to the correct diagnosis.

REFERRAL/CONSULTATION GUIDELINES

The management of large congenital moles requires a multidisciplinary approach and includes not only surgeons trained in the techniques of tissue expanders, grafts, and flaps but also psychologists who can help the patient and the family deal with the cosmetic burden of the condition.

Individuals with multiple or atypical moles, those with a family history of melanoma, and others at extreme risk for melanoma are best assessed and followed by physicians who deal with pigmented lesions on a daily basis.

Finally, melanoma patients with thick primary tumors are at high risk to develop systemic disease. A specialized clinic for pigmented lesions, if available, is ideally suited for the follow-up of these individuals, as it provides the trained personnel (dermatologists, surgeons, and radiation and medical oncologists) who can quickly intercede on behalf of the patient, should the need arise.

REFERENCES

1. Williams ML, Pennella R: Melanoma, melanocytic nevi, and other melanoma risk factors in children. J Pediatr 1994; 124:833–845.
2. Kelly JW, Rivers JK, MacLennan R, et al: Sunlight: A major factor associated with the development of melanocytic nevi in Australian schoolchildren. J Am Acad Dermatol 1994; 30:40–48.
3. Johnson TM, Smith JW II, Nelson BR, et al: Current therapy for cutaneous melanoma. J Am Acad Dermatol 1995; 32:689–707.
4. Coates AS, Ingvar CI, Petersen-Schaefer K, et al: Elective lymph node dissection in patients with primary melanoma of the trunk and limbs treated at the Sydney Melanoma Unit from 1960 to 1991. J Am Coll Surg 1995; 180:402–409.

CHAPTER 35

Molluscum Contagiosum

Adelaide A. Hebert and Michelle M. Goller

CLINICAL APPEARANCE

Definition

Molluscum contagiosum, a common viral disease of the skin and mucous membranes, manifests as discrete, umbilicated papules over the face, trunk, and extremities. The infection most often occurs in children; however, adults may be affected, with lesions commonly developing in the genital region. Distribution of lesions also depends on the immune status of the host as is evidenced by widespread eruptions in immunocompromised patients.

Typical Lesions and Symptoms in Children

Children tend to have lesions on the face, trunk, and extremities. Boys are affected more often than girls. Lesions are flesh-colored, occasionally translucent, dome-shaped papules that range in size from 3 to 6 mm (see Fig. 35–1 on Color Plate 14). Papules have a central umbilication or depression and an erythematous base. A white, curdlike material can be expressed from underneath the central depression. Most lesions are grouped, and generally fewer than 20 to 30 lesions are present at one time. Most cases are asymptomatic, although a few patients may experience itching or tenderness. Molluscum contagiosum may affect the eyelids and conjunctivae as well as the perioral skin and labial mucosa. Less commonly, children may be affected in the axillae, groin, perianal, perineal, and scrotal areas.

A minority of patients may have an inflammmatory reaction surrounding the lesion consisting of erythema and scaling.[1] Occasionally, papules may become inflamed either spontaneously or as a result of trauma (see Fig. 35–2 on Color Plate 14). These inflamed lesions may appear atypical with increased erythema and size and may become tender and painful. In individuals with atopic dermatitis and widespread molluscum contagiosum, lesions may become secondarily infected.

Typical Lesions in Adults

Adults with molluscum contagiosum generally have involvement of the groin area and lower abdomen. Lesions are likely to be transmitted through sexual contact. Lesion appearance is the same as in children.

Atypical Presentation or Alternative Forms

Lesions in patients with human immunodeficiency virus (HIV) infection can have an atypical appearance and a much wider distribution on the body compared with those in immunocompetent patients. In fact, the severity of molluscum contagiosum tends to be inversely related to a patient's CD4+ T-lymphocyte count.[2] Lesions commonly occur on the face (see Fig. 35–3 on Color Plate 14), trunk, and extremities. Giant lesions up to 1.5 cm may occur in immunocompromised individuals. Eruptive widespread molluscum contagiosum may occur in patients with sarcoid, leukemia, or atopic dermatitis, as well as in patients undergoing treatment with immunosuppressive agents after organ transplantation or therapeutically for various other conditions. Lesions in all these cases tend to be resistant to therapy as long as the immune system remains suppressed.

DESCRIPTION OF DISEASE

Molluscum contagiosum virus is a poxvirus, a large DNA virus that replicates in the cytoplasm of infected cells. The infection has a worldwide distribution with an incidence ranging from 2 to 8%.[3] Children are most commonly affected, boys more often than girls, with a peak incidence under 10 years of age.[3–5] One recorded outbreak had a maximal incidence at ages 3 to 6 years.[5]

Individual lesions tend to resolve spontaneously within 2 to 4 months. However, autoinoculation is common, and lesions may continue to occur from 6 months to 3 years after initial appearance. Increased numbers of lesions have been reported in children who swim frequently in public pools.[4] Lesions in immunocompromised individuals tend to persist longer and are often resistant to therapy. Unless secondarily infected, lesions resolve without scarring.

Viral particles can be seen in the infected keratinocytes on light microscopy. These are referred to as *molluscum bodies* or *Henderson-Patterson bodies* and contain cellular debris along with the viral particles. Molluscum bodies appear as ovoid eosinophilic structures in the lower cells of the stratum malpighii, increasing in size as the infected cells move toward the surface. In the horny layer, large basophilic molluscum bodies, up to 35 μm, are present. These intracytoplasmic inclusions push the nucleus to the periphery of the cell. The lesion may have a central crater where the stratum corneum has disintegrated in the center of the lesion. Intact lesions have little to no inflammation; however, in ruptured lesions, a dense mixed inflammatory response may be present that includes multinucleated giant cells.

Viral growth is confined to the epidermis, and infected cells have an increased turnover rate as they move toward the superficial epidermis. The incubation period for the virus is approximately 3 weeks to 3 months after exposure.

TREATMENT

Therapeutic Expectations

Although spontaneous resolution is the natural course of the disease, treatment of individual lesions helps to prevent autoinoculation as well as person-to-person spread. In adults with genital lesions, sexual partners should be examined and treated, if necessary. Appropriate evaluation for other sexually transmitted diseases is recommended. Molluscum contagiosum responds to local therapy in most immunocompetent individuals. Immunosuppressed individuals present a therapeutic challenge.

First-Line Therapy

Therapy is localized and aimed at destruction of individual lesions. Cryotherapy with liquid nitrogen either in a spray or on a cotton-tipped swab is used directly on the lesion. An alternative therapy involves removing the entire lesion with a curette or enucleating the central core with a curette and then treating with a caustic agent such as cantharidin. Cantharidin 0.7% (Canthacur, Pharma Science) can be applied alone, a single drop directly to each lesion. A blister will form within a day, and the lesion will subsequently slough off. This preparation may need to be repeated at 2- to 3-week intervals if lesions do not respond initially. Mucous membrane lesions, including those close to the eyes, should not be treated with cantharidin or other caustic agents. Patients should be seen within 2 to 6 weeks after initial removal in order to treat any new lesions. This period corresponds to the viral incubation period.[6]

Age Considerations

Children may require topical anesthesia in the form of lidocaine and prilocaine cream (EMLA, Astra Pharmaceuticals) applied to lesions 1 to 2 hours prior to curettage.[7] Liquid nitrogen therapy is poorly tolerated by children below the ages of 10 to 12 years, and topical blistering agents are preferred in this age group.

Alternative Therapeutic Options

1. Electrodesiccation at the center of the lesion may be effective.
2. Topical retinoic acid (Retin-A 0.05%) may resolve lesions.
3. Trichloroacetic acid 25 to 50% applied to lesions may be used as a caustic agent alone or in combination with liquid nitrogen freezing. Trichloroacetic acid 25 to 50% peel may reduce the lesion counts in patients with widespread lesions.
4. Removal of the molluscum body by one of the following techniques may be effective.
    a. Split a wooden tongue blade in half and use each half to pinch the core from the molluscum.
    b. Use a large-gauge needle to pluck out the core of the molluscum.

PITFALLS AND PROBLEMS

1. During spontaneous regression, lesions may become inflamed, resembling staphylococcal folliculitis, pyogenic granuloma, or basal cell carcinoma. Large lesions, more common in HIV-infected individuals, may resemble keratoacanthoma.
2. Lesions of cryptococcosis and histoplasmosis in HIV-infected individuals may resemble molluscum contagiosum. Any lesion with a mucoid discharge should be biopsied, and special stains should be requested.
3. Eyelid lesions and those unresponsive to topical applications are best treated with simple curettage.
4. Complications include secondary infection as well as abscess formation if the molluscum body ruptures into the dermis. Conjunctivitis and keratitis may complicate lesions involving the eyelids.
5. Therapy should be used judiciously to avoid scarring.

REFERRAL AND CONSULTATION GUIDELINES

Rarely, widespread eruptive lesions in children may require conscious sedation or even general anesthesia. The differential diagnosis for molluscum contagiosum (Table 35–1) is extensive and includes inflammatory, infectious, and malignant disorders. Improper diagnosis may result in persistent lesions unresponsive to therapies directed at molluscum contagiosum.

TABLE 35–1
Differential Diagnosis for Molluscum Contagiosum

Warts
Chickenpox (varicella)
Basal cell carcinoma
Lichen planus
Staphylococcus aureus folliculitis
Pyogenic granuloma
Keratoacanthoma
Furuncle
Cryptococcosis (immunocompromised)
Histoplasmosis (immunocompromised)

REFERENCES

1. DeOre GA, Johnson HH, Binkley GW: An eczematous reaction associated with molluscum contagiosum. Arch Dermatol 1956; 74:344–348.
2. Koopman RJJ, Van Merrienboer FCJ, Vreden SGS, Dolmans WMV: Molluscum contagiosum: A marker for advanced HIV infection. Br J Dermatol 1992; 126:528–529.
3. Gellis SE: Warts and molluscum contagiosum in children. Pediatr Ann 1987; 16:69–76.
4. Niizeki K, Kano O, Kondo Y: An epidemic study of molluscum contagiosum. Relationship to swimming. Dermatologica 1984; 169:197–198.
5. Oren B, Wende SO: An outbreak of molluscum contagiosum in a kibbutz. Infection 1991; 19:159–161.
6. Gottlieb SL, Myskowski PL: Molluscum contagiosum. Int J Dermatol 1994; 33:453–461.
7. Rosdahl I, Edmar B, Gisslen H, et al: Curettage of molluscum contagiosum in children: Analgesia by topical application of lidocaine/prilocaine cream (EMLA). Acta Derm Venereol (Stockh) 1988; 68:149–153.

CHAPTER 36

Nummular Dermatitis

Arnold W. Gurevitch

CLINICAL APPEARANCE

Definition

Nummular dermatitis is characterized by coin-shaped (discoid) patches that may vary from papulovesicular and exudative to red and scaly. This idiopathic eruption preferentially affects the extensor extremities but may be seen on the trunk.

Typical Lesions and Symptoms

The eruption characteristically begins with bright red, often edematous papules or tiny vesicles.[1] These individual lesions coalesce into small, round patches that vary in size from 1 to several centimeters. The surface may become exudative and crusted (see Fig. 36–1 on Color Plate 14). The extent of cutaneous involvement varies from a few to many such lesions, usually symmetrically distributed. The favored sites are the extensor surfaces of the lower legs and the dorsum of the feet, especially in middle-aged and elderly men. However, the upper extremities, dorsal hands, trunk, and thighs may be involved as well. With time, the acute papular and vesicular patches may develop into drier, less red, scaling patches (see Fig. 36–2 on Color Plate 14). In some patients, the initial lesions are of the latter, more chronic-appearing variety. The borders of the discoid patches are well defined. Pruritus is variable but is most often moderate to severe, leading to the presence of excoriations. Persistent scratching of the lesions may lead to hyperpigmentation and lichenification. As the eruption resolves, the erythematous component disappears first, leaving dry, scaling patches that ultimately clear.

Atypical Presentation or Alternate Forms

Occasionally, central clearing develops, and the lesions may assume an annular configuration. In 1937, Sulzberger and Garbe described a "distinctive exudative discoid and lichenoid chronic dermatosis."[2] This pruritic eruption consists of lesions varying from exudative and discoid to lichenoid to infiltrative and even urticarial. The eruption may be extensive but characteristically involves the penis and scrotum and predominates in older Jewish men. Although some of these features are somewhat distinctive, the Sulzberger-Garbe syndrome probably represents a variant of nummular dermatitis.

DESCRIPTION OF DISEASE

Idiopathic nummular dermatitis occurs in both men and women and seems to be most common over the age of 50 years. Its occurrence in younger women is noted in some reports, but these patients almost always have a nummular form of hand dermatitis, which may be a different entity. Nummular dermatitis usually responds to appropriate treatment but may recur. The pathologic changes in nummular dermatitis are those of a spongiotic dermatitis and are not specific. Therefore, skin biopsy is not usually helpful.

Some authors include a variety of disparate dermatoses, all of which may have discoid lesions, under the overall heading of *nummular dermatitis*. Others exclude those cases with a specific etiology from this category. The fact that other dermatoses may, on occasion, have discoid lesions has been a source of some confusion. Is nummular dermatitis an eczematous reaction pattern with various causes, or is it a clinical entity of unknown cause? Given the current state of our knowledge on this subject, it seems reasonable to exclude specific disorders that present with nummular lesions. Thus, atopic dermatitis with round, scaling lesions is still atopic, rather than nummular, dermatitis. However, nummular dermatitis often does occur in association with dry skin, and there may be a relationship between nummular and xerotic (asteatotic) eczema.[3, 4] An increase in bacterial colonization has also been reported in nummular dermatitis. This most likely represents a secondary event on eczematized skin rather than a primary cause.

TABLE 36–1

Treatment of Nummular Dermatitis

General Measures
Short (5–7 minutes), lukewarm bath or shower every 1–2 days
Mild cleansing agent (Dove)
Emollient over entire body (Eucerin lotion)
Avoid irritants
Avoid low humidity if possible
Specific Therapy
Milder cases—mid-potency steroid ointment twice daily
Severe or unresponsive cases—high-potency steroid ointment twice daily
Extensive involvement—systemic corticosteroid
Prednisone 40 mg/day, tapered over 3 weeks
Triamcinolone acetonide IM—40–60 mg
H_1 antihistamine (hydroxyzine, diphenhydramine) 25–50 mg BID-QID
Secondary infection—dicloxicillin, erythromycin, cephalexin monohydrate

Abbreviations: IM, intramuscular; bid, twice a day; qid, four times a day.

TREATMENT

Therapeutic Expectations

Marked improvement or total clearing of the eruption may be expected in 3 to 4 weeks. However, recurrences are common, especially if the patient does not continue to adhere to an emollient regimen.

First-Line Therapy

Treatment of nummular dermatitis involves both general and specific measures (Table 36–1). Successful therapy must take into account the patient's xerotic skin by utilizing short, lukewarm baths or showers every day to every other day. Baths are most effective. A mild skin cleansing agent, such as Dove, is recommended. Drying soaps are to be avoided. Following the bath or shower, emollient lotions should be applied over the entire skin surface. Application of emollients may be repeated as needed throughout the day. Light, thin emollients are less beneficial than thicker lotions (Eucerin lotion). If possible, irritants should be avoided, as should conditions of low humidity. Humidifying the bedroom or the entire living area is helpful during dry, cold seasons.

The most effective treatment in the majority of cases is a midpotency topical corticosteroid (triamcinolone, fluocinolone, fluticasone, or betamethasone valerate) in an ointment vehicle, applied twice daily. In severe or resistant cases, a high-potency corticosteroid ointment (amcinonide, betamethasone dipropionate, mometasone, or fluocinonide) may be used until improvement is seen. If skin involvement is extensive, topical treatment may be impractical and excessively expensive. In that event, use of a systemic corticosteroid (prednisone 40 mg per day or intramuscular triamcinolone 40 to 60 mg) is advisable. The oral steroid should be tapered off over a 3-week period, while attempting to maintain the improvement with a topical agent. In addition, H_1 antihistamines (hydroxyzine or diphenhydramine) are extremely important in attempting to control pruritus. Either of these agents may be given in doses ranging from 25 to 50 mg 2 to 4 times a day. Occasionally, especially in the elderly, even smaller doses must be utilized to avoid excessive drowsiness. In the presence of secondary infection, an antistaphylococcal antibiotic (dicloxicillin, cephalexin monohydrate, or erythromycin) is necessary.

PITFALLS AND PROBLEMS

Diagnosis is made on clinical grounds, based on the characteristic appearance and distribution of lesions. However, several other dermatoses may have nummular-appearing lesions (Table 36–2). Atopic dermatitis with discoid lesions is not infrequent in infants and children and may be excluded by the presence of a personal or familial atopic history as well as the presence or history of typical atopic dermatitis in other areas. Allergic contact dermatitis tends to be less symmetric, and the lesions are usually not as round. A history of contact exposure may often be elicited. Num-

TABLE 36-2

Differential Diagnoses of Nummular Dermatitis

Common	Uncommon
Atopic dermatitis, nummular type	Mycosis fungoides
Allergic contact dermatitis	Lichen planus
Irritant contact dermatitis (nummular hand eczema)	Dermatitis herpetiformis
Psoriasis	Parapsoriasis en plaques
Tinea corporis	Bowen's disease
Autoeczematization (ID reaction)	Superficial basal cell carcinoma
	Herald spot, pityriasis rosea

mular eruptions limited to the hands are frequently forms of irritant dermatitis. Psoriasis is more sharply marginated, with a thicker white scale and less pruritus. Tinea corporis may be excluded by a negative potassium hydroxide preparation of scales. Autoeczematization is an acute eruption, sometimes discoid in shape, that is secondary to a preexisting localized severe dermatitis, most commonly stasis dermatitis. Bowen's disease, an in situ form of squamous cell carcinoma, usually presents with a solitary erythematous scaling patch that enlarges slowly and does not respond to either topical corticosteroids or antifungals. Superficial basal cell carcinomas are also well-defined red, scaling patches and may be single or multiple. There is usually a fine, threadlike pearly border. The herald spot of pityriasis rosea may be mistaken for nummular dermatitis.

REFERRAL AND CONSULTATION GUIDELINES

A lack of response to therapy may indicate an improper diagnosis. The differential diagnosis is extensive and includes other eczematous and inflammatory eruptions, as well as tinea corporis, mycosis fungoides (cutaneous T-cell lymphoma), and forms of skin cancer. If the eruption has not responded after 1 month of treatment, additional tests including a biopsy may be necessary.

REFERENCES

1. Weidman AI, Sawicky HH: Nummular eczema. Arch Dermatol 1956; 73:58–65.
2. Sulzberger MB, Garbe W: Nine cases of a distinctive exudative discoid and lichenoid chronic dermatosis. Arch Dermatol Syphilol 1937; 36:247–272.
3. Gross P: Nummular eczema: Its clinical picture and successful therapy. Arch Dermatol Syphilol 1941; 44:1060–1077.
4. Bettoli V, Tosti A, Varotti C: Nummular eczema during isotretinoin treatment [Letter]. Arch Dermatol 1987; 16:617.

CHAPTER 37

Perioral Dermatitis

Steven M. Manders

CLINICAL APPEARANCE

Definition

Perioral dermatitis is an acute or subacute inflammatory disorder characterized by erythematous papules and pustules distributed periorally, paranasally, or periorbitally. It may arise de novo or can be associated with the use of mid- to high-potency topical corticosteroids on the face. Perioral dermatitis affects both men and women but is most frequent in females in the third and fourth decades of life. Pediatric cases are not uncommon in both sexes.

Typical Lesions and Symptoms

Perioral dermatitis presents with erythematous micropapules and vesicopustules on a variably present background of erythema and scale. The distribution is typically perioral (Fig. 37–1), with a margin of normal skin between the vermilion border and the affected skin. Although classically described around the mouth, lesions are often present adjacent to the nose and eyes.[1] Pruritus is absent; however, a burning sensation may be described.

Atypical Forms

Although the presentation of perioral dermatitis in childhood is similar to that of the adult form, a granulomatous variant has been described in children. This form is characterized by skin-colored ''micronodules,'' histologically by granuloma formation, and therapeutically by a variable response to treatment.[2]

DESCRIPTION OF DISEASE

Demographics

Perioral dermatitis occurs primarily in young women, with an average age of onset between 25 and 35 years of age. In childhood, the gender preference is not as strong.[1]

Natural History

Perioral dermatitis is usually self-limited, but it may take months to years to resolve without treatment.

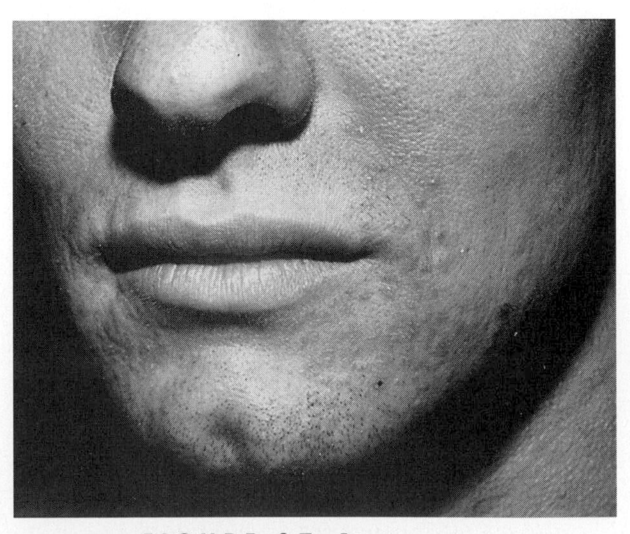

FIGURE 37–1
Micropapules in a perioral distribution.

Pathology

The histopathology of the common form of perioral dermatitis is not specific, and skin biopsy is rarely necessary. As the granulomatous form may mimic sarcoidosis clinically, biopsy can be helpful. Granulomas in perioral dermatitis are characterized by a more prominent lymphocytic component, whereas sarcoidal granulomas usually have few lymphocytes.

Etiology/Pathogenesis

Multiple etiologies for perioral dermatitis have been proposed. The best documented etiology has been the application of potent topical corticosteroids to the face, directly analagous to ''steroid rosacea.'' Mid- to high-potency topical steroids are often initially applied to a mild preexisting eruption, such as an irritant dermatitis, with initial improvement. However, with repeated application, the continued use of topical corticosteroid then leads to the secondary side effect of perioral dermatitis. Other etiologic factors that may be important in certain cases include the use of tartar-control toothpaste.[3]

TREATMENT

Therapeutic Expectations

Perioral dermatitis usually requires 1 to 3 months of topical, oral, or combination therapy. An early rebound flare is common during treatment if a potent topical steroid must be discontinued. The granulomatous variant may take months to years to resolve. Resolution of perioral dermatitis is usually, but not always, long-lasting.

First-Line Therapy

Prompt discontinuation of mid- to high-potency topical corticosteroids is fundamental to treatment. Mild to moderate cases may be treated with topical metronidazole (MetroGel, MetroCream) twice daily. Resistant, or more severe, cases of perioral dermatitis in persons over the age of 8 years may be treated with tetracycline, 250 to 500 mg two to three times daily, or minocycline (Minocin, Dynacin), 50 to 100 mg twice daily.

Age Considerations

In children, the preferred treatment is topical metronidazole. If oral treatment is necessary in a child younger than 8 years of age, erythromycin, 125 to 250 mg twice daily, is suggested.

Alternative Therapeutic Options

1. *Low*-potency steroid creams (hydrocortisone [Hytone 2.5%], alclometasone [Aclovate], desonide [DesOwen]), twice daily.
2. Erythromycin gel (Erygel, Emgel, A/T/S), twice daily.
3. Oral erythromycin (E-Mycin, ERYC, Ery-Tab PCE), 250 to 333 g twice daily.

PITFALLS AND PROBLEMS

Perioral dermatitis may look clinically similar to the micropapular form of sarcoidosis. In addition, cutaneous T-cell lymphoma may rarely resemble perioral dermatitis.[4]

For the large subset of patients in whom perioral dermatitis is due to potent topical steroids, patient education is often necessary to avoid a return to self-medication with steroids during the expected rebound period. Despite temporary improvement with stronger or more frequent topical steroid use, the patient needs to be made aware of the eventual permanent side effects of continued use (atrophy, telangiectasia, and striae).

An uncommon, but important, simulant of perioral dermatitis (especially with a prominent scaling and erythematous component) in children is seen in the setting of nutritional deficiency, such as zinc deficiency (acrodermatitis enteropathica). Determination of serum zinc levels may be necessary to distinguish among these conditions.

TABLE 37-1

Differential Diagnosis of Perioral Dermatitis

Acne rosacea
Acne vulgaris
Acrodermatitis enteropathica
Bockhart's impetigo
Candidiasis
Contact dermatitis
Cutaneous T-cell lymphoma
Demodicosis
Eosinophilic pustular folliculitis
Sarcoidosis
Seborrheic dermatitis

REFERRAL/CONSULTATION GUIDELINES

Lack of therapeutic response may be due to occasional treatment resistance, continued surreptitious topical steroid use, or misdiagnosis. The differential diagnosis includes inflammatory, infectious, neoplastic, and nutritional disorders (Table 37–1), each of which has a distinct therapy.

REFERENCES

1. Manders SM, Lucky AW: Perioral dermatitis in childhood. J Am Acad Dermatol 1992; 27:688–692.
2. Frieden IJ, Prose NS, Fletcher V, et al: Granulomatous perioral dermatitis in children. Arch Dermatol 1989; 125:369–373.
3. Beacham BE, Kurgansky D, Gould WM: Circumoral dermatitis and cheilitis caused by tartar control dentifrices. J Am Acad Dermatol 1990; 22:1029–1032.
4. Amann U, Mielke V, Metze D, et al: Perioral eczema as a manifestation of cutaneous T-cell lymphoma. Br J Dermatol 1995; 132:671–673.

CHAPTER 38

Pityriasis Rosea

Daniella Duke

CLINICAL APPEARANCE

Definition

Pityriasis rosea (PR) is an acute, benign inflammatory skin disease of unknown etiology that has a distinctive clinical appearance. The eruption starts with one plaque and then secondarily becomes generalized, may have prodromal symptoms, resolves after several weeks, has no long-term sequelae, and has lifelong immunity in 98% of patients.

Typical Lesions and Symptoms

For many patients, PR is preceded by prodromal symptoms such as sore throat, malaise, joint pain, fever, nausea, loss of appetite, headache, or gastrointestinal upset. In 50 to 90% of patients, a primary lesion, or herald patch, is present (see Fig. 38–1 on Color Plate 15). The herald patch, larger than the lesions of the secondary eruption, is usually located on the trunk. It is a few centimeters in diameter, salmon-pink, oval to round, with a fine collarette of scale at the periphery of the lesion. Some lesions are more inflamed and therefore appear papulovesicular and eczematous.

Two to 10 days after the herald patch, smaller but similar-appearing lesions develop in crops on the trunk, neck, and extremities. Lesions distal to the knees and elbows are less common, and the face is usually spared. The lesions are arranged in a "Christmas-tree" distribution, following the natural skin lines. The duration of the rash is 2 to 10 weeks. Either hypopigmentation or hyperpigmentation may persist after the rash has resolved. In addition to the prodromal symptoms, pruritus is present in up to 50% of patients.

Atypical Presentation

Several variations in the presentation of PR exist. Atypical lesions have minimal to no scale, resemble erythema multiforme or psoriasis, involve the palms and soles, or are urticarial, vesicular, follicular-based, papular, pustular, or purpuric. The herald patch may be absent or may be the only manifestation of the disease. Facial, oral, and vulvar lesions are uncommon yet have been reported. Oral lesions consist of red patches and plaques, hemorrhagic puncta, confluent white erosions, annular lesions, and desquamation. In PR inversa, patients have more peripheral than central lesions. Localized PR, or pityriasis circinata et marginata of Vidal, occurs on limited parts of the body.

DESCRIPTION OF DISEASE

Epidemiology

Most patients with PR are between the ages of 10 and 43 years, although PR has been reported in the very young (3 months) and the elderly. Total population incidence is estimated at 0.13 to 0.14%. PR is equally common in men and women, although PR incidence ratios of men to women vary from 2:1 to 0.55:1.[1] PR occurs in any climate or season yet has an increased incidence during the spring and autumn.

Etiology

The etiology of PR is unknown. Because the disease course is similar to that of a viral exanthem, several researchers have studied the possibility that PR is an infectious disease. Furthermore, clustering studies suggest that PR occurs at a higher incidence in groups of people who live or work together. Researchers have looked for evidence of a viral or bacterial infection: picornavirus-like particles, mycoplasma-like structures, Epstein-Barr virus, adenovirus, streptococci, spirochetes, and other species, yet no data are definitive.[2]

A hypersensitivity reaction is another proposed pathogenic process of PR. Certain drugs have been associated with a PR-like eruption: captopril, gold, arsenicals, bismuth compounds, clonidine, mercury, barbiturates, D-penicillamine, isotretinoin, and others.[3]

TREATMENT

Therapeutic Expectations

PR is a self-limited disease, and no treatment is usually necessary. The duration of the disease is 2 to 10 weeks. Postinflammatory pigmentary changes may persist beyond activity of the disease.

First-Line Therapy

If the patient is very itchy and uncomfortable, the pruritus can be treated with topical antipruritic therapies such as calamine lotion, topical antihistamines (doxepin [Zonalon]), or a mentholated lotion (Sarna). A brief course of topical potent steroids can be used to treat inflammation, if necessary. Other therapies useful in more severe instances include ultraviolet B light therapy for more extreme pruritus,[4] oral corticosteroids (15-day prednisone taper, starting with 40 to 60 mg/day) for severely inflammatory or vesicular PR, and on occasion, dapsone. Irrespective of the type of treatment used, postinflammatory hyperpigmentation may take weeks to months to clear.

PITFALL AND PROBLEMS

The importance of establishing the diagnosis of PR is that other cutaneous diseases that resemble PR have different etiologies, long-term consequences, and treatments. The diagnosis of PR curtails an extensive workup and unnecessary therapeutic trials.

Other diseases that may occur in a Christmas-tree distribution include erythema dyschromicum perstans, lichen planus, pityriasis lichenoides, and Kaposi's sarcoma. Other PR-like rashes include: drug eruption, Gianotti-Crosti syndrome, guttate psoriasis, secondary syphilis, pityriasis lichenoides varioliform et acuta, erythema annulare centrifigum, eczema, scabies infestation, seborrheic dermatitis, and tinea corporis. The workup of a rash suspected of being PR should include a potassium hydroxide preparation completed to exclude dermatophyte infection; when relevant, a Venereal Disease Research Laboratory (VDRL) test to rule out secondary syphilis; and a thorough drug history.

REFERRAL GUIDELINES

A patient should be referred to a dermatologist if the diagnosis of PR is uncertain, if PR is the working diagnosis but the patient is getting worse or not improving over several weeks, or if phototherapy is the treatment of choice.

REFERENCES

1. Bjornberg A, Hellgren I: Pityriasis rosea: A statistical, clinical and laboratory investigation of 826 patients and matched healthy controls. Acta Derm Venereol 1962; 42(Suppl 50):1–68.
2. Parsons JM: Pityriasis rosea update: 1986. J Am Acad Dermatol 1986; 15:159–167.
3. Wilkin JK, Kirkendall WM: Pityriasis rosea–like rash from captopril. Arch Dermatol 1982; 118(3):186–187.
4. Arndt KA, Paul BS, Stern RS, Parrish JA: Treatment of pityriasis rosea with UV radiation. Arch Dermatol 1983; 119(5):381–382.

CHAPTER 39

Pregnancy Rashes

Lisa M. Cohen

During pregnancy, a number of cutaneous changes occur. Hyperpigmentation of the nipples, areolae, vulva, and linea alba, the latter producing the linea nigra, is common. Melanocytic nevi often darken, and patchy brown pigmentation may develop on the malar cheeks, known as *melasma* (''the mask of pregnancy'') (Fig. 39–1). Patients may experience striae distensae (stretch marks), hirsutism, acne, hair loss, increased sweating, and flushing. Vascular changes include the development of spider hemangiomas, palmar erythema, varicosities, hemorrhoids, and pyogenic granulomas (a benign granulation tissue–like growth, also called *granuloma gravidarum*). Certain skin diseases may be aggravated by pregnancy (Table 39–1).[1]

The specific dermatoses of pregnancy include pruritic urticarial papules and plaques of pregnancy (PUPPP), herpes gestationis (HG), and intrahepatic cholestasis of pregnancy (ICP). The clinical features, pathophysiology, histopathology, treatment, and prognosis of each of these entities are discussed.

PRURITIC URTICARIAL PAPULES AND PLAQUES OF PREGNANCY

CLINICAL APPEARANCE

Definition

PUPPP, also called *toxic erythema of pregnancy* and *polymorphic eruption of pregnancy,* is an eruption that occurs predominantly in primigravidas in their third trimester. Resolution occurs spontaneously soon after delivery.

Typical Lesions and Symptoms

Patients often present with pruritus and erythema within the striae. As the name implies, the primary lesions are urticarial papules and plaques that occur initially on the lower abdomen, often within the striae, and may spread

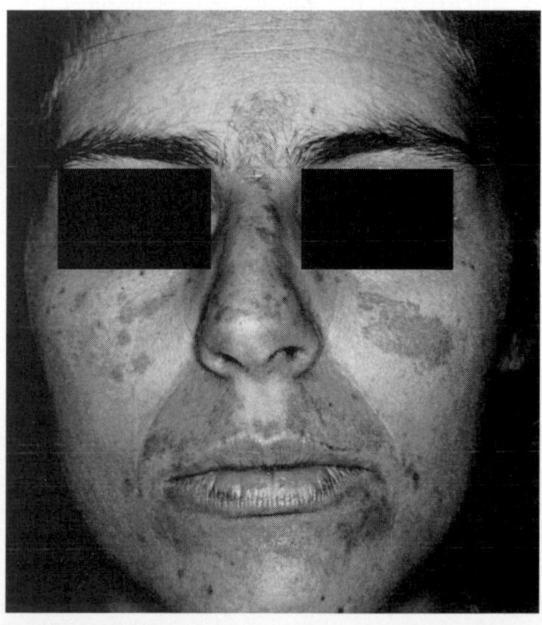

FIGURE 39–1
Macular hyperpigmentation of the glabella, cheeks, upper lip, and chin, characteristic for melasma.

TABLE 39-1

Skin Diseases Aggravated by Pregnancy

Infections
Candida vaginitis
Trichomoniasis
Condylomata acuminata
Herpes simplex
Varicella zoster
Acquired immunodeficiency syndrome
Immunologic Diseases
Collagen vascular diseases
Pemphigus
Erythema nodosum
Metabolic Diseases
Porphyria cutanea tarda
Acrodermatitis enteropathica
Miscellaneous
Mycosis fungoides
Neurofibromatosis
Malignant melanoma

Modified from Winton GB. Skin diseases aggravated in pregnancy. J Am Acad Dermatol 1989; 20:1–13.

to involve the chest, breasts, back, and extremities (Fig. 39–2). Perilesional halos are common. Moderate to severe pruritus is a constant feature. The palms, soles, face, and mucous membranes are spared.

Atypical Lesions

Only 10 to 15% of patients have umbilical lesions. Pinpoint vesicles are seen in about one third of cases, but the presence of bullae (blisters larger than 5 mm) rules out a diagnosis of PUPPP. Target lesions and polycyclic erythema each may be present in 10 to 20% of patients. Excoriations are uncommon despite severe pruritus.

DESCRIPTION OF DISEASE

Population/Demographics

The reported incidence of PUPPP is approximately 1 in 300 pregnancies. In 70 to 80% of cases, patients are primigravidas. Most cases begin in the third trimester, in the 35th week on average. The lesions begin in the postpartum period in 10 to 15% of patients, and occasionally, the eruption flares after delivery. The incidence of twin pregnancies is 10 to 20% in patients with PUPPP, as compared with 1.2% in the general population.[2, 3]

Natural History

The eruption typically resolves spontaneously within days of delivery, and symptoms may improve in the immediate postpartum period. There is no risk to the mother or infant. Recurrence in subsequent pregnancy is uncommon.

Pathology

The histopathology of PUPPP is nonspecific, and most patients are not subjected to skin biopsy to confirm the

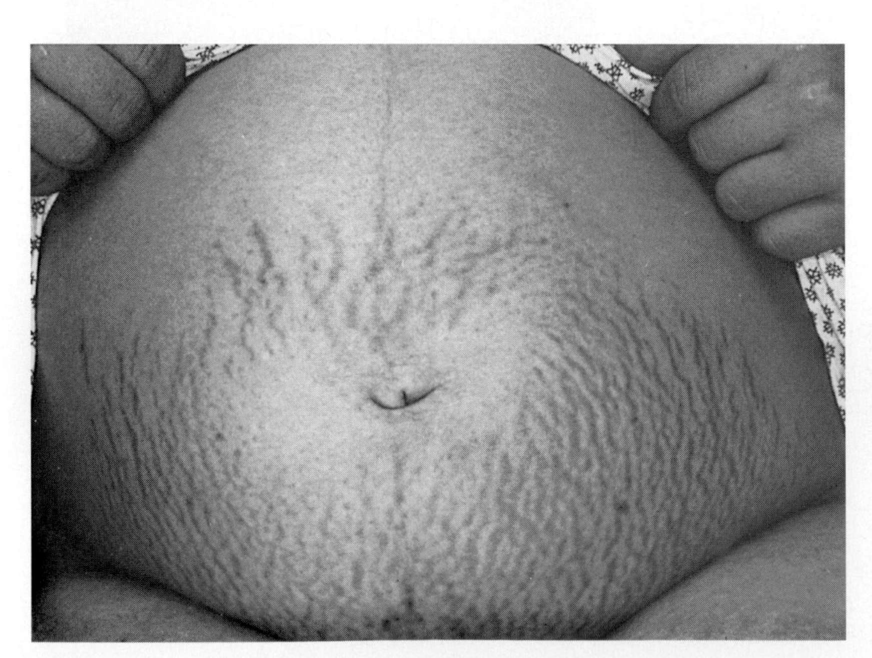

FIGURE 39-2

Urticarial papules, confluent plaques, and prominent striae of the abdomen, with sparing of the periumbilical area, characteristic for pruritic urticarial papules and plaques of pregnancy. Note also the linea nigra.

diagnosis. Papillary dermal edema and a perivascular, dermal lymphohistiocytic infiltrate with eosinophils are the most constant histopathologic features in PUPPP. Epidermal changes, such as spongiosis, parakeratosis, and crust, may also be seen. Direct immunofluorescence (IF) is negative.

Etiology/Pathogenesis

The etiology of PUPPP is unknown. Abdominal distention has been suggested in the pathogenesis of PUPPP, because the disease occurs in the third trimester of primigravidas, with a predilection for the striae, and because of the increased maternal weight gain, fetal birth weight, and rate of twinning.[2] There is no known association with hormone levels (β–human chorionic gonadotropin, estradiol, cortisol, urinary estriol) or human leukocyte antigen (HLA) type, and autoantibodies have not been detected.

TREATMENT

Since PUPPP resolves spontaneously after delivery, the treatment is conservative. Many patients derive symptomatic relief from emollients and lotions, midpotency topical corticosteroids, and oral antihistamines. Over-the-counter preparations that may be soothing include 1% hydrocortisone cream, camphor and menthol (Sarna) lotion, and colloidal oatmeal (Aveeno) baths. Pramoxine (Prax cream or lotion) alone or in combination with hydrocortisone (Pramosone cream, 0.5%, 1.0%, or 2.5%) may be applied three to four times daily. Midpotency topical corticosteroids such as triamcinolone (Aristocort cream 0.1%) or fluocinonide (Lidex cream 0.05%) may be used twice daily. Chorpheniramine (Chlor-Trimeton Allergy, 1 tablet every 4 to 6 hours), hydroxyzine (Atarax 10 to 25 mg every 6 hours), or diphenhydramine (Benadryl 25 mg every 6 hours) are useful oral antihistamines but may cause sedation. For severe, recalcitrant cases, oral prednisone (20 to 40 mg per day) may be required.

PITFALLS AND PROBLEMS

It is extremely important to rule out herpes gestationis (HG), a less common dermatosis of pregnancy. Although most patients with HG have bullae, some women present with urticarial lesions indistinguishable from PUPPP. Skin biopsies from lesional skin for light microscopy and perilesionally for direct IF (negative in PUPPP but positive in HG) confirm the diagnosis. Although some authors feel that IF confirmation in all cases is prudent, this author believes that, in most cases, PUPPP and HG can be distinguished by history, demographic characteristics, and physical examination.

In addition to HG, the differential diagnosis includes eczematous dermatitis, such as contact or atopic dermatitis (although the latter often improves in pregnancy); drug eruption; arthropod bites; scabies; idiopathic urticaria; and viral exanthem.

The benefits of symptomatic relief to the mother must be balanced with possible risks of therapy to the fetus. Oral antihistamines such as diphenhydramine and chlorpheniramine are generally considered safe during pregnancy. Corticosteroids applied topically to extensive areas or taken orally can lead to adrenal axis suppression in the newborn.

REFERRAL AND CONSULTATION GUIDELINES

Any woman who has vesiculobullous lesions or an atypical presentation should have a biopsy for light microscopy and IF to rule out a diagnosis of HG.

HERPES GESTATIONIS

CLINICAL APPEARANCE

Definition

HG is a pruritic eruption of pregnancy that is characterized primarily by vesicles and bullae. The lesions often begin at the umbilicus and spread to the trunk and extremities. Antibodies are directed against the basement membrane zone (BMZ). Hence, HG is an immune-mediated bullous disease with many similarities to bullous pemphigoid (BP) and bears no relationship to herpesvirus.

Typical Lesions and Symptoms

Patients often have urticarial papules and plaques at onset, but 95% will develop tense vesicles and bullae as the disease advances. Polycyclic erythema and target lesions are common, but prominent striae are extremely rare. Lesions commonly involve the umbilicus, and in many patients, it is the first site of involvement (Fig. 39–3). Most patients develop severely pruritic, generalized vesiculobullous lesions as the eruption progresses.

Atypical Forms

In about 5% of cases, patients have only pruritic papules and plaques, and thus, the disease is indistinguishable from PUPPP. Although most patients with HG are truly pregnant, women with hydatidiform moles (molar pregnancies) occasionally develop the disease.

DESCRIPTION OF DISEASE

Population/Demographics

HG occurs in 1 in 40,000 pregnancies. Unlike PUPPP, only 30% of patients are primigravidas. The mean onset is 21 weeks, and whereas most patients develop lesions during the late second or early third trimester, the eruption may begin at any time during pregnancy or postpartum.[4]

Natural History

A postpartum flare occurs in about 75% of patients. Unlike PUPPP, the disease does not regress immediately postpartum and can persist for more than 1 year after delivery.[5] Exacerbation may recur with menstruation and use of oral contraceptives, and more than 90% of patients have recurrence in subsequent pregnancies. The disease often recurs earlier and more severely with each pregnancy.

Although early studies reported an increased risk of fetal death, stillbirth, and spontaneous abortion, the largest study found only an increase in prematurity and a tendency for small-for-gestational-age babies.[6] Blisters are present in about 5% of newborns but heal shortly after birth without sequelae.[5]

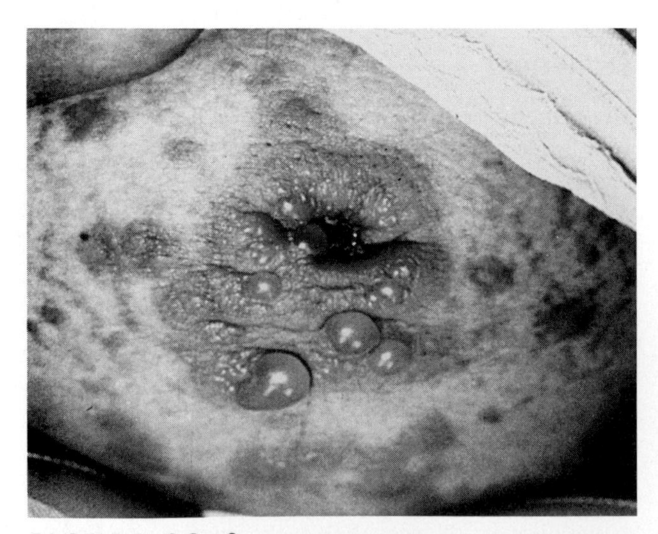

FIGURE 39-3
A patient with herpes gestationis, showing the periumbilical plaques and tense bullae typical of this disease.

Pathology

The biopsy from a patient with HG shows marked papillary dermal edema and a perivascular infiltrate with eosinophils. Eosinophils are commonly seen within the epidermis (eosinophilic spongiosis). If a vesicle is biopsied, it may be subepidermal or intraepidermal. Direct IF reveals linear C3 along the BMZ in 100% of cases, and immunoglobulin G (IgG) in about 25%. Using indirect, complement-added techniques, IgG may be identified in the majority of cases.

Etiology/Pathogenesis

HG is characterized by a circulating IgG1 (''HG factor'') that binds a 180-kd protein (BP minor antigen) in the lamina lucida of the BMZ. This triggers the classic complement pathway, eosinophil chemotaxis and deposition of complement along the BMZ. Eosinophils degranulate and release proteolytic enzymes, leading to epidermal-dermal separation and blister formation. The IgG1 is capable of crossing the placenta and fixing complement.

Although the etiology is unknown, genetic and immunologic mechanisms, paternal antigens and abnormalities of the amniotic BMZ have all been proposed. Patients with HG are much more likely than controls to have the combination of HLA-DR3 and -DR4 (relative risk = 23.5).[7] Patients with HG have a 10% incidence of Graves' disease, and 25% of their families have thyroid disease.[8] The same 180-kd protein found in the skin is found in the BMZ of the placental amnion and chorion.

TREATMENT

Topical corticosteroids and oral antihistamines are ineffective at reducing blister formation or pruritus. The first line of therapy is systemic corticosteroids such as oral prednisone, starting at 0.5 to 1.0 mg/kg/day. The goal is to treat with the lowest dosage that suppresses lesions and to taper gradually as tolerated. Since many patients have postpartum exacerbations, an increased dose after delivery should be anticipated. Dapsone, plasmapheresis, pyridoxine, gold, methotrexate, and cyclophosphamide have also been used with variable results.

PITFALLS AND PROBLEMS

The differential diagnosis of an urticarial or papulovesicular eruption includes PUPPP, urticarial drug eruption, contact dermatitis, arthropod bite reaction, scabies, or a viral exanthem. The presence of bullae is helpful in establishing a diagnosis of HG, but IF is required for confirmation. The differential diagnosis in a patient with bullae includes BP, linear immunoglobulin A (IgA) bullous dermatosis, epidermolysis bullosa acquisita, bullous drug eruption, generalized herpesvirus infection, and pemphigus vulgaris. Although patients with BP are older, HG is otherwise indistinguishable from BP.

One must weigh the risks and benefits of therapy. Systemic corticosteroids can cause adrenal axis suppression in the newborn.

REFERRAL AND CONSULTATION GUIDELINES

Once the diagnosis of HG is established, the patient should be continued on systemic corticosteroids until resolution of vesiculobullous lesions. Patients may require treatment for weeks to months after delivery. The disease usually recurs in subsequent pregnancies. The patient should be referred if the diagnosis is in doubt or if therapy fails to clear the eruption.

INTRAHEPATIC CHOLESTASIS OF PREGNANCY

CLINICAL APPEARANCE

Definition

ICP produces severe generalized pruritus owing to elevated serum bile acids. Symptoms may begin at any time during pregnancy and resolve within 48 hours of delivery. A patient with ''pruritus gravidarum'' has a similar disorder but has a normal bilirubin.

Typical Lesions and Symptoms

There are no primary lesions, and the clinical presentation consists of generalized excoriations. Symptoms may begin on the hands and feet and spread centripetally, sparing only the mucous membranes. Pruritus is typically severe, most severe at night, and correlates with the level of serum bile acids. Mild jaundice occurs in about 20% of patients.[9] Patients may develop nausea and vomiting.

DESCRIPTION OF DISEASE

Population/Demographics

The incidence of ICP is significantly higher in Chile and the Scandinavian countries (3 to 14%) than in North America (1 in 1293 pregnancies), which may be attributed to genetic or cultural differences. There is a family history in one third of cases. Patients may develop symptoms as early as their second or third month of pregnancy, but 80% develop pruritus only after 30 weeks.[9]

Natural History

There is no effective treatment, and symptoms abate within 48 hours of delivery. Abnormal serum bile acids and liver function tests normalize within 4 weeks. In about 50% of patients, the disease recurs in subsequent pregnancy. Rarely, recurrence occurs with use of oral contraceptives.

The fetal risk is controversial, but some authors report an increased risk of stillbirth or premature birth. Patients with ICP are two to three times more likely to develop cholelithiasis. Postpartum hemorrhage may occur, perhaps owing to vitamin K deficiency.

Pathology/Laboratory Abnormalities

Skin biopsy is usually not necessary and will show only nonspecific excoriation. There is an elevation in fasting total serum bile acids (150 to 4000 μg/100 ml; normal ≤60), cholesterol, other lipids, alkaline phosphatase, and transaminases. Bilirubin is mildly to moderately elevated. Liver biopsy reveals mild cholestasis, showing intracellular bile pigment and canalicular bile plugs. Examination of the placenta may reveal edematous villi, degenerative changes, or infarcts, thus causing fetal hypoxia or malnutrition.

Etiology/Pathogenesis

Elevated serum bile acids and, thus, increased bile acids in the skin lead to severe pruritus. Although the etiology is unknown, genetic factors are thought to be important. Increased estrogen production or abnormal hepatic response to a physiologic increase of estrogens may contribute to cholestasis by decreasing bile flow. In addition, there may be decreased estrogen or progesterone excretion in the bile.

TREATMENT

Treatment is usually ineffective, and symptoms abate within hours to days of delivery. Phenobarbital, cholestyramine, sulfathiazole, ursodeoxycholic acid, and ion exchange resin have all been used with variable success. Emollients, camphor and menthol lotion, and colloidal oatmeal baths are over-the-counter preparations and may be used two to three times daily for symptomatic relief. Pramoxine (Prax cream or lotion) alone or in combination with hydrocortisone (Pramasone cream, 0.5%, 1.0%, or 2.5%) may be applied three to four times daily. Oral antihistamines, such as chorpheniramine (Chlor-Trimeton Allergy, 1 tablet every 4 to 6 hours), hydroxyzine (Atarax 10 to 25 mg every 6 hours), or diphenhydramine (Benadryl 25 mg every 6 hours) may be useful.

PITFALLS AND PROBLEMS

The goal is to keep the patient as comfortable as possible until delivery and to minimize the risk to the fetus. The benefits of therapy should be weighed against its risks. The differential diagnosis includes viral hepatitis, acute fatty liver of pregnancy, biliary tract obstruction, primary biliary cirrhosis, and other cholestatic disorders.

REFERRAL AND CONSULTATION GUIDELINES

Patients with elevated liver function tests in whom the diagnosis is in question should be referred to a gastroenterologist for evaluation.

REFERENCES

1. Winton GB: Skin diseases aggravated in pregnancy. J Am Acad Dermatol 1989; 20:1–13.
2. Cohen LM, Capeless EL, Krusinski PA, et al: Pruritic urticarial papules and plaques of pregnancy and its relationship to maternal-fetal weight gain and twin pregnancy. Arch Dermatol 1989; 125:1534–1536.
3. Yancey KB, Hall RP, Lawley TJ: Pruritic urticarial papules and plaques of pregnancy. Clinical experience in twenty-five patients. J Am Acad Dermatol 1984; 10:473–480.
4. Shornick JK, Bangert JL, Freeman RG, et al: Herpes gestationis: Clinical and histologic features of twenty-eight cases. J Am Acad Dermatol 1983; 8:214–224.
5. Holmes RC, Black MM, Dann J, et al: A comparative study of toxic erythema of pregnancy and herpes gestationis. Br J Dermatol 1982; 106:499–510.
6. Shornick JK, Black MM: Fetal risks in herpes gestationis. J Am Acad Dermatol 1992; 26:63–68.
7. Shornick JK, Stastny P, Gilliam JN: High frequency of histocompatibility antigens HLA-DR3 and -DR4 in herpes gestationis. J Clin Invest 1981; 68:553–555.
8. Shornick JK, Black MM: Secondary autoimmune diseases in herpes gestationis (pemphigoid gestationis). J Am Acad Dermatol 1992; 26:563–566.
9. Reyes H: The spectrum of liver and gastrointestinal disease seen in cholestasis of pregnancy. Gastroenterol Clin North Am 1992; 21:905–921.

CHAPTER 40

Psoriasis

Robert S. Stern

CLINICAL APPEARANCE

Definition

Psoriasis is a chronic, inflammatory, scaling disorder of the skin that may also occasionally involve mucous membranes. These scaling plaques are due to epidermal hyperproliferation. Immunologic factors may play an important role in this chronic cutaneous disorder. The severity of psoriasis can vary greatly from a few small red scaling patches to whole-body erythroderma (see Chapter 55: Erythroderma. Psoriasis is a genetically determined disease, but not all affected patients have affected relatives. Early onset is associated with more severe disease and a higher risk of developing arthritis. Psoriatic arthritis is an inflammatory oligoarthritis that may be disabling.

Typical Lesions

Psoriasis may vary in morphology and distribution. By far, the most common psoriasis is plaque-type. This is characterized by erythematous, well-demarcated scaling plaques that may occur anywhere on the body (see Figs. 40–1 through 40–3 on Color Plate 15). Areas of predilection include elbows, knees, and buttocks. In addition, scaling plaques on the scalp (see Fig. 40–4 on Color Plate 15) as well as the red plaques in intertriginous areas and on the central face, which may be indistinguishable from those of seborrheic dermatitis (see Chapter 44: Seborrheic Dermatitis), often occur. Nail changes, as described later, are common to all types of psoriasis.

The lesions may be asymptomatic or pruritic. When they become dried and fissured, they may be painful and secondary infection can be a problem. Bleeding can also occur as scale is removed. The plaques can become very hyperkeratotic and have an asbestos-like quality (see Fig. 40–2 on Color Plate 15). Nail changes in psoriasis range from small pits, small indentations in the nail plate, to onycholysis (separation of the nail plate from nail bed), as well as accumulation of subungual debris and general nail dystrophy (see Fig. 40–5 on Color Plate 15). Yellow discoloration of the nail, known as *oil streaks,* may also occur. Nail changes are common to all types of psoriasis.

Alternative Forms

Guttate Psoriasis

Patients with no past history of psoriasis or mild psoriasis may suddenly have eruptions of hundreds to thousands of small, red, scaly papules. This is known as *guttate psoriasis,* and it often follows a streptococcal infection. Once cleared, many patients who experience acute guttate psoriasis usually have limited or no evidence of psoriasis for prolonged periods of time.

Pustular Psoriasis

Although classic psoriasis presents as scaling plaques, occasionally patients may develop sterile pustules on a background of erythema (see Fig. 40–6 on Color Plate 16). This may be generalized (acute von Zumbush's generalized pustular psoriasis) or localized pustular psoriasis that most commonly involves the palms and soles. This latter condition is often termed *palmoplantar pustulosis.* Patients with acute generalized pustular psoriasis often have fever and may be acutely ill and require hospitalization. Withdrawal of systemic steroids may trigger pustular psoriasis in an individual who previously suffered from plaque-type psoriasis.

Erythrodermic Psoriasis

Erythrodermic psoriasis is characterized by whole-body redness and scaling. The affected individual may have a fever, chills, and an electrolyte imbalance and is often acutely ill. This may be a presenting form of psoriasis, but it occurs more often in individuals with chronic psoriasis following infection or exposure to certain drugs, including withdrawal of systemic steroids.

Psoriatic Arthritis

Psoriatic arthritis occurs in 15 to 25% of affected individuals. It is a seronegative spondyloarthropathy. Most often, the fingers, toes, knees, and ankles are involved. Spondylitis is also often noted. During acute flares, swelling of affected digits (sausage digits) occurs. Characteristic radiographic findings including the ''pencil-in-cup'' deformity may be seen.

DESCRIPTION OF DISEASE

Demographics

One to 2% of adults of European ancestry have psoriasis. The frequency of this disease is substantially lower among Asian, Native American, and most African populations. The onset of disease may occur at any age, but the typical age of onset is between ages 15 and 50 years. Early onset is associated with more severe disease and a stronger family history of the disease.

Natural History of the Disease

Once the disease develops in an individual, it is likely to wax and wane over the remainder of that person's lifetime. Most individuals affected by the disease will have plaque-type psoriasis covering less than 5% of the body area, but some persons may develop involvement of entire body surfaces or erythroderma. Although individual lesions will often respond to therapy, recurrences are the rule.

Pathology

The histologic changes seen in psoriasis reflect its pathophysiology. There is epidermal thickening as well as elongation of rete ridges. There is change in epidermal maturation with loss of the granular layer and extensive parakeratotic scale. The papillary dermal vessels proliferate and there is perivascular infiltrate composed chiefly of lymphocytes. Polymorphonuclear leukocytes are also seen within dermal vessels and may form intraepidermal spongiform pustules.

Etiology

The predilection to develop psoriasis is almost certainly genetically determined, but the precise mode of inheritance or other factors that trigger the expression of this disease are not known. Lithium, systemic steroid withdrawal, and beta blockers may exacerbate all forms of the disease.

TREATMENT

Therapeutic Expectations

Psoriasis is a chronic disease that is likely to be apparent for the rest of the patient's life when the patient is not under active treatment. Often, the disease is not completely cleared even with therapy. The choice of treatment and likelihood of response to therapy depend on the severity and type of disease and the sites involved. In prescribing therapy, it is important to consider the type of psoriasis, extent of lesions, patient risk factors for side effects, sites involved (e.g., skin, scalp, and nails). Most importantly, the level of improvement the patient hopes to achieve and the burden of the disease on the patient should be considered.

Therapy

Plaque-Type Psoriasis

For limited plaque disease, topical therapy is most often the first line of treatment. The two principal topical therapies of limited cutaneous disease are topical corticosteroids and topical vitamin D preparations. Emollients and keratolytics are also very helpful in removing scale and reducing itching, fissuring, and bleeding from psoriatic plaques. Nail disease does not generally respond to topical therapy. Limited plaque disease, especially of elbows and knees and in the scalp, that does not respond to topical steroids may sometimes benefit from intralesional steroids (triamcinolone, 3 to 5 mg/ml intradermally administered). Systemic corticosteroids may be initially helpful, but their usual risks as well as the risk of triggering a severe flare of psoriasis after withdrawal argues strongly against their use in most circumstances.

The first principle in treating plaque psoriasis is gentle removing of the scale. This can be done with baths, which are generally tolerated if used in conjunction with a bath oil or powder such as colloidal oatmeal and mineral oil (Aveeno) or coal tar (Balnetar bath oil). Keratolytics that contain salicylic acid or alpha-hydroxy acids (Lac-Hydrin) are also sometimes helpful for removing scale.

Topical steroids are most widely used in the treatment of limited disease. The potency of the steroid to be used and its dosage form chosen (ointment, cream, lotion, and solution) depend on the location and extent of disease. A clinician should become familiar with the use of very high, high-, medium-, and low-potency steroids. Many brands are available for each potency level.

The choice of topical corticosteroids depends on the site of the disease, the extent of involvement, and patient preferences. Although somewhat more effective, very high potency topical corticosteroids (Class I steroids such as clobetasol [Temovate cream], betamethasone in an optimized vehicle [Diprolene cream]) are usually most appropriate for short-term or intermittent use. The problems associated with long-term use of very high potency topical steroids include cutaneous atrophy and, with widespread application, sufficient systemic absorption to induce the risks of systemic steroids. In general, very high potency topical corticosteroids should not be used on the face and intertriginous areas, and their use in any other location should be limited to 4 weeks of twice-daily therapy and only intermittent therapy for 1 month (i.e., twice per week before reinitiating more intensive therapy for another 2-week period of regular use). Further, if large quantities per week (>30 g) are used chronically, adrenal suppression becomes a real risk. Therefore, for chronic use on open areas of skin, moderate-potency to moderately high potency corticosteroids (e.g., triamcinolone) are most appropriate. Even steroids of this potency should not be used in large quantities chronically or for extended periods in intertriginous areas or on the face. On these more sensitive sites, low-potency topical steroids (2.5% hydrocortisone cream) should be the mainstay of treatment.

The choice of vehicle is also important. In hairy areas, lotions and gels are more acceptable. Although ointments help to remove scale and keep plaques from cracking better than creams do, many patients find ointments cosmetically unacceptable. Therefore, creams are most often prescribed.

First available in 1994 in the United States, topical calcipotriene (Dovonex ointment) is helpful for plaque psoriasis on open body areas. Response is often slower than with topical steroids. In December 1995, this product was available only as an ointment. Irritancy of normal skin is the main problem. For this reason, intertriginous areas and the face should also be avoided. Use should be limited to 100 g/week to avoid problems of hypercalcemia.

The cost of topical medications varies widely according to dosage form and whether the agent is available as a generic preparation. Higher-potency branded topical corticosteroids and calcipotriene (Dovonex) are expensive and cost in excess of $1/g wholesale. Generic preparations may cost as little as $0.05 to $0.10/g. Therefore, in choosing a product and strategy, those costs that may become substantial (e.g., a person using only 30 g of topical calcipotriene per week would spend more than $2,500 per year) should be considered.

In addition to the use of topical corticosteroids (usually lotions or solutions), medicated shampoos are helpful for scalp and beard psoriasis (see Chapter 44: Seborrheic Dermatitis).

Extensive Plaque Psoriasis

For psoriasis that is too extensive for topical corticosteroids to be either practical or safe or that does not respond to topical corticosteroids or other topical therapies, there are a variety of more effective but also more toxic therapies. These include ultraviolet B (UVB) phototherapy, psoralens plus ultraviolet A radiation (PUVA), oral methotrexate, and systemic retinoids (etretinate). Immunosuppressive therapies (such as cyclosporine and FK-506) have also been advocated.

UVB is especially helpful for chronic moderate-plaque psoriasis and guttate psoriasis. UVB utilizes that part of the sunburn spectrum of solar radiation (300 to 320 nm) not present in substantial quantity in most suntan salon sources. For this therapy to be effective, doses of ultraviolet radiation close to that which will make a patient pink must be used. Therefore, the individual or institution administering therapy should be familiar with this treatment. Guttate psoriasis usually responds especially well to UVB therapy.

Sunlight may also be helpful for psoriasis. It is essential that scale be removed (see earlier) prior to UVB or sun exposure and that sunscreens not be used on affected areas, but they can be used on other sun-exposed sites. The risks of UVB therapy include acute sunburn reactions that may exacerbate psoriasis, exacerbation of photosensitive disorders such as lupus and polymorphic light eruption, and changes associated with long-term exposure to UVB including photoaging and perhaps an increased risk of skin cancer.

PUVA is a highly effective treatment for psoriasis. Only experts should administer this therapy. Acute problems are similar to those seen with UVB radiation. In addition, some patients experience nausea and headache from the tablets. PUVA is substantially more effective than UVB therapy, but with long-term use, there is a substantial increase in the risk of squamous cell carcinoma of the skin.

Methotrexate has been used since the early 1960s in the treatment of severe psoriasis. It is especially helpful in patients who also have severe nail disease that is unlikely to respond to other types of therapy and in patients with psoriatic arthritis. Weekly doses of 7.5 to 22.5 mg are typically used. In addition to the many acute risks of methotrexate (leukopenia and pulmonary hypersensitivity reactions), long-term low-dose methotrexate therapy is associated with an increased risk of hepatic fibrosis, even among patients who show no evidence of abnormal liver function on repeated laboratory testing, which is required in these individuals. Bone marrow suppression is a potential problem in all patients. The elderly and patients with diminished renal function are especially susceptible to the acute side effects of methotrexate.

Etretinate is an aromatic retinoid that is orally administered. It is especially useful for the treatment of severe pustular and erythrodermic psoriasis. Etretinate is a teratogen with a very long half-life. Therefore, it should not be used in women who still have child-bearing potential. Its administration should be restricted to experts.

Immunomodulators such as cyclosporine and FK-506 have enjoyed great attention in the clinical literature, but their long-term safety limits their use to special circumstances.

PITFALLS AND PROBLEMS

Diagnosis

The differential diagnosis of psoriasis includes cutaneous T-cell lymphoma, chronic eczema, and pityriasis rubra pilaris. In addition, patients with erythrodermic psoriasis may develop this condition as a result of the conditions previously discussed or other types of lymphoma or as a result of a drug reaction. For patients with atypical disease or those who do not respond to therapy, these diagnoses should also be considered and investigated. Chronic eczema may be difficult to distinguish from psoriasis, especially after partial treatment or in the patient who picks or rubs. Skin biopsy is probably the single most useful diagnostic test if the clinical diagnosis is not certain.

Exacerbating Factors

Streptococcal infections often induce flares of psoriasis, especially guttate flares. Certain drugs, especially beta blockers and lithium, worsen psoriasis. Systemic steroid withdrawal may also trigger acute exacerbations. Trauma to the skin can induce localized disease (the Koebner phenomenon).

Patient Counseling

In treating patients with psoriasis, it is important to educate them about the chronic nature of the disease and the lack of a cure. It is important that agreement exists between the treating practitioner and the patient about the goals of therapy (e.g., what extent of clearing to expect and at what cost and risk). A clear understanding that treatment now will not cure the disease and, even if successful, may lead to incomplete clearing is essential. Patients should be educated about the potential toxicity of the treatments they receive.

REFERRAL AND CONSULTATION GUIDELINES

Generally, patients with erythrodermic and pustular as well as widespread plaque psoriasis are better treated in specialty settings that offer specialized therapy such as etretinate and PUVA and UVB phototherapy. Similarly, people with severe psoriatic arthritis are most likely to benefit from care in a facility experienced in using methotrexate. When patients have acute exacerbations or do not respond to topical therapy, consultation is often justified.

REFERENCES

1. Meol T, Soter NA, Lim HW: Are topical corticosteroids useful adjunctive therapy for the treatment of psoriasis with ultraviolet radiation? A review of the literature. Arch Dermatol 1991; 127:1708–1713.
2. Wolverton SE: Systemic drug therapy for psoriasis. The most critical issue. Arch Dermatol 1991; 127:565–568.
3. Greaves MW, Weinstein GD: Treatment of psoriasis. N Engl J Med 1995; 332:581–588.
4. Epstein JH: Phototherapy and photochemotherapy. N Engl J Med 1990; 322:1149–1151.

CHAPTER 41

Raynaud's Disease/ Phenomenon

Hensin Tsao

CLINICAL APPEARANCE

Definition

Raynaud's name has been associated with two distinct entities—Raynaud's disease and Raynaud's phenomenon. *Raynaud's disease* refers to episodic attacks of vasospasm, on exposure to cold temperature, leading to cyanosis of one or more digits. When these vasospastic attacks are secondary to an underlying etiology, the disorder is termed *Raynaud's phenomenon.*

Typical Symptoms and Lesions

The history is essential in the diagnosis of Raynaud's disease/phenomenon. Patients will typically complain of cold intolerance. This intolerance can manifest as "white" or "blue" fingers when outdoors, in cold water, or working in refrigeration. The attacks can last from minutes to hours and may produce a numb sensation. However, when severe pain occurs, other causes of ischemia should be investigated.

More often than not, there will be no specific findings on physical examination in the absence of vasospasm. In between episodes, the fingers and toes may be cool and may perspire excessively. However, examination during an attack will typically reveal sharply delineated, blanching, white pallor extending from the tips of the fingers to various distances proximally. The skin proximal to the line of demarcation will usually be pink and warm. In approximately 40% of patients, the toes may also be involved. Given time and thermal encouragement, the white digits will turn cyanotic blue and then hyperemic red. These transitional phases usually elicit sensations of throbbing or pain. Although the sequence of white-blue-red is characteristic of Raynaud's disease/phenomenon, not all patients will experience the entire triphasic response. Rarely, the earlobes and the tip of the nose may be affected.

In patients with longstanding disease, trophic changes may be seen. Repeated ischemic assaults may lead to thinned skin over the digits, dystrophic nails, and sclerodactyly. The nail cuticle may fuse with the proximal nail fold forming a pterygium. Fixed ischemic discoloration usually suggests a secondary cause of Raynaud's and may lead to distal gangrene and autoamputation (see Fig. 41–1 on Color Plate 16).

The general physical examination is usually normal unless stigmata of an underlying disease gain prominence in the setting of Raynaud's phenomenon. For example, the patient may exhibit pursed lips from scleroderma or a malar rash from systemic lupus. The radial, ulnar, and pedal pulses are usually normal.

DESCRIPTION OF DISEASE

Raynaud's disease usually occurs in patients between 15 and 40 years old, and women are four times as likely as men to experience these attacks. Over half of the patients will not have an underlying etiology (Table 41–1 contains a list of causes of Raynaud's). An obvious worsening during the winter months can be expected.

In primary Raynaud's disease, approximately 33% of patients will stabilize over time, and another 33% will improve. Approximately 10% of the patients experience complete resolution, and 16% will worsen. Less than 5% of the patients will develop sclerodactyly, and less than 1% will autoamputate their digits. In secondary Raynaud's phenomenon, the course of the disease will reflect the progression of its underlying disorder.

The pathology of Raynaud's disease is not specific—findings may range from normal histology in mild disease to intimal hyperplasia with narrowing of vessels or thrombi in severe disease. Digital angiography for diagnostic purposes is usually not indicated.

The pathogenesis of primary Raynaud's disease is still controversial. Increased local hypersensitivity to cold rather than sympathetic overactivity has been proposed. During cold exposure, low digital arterial systolic pressures may lead to vasocollapse and subsequent ischemia. There is also some evidence that an abnormality in serotonin metabolism may play a role in the dysregulation of vasotone.

The etiologies of Raynaud's phenomenon are numerous. Eighty to 90% of scleroderma patients complain of Raynaud's symptoms, and approximately 33% of these patients present with these symptoms. Approximately 10 to 35% of patients with systemic lupus and 30% of patients with dermatomyositis experience Raynaud's phenomenon. Atherosclerosis is a frequent etiology in men over 50 years of age. Blood dyscrasias, such as abnormalities in plasma fibrinogen, cold agglutinins, cryoglobulins, or hyperviscosity syndromes associated with myeloproliferative disorders, have also been associated with Raynaud's phenomenon. Occupational-induced disease occurs in workers using vibratory tools, chainsaws, and jackhammers and in pianists. Finally, drugs such as methysergide, beta blockers, and chemotherapeutic agents including bleomycin, cisplatin, and vinblastine have all been implicated.

TABLE 41–1

Classification of Raynaud's Disease/Phenomenon

Primary Raynaud's Disease	***Blood Dyscrasias***
Secondary Raynaud's Phenomenon	Polycythemia vera
Rheumatologic Disorders	Cryoglobulinemia
Scleroderma	Cold agglutinins
Systemic lupus erythematosus	Macroglobulinemia
Dermatomyositis and polymyositis	Cryofibrinogenemia
Mixed connective tissue disease	***Drugs***
Rheumatoid arthritis	Ergot derivatives
Polyarteritis and vasculitis	Methysergide
Sjögren's syndrome	Beta blockers
Arterial Occulsive Disease	Bleomycin
Arteriosclerosis obliterans	Vincristine
Thromboangiitis obliterans	Cisplatin
Arterial embolism	Cyclosporine
Pulmonary Hypertension	Clonidine
Neurologic Disorders	Bromocriptine
Thoracic outlet syndrome	***Trauma***
Hemiplegia	Vibration injury
Carpal tunnel syndrome	Hammer hand syndrome
Poliomyelitis	Electric shock
Syringomyelia	Cold injury
Multiple sclerosis	Typing
Reflex sympathetic dystrophy	Piano playing
	Meat cutting
	Others
	Hypothyroidism
	Vinyl chloride exposure
	Intraarterial injections
	Neuroendocrine tumors

TREATMENT

Many patients have mild disease and do not need systemic therapy. General considerations include avoidance of cold exposure and the use of warm clothing over the entire body in addition to other thermal insulation such as heated gloves and socks. Patients should be instructed to stop smoking and minimize stress, as emotional turmoil may precipitate attacks. If a specific vocation has been implicated in the genesis of the disease, changing occupations may help. Similarly, if a drug has been implicated, cessation of therapy may ameliorate symptoms. Traumatic insults to the digits should be minimized, especially if atrophic skin changes are prominent. Finally, many people experience improvement after moving to warmer climates.

Drug therapy should be reserved for moderate to severe cases.

- The calcium channel blockers, especially diltiazem (30 to 60 mg qid) or nifedipine (10 to 30 mg tid), reduce peripheral vascular resistance and have been found to be effective. Verapamil does not seem to be as efficacious.
- Glycerol trinitrate ointment applied topically qd may help in conjunction with other therapies.
- In some cases, α-adrenergic blocking agents may be helpful. These agents do not reliably prevent Raynaud's phenomenon. Phenoxybenzamine (10 to 60 mg qd) and prazosin (2 to 8 mg qd) may offer some benefit to patients.

Alternative therapies including stanozolol, serotonin antagonists, plasmapheresis, and biofeedback have all been reported to help. Surgical approaches include upper extremity and lumbar sympathectomy. These procedures are often short-lived and accompanied by significant morbidity.

PITFALLS AND PROBLEMS

Diagnosis of Raynaud's disease and phenomenon is usually made on the basis of occupational, medical, and drug histories as well as physical examination. Laboratory studies to evaluate for hyperviscosity (complete blood count, serum protein electrophoresis, cryoglobulins, cold agglutinins) and collagen vascular diseases (antinuclear antibodies, rheumatoid factor, anti-Scl 70) may be helpful. The major differential diagnoses include acrocyanosis, chilblains, and erythromelalgia. In acrocyanosis, a bluish discoloration is usually persistent and not episodic, and both hands and feet are involved in addition to the digits. Chilblains is an inflammatory response to the cold, affecting more proximal phalanges, plantar surfaces, heels, nose, and ears. Erythromelalgia is characterized by paroxysmal attacks of pain and redness of the hands and feet, often precipitated by heat instead of cold.

Although a patient may not have evidence of an underlying disorder at the time of presentation, Raynaud's phenomenon may precede the development of systemic illnesses. It is imperative to follow patients with Raynaud's symptoms for future problems.

Therapeutically, Raynaud's disease is more amenable than Raynaud's phenomenon to treatment with calcium channel blockers. Potential side effects of calcium channel blocker therapy include hypotension, central nervous system toxicity, exacerbation of esophageal reflux, peripheral edema, and reflex tachycardia.

REFERRAL/CONSULTATION GUIDELINES

Primary Raynaud's disease will rarely lead to serious systemic or cutaneous morbidity. However, with secondary Raynaud's phenomenon, consultation with the appropriate specialists defined by the etiology may be necessary. Patients with evidence of connective tissue disease would benefit from a rheumatology consult. Similarly, a neurologist or hematologist becomes indispensable in the management of other patients.

BIBLIOGRAPHY

General

Berger TM, Elias PM, Wintroub BU: Raynaud's phenomenon/disease. *In* Manual of Therapy for Skin Disease. New York: Churchill Livingstone, 1990; pp 260–262.

Coffman JD: Cutaneous changes in peripheral vascular disease. *In* Fitzpatrick TB, Eisen AZ, Wolff K, et al (eds): Dermatology in General Medicine. 4th ed. New York: McGraw-Hill, 1993; pp 2084–2090.

Specific

Kahan A, Amor B, Menles CJ: A randomized double-blind trial of diltiazem in the treatment of Raynaud's phenomenon. Ann Rheum Dis 1985; 44:30–33.

Krahenbuhl B, Nielsen SL, Lassen NA: Closure of digital arteries in high vascular tone states as demonstrated by measurement of systolic blood pressure in the fingers. Scand J Clin Lab Invest 1977; 31(1):71–76.

Rodeheffer RJ, Rommer JA, Wigley F, Smith CR: Controlled double-blind trial of nifedipine in the treatment of Raynaud's phenomenon. N Engl J Med 1983; 308:880–883.

CHAPTER 42

Rosacea

Diane M. Thiboutot

CLINICAL APPEARANCE

Definition

Rosacea is a cutaneous vascular disorder that occurs in genetically predisposed individuals. It is characterized by a constellation of skin findings including facial telangiectasia, malar erythema, inflammatory papules and pustules, or rhinophyma (bulbous enlargement of the tip of the nose). Although it is most common in adults 30 to 50 years of age, rosacea has also been reported in younger patients. Rosacea has been classified into various stages based on its clinical appearance.[1] These include prerosacea, vascular rosacea, inflammatory rosacea, and late rosacea. The severity of the symptoms of rosacea varies greatly among individuals.

Typical Lesions and Symptoms

Flushing

Rosacea-prone individuals demonstrate increased susceptibility to flushing and blushing, which occur in response to a variety of emotional, physiologic, and environmental stimuli. This recurrent flushing and blushing has been termed *prerosacea.*[1] Rosacea has developed in cases of flushing associated with diseases such as carcinoid syndrome and mastocytosis.

Erythema and Telangiectasia

Persistent erythema and facial telangiectasia often develop in individuals with a longstanding history of flushing reactions. Erythema most often involves the cheeks, nose, forehead, and chin and is exacerbated by heat, sunlight, and ingestion of hot beverages, spicy foods, or alcohol. Telangiectasia are seen as fine, dilated superficial blood vessels most often observed on the cheeks of rosacea patients. Paranasal telangiectasia are commonly found in many individuals, but they are not necessarily indicative of rosacea.

Inflammatory Papules and Pustules

With time, inflammatory erythematous papules, pustules, and nodules can develop within the erythematous skin of rosacea patients (see Figs. 42–1 and 42–2 on Color Plate 16). The inflammatory lesions of rosacea are indistinguishable from those of acne vulgaris. In rosacea, however, the inflammatory lesions are neither preceded by nor associated with open or closed comedones, as they are in cases of acne vulgaris. Comedones are not a feature of rosacea.

Rhinophyma

Rhinophyma is a bulbous enlargement of the nose that occurs late in the course of rosacea. It is found most commonly in males and results from proliferation of connective tissue, blood vessels, and sebaceous glands.

Ocular Symptoms

The ocular symptoms of rosacea consist of blepharoconjunctivitis, keratitis, scleritis, and episcleritis (see

Fig. 42–3 on Color Plate 16).[2] These symptoms occur most commonly in association with the cutaneous findings of rosacea, but they may represent the only, or the most bothersome, symptom of rosacea in a small number of patients.

Atypical Presentation or Alternative Forms

Steroid Rosacea

Use of potent topical corticosteroids on the face can induce the signs of rosacea. Steroid-induced rosacea often develops as a secondary phenomenon during treatment of facial conditions such as eczematous or seborrheic dermatitis. It presents as an increase in facial erythema and the development of inflammatory papules and pustules. It may be localized to discrete regions where the steroids were applied. Rosacea is rarely induced by the use of systemic steroids.

Granulomatous Rosacea

Granulomatous rosacea is a rare variant of rosacea characterized by inflammatory lesions that appear as granulomatous dermal papules whose color resembles that of ''apple jelly.'' Granuloma formation in the dermis is noted histologically. Clinically, this form of rosacea can resemble other conditions associated with granulomatous inflammation such as sarcoid, tuberculosis, and leprosy.

Localized Rosacea

Localized rosacea is most commonly steroid-induced. There are cases, however, without a history of steroid use where persistent erythema, telangiectasia, or inflammatory papules or pustules are localized to focal regions on the cheek, chin, or forehead. These cases often respond to conventional therapy for rosacea, as outlined later.

Persistent or Solid Facial Edema

Varying degrees of facial edema have been reported in cases of rosacea. In more severe forms, a persistent solid edema of the forehead, nasal bridge, and cheeks can occur, and the face may take on a leonine appearance. Solid facial edema can also be associated with acne.

DESCRIPTION OF DISEASE

Rosacea is a fairly common condition among those with a skin phenotype characterized by light skin, hair, and eye color and frequent blushing or flushing reactions. It is most common in those with Celtic ancestry.

The etiology of the vascular changes leading to rosacea is unknown. Repeated facial blushing and flushing are thought to lead to persistent erythema and the development of ocular symptoms. The widening of the vascular lumen, characteristic of telangiectasia formation, is thought to be facilitated by damage to the integrity of the dermis by factors such as sun exposure and chronic dermal inflammation.

A pathogenic role for bacteria has not been found in the inflammatory lesions of rosacea, as it has been in the inflammatory lesions of acne vulgaris. Rather, it is thought that the mite *Demodex folliculorum* may play a pathogenic role in the inflammatory lesions of rosacea. This mite resides within pilosebaceous follicles and utilizes cellular keratin debris as a nutrient source. Although a direct role for *Demodex* in the pathogenesis of rosacea has not been shown, several studies have demonstrated increased numbers of mites in facial skin from rosacea patients compared with that of controls. Interestingly, the improvement in rosacea symptoms following a 1-month course of tetracycline was not associated with a reduction in mite counts, however.[3]

TREATMENT

Therapeutic Expectations

Since the facial phenotypic features characteristic of rosacea patients are genetically determined, patients should understand that this condition cannot be cured. With avoidance of provocative factors and appropriate treatment, however, symptoms can usually be controlled. Improvement is generally noted after 6 to 8 weeks of therapy with topical or oral antibiotics. Oral antibiotics may be tapered over 1 or 2 months, and patients may often be successfully maintained on topical agents for several years. Of all the symptoms of rosacea, facial erythema is the least responsive to treatment.

First-Line Therapy

Facial Erythema and Telangiectasia

Avoidance of factors that provoke flushing such as heat, sunlight, and ingestion of hot beverages, spicy foods, and alcohol is important in helping to improve the facial erythema of rosacea patients. Oral and topical antibiotics have a marginal effect on reducing facial erythema. Clonidine 0.05 mg once or twice daily has been prescribed in an effort to reduce flushing episodes.

Many female patients have successfully masked the facial erythema of rosacea with the use of a green-tint cover-up cosmetic product. These come in a cream or liquid form and are widely available at cosmetic counters. Application of this product neutralizes the red skin tone characteristic of rosacea and greatly enhances the camouflaging action of routine facial foundations.

Surgical treatments of facial telangiectasia include electrodessication at a very low setting or use of continuous wave or pulsed dye lasers.

Inflammatory Lesions

The inflammatory lesions of rosacea are the most amenable to treatment. Mild cases can be treated topically once or twice daily with metronidazole gel 0.75% (MetroGel), clindamycin lotion 1% (Cleocin T), or sodium sulfacetamide (Sulfacet-R, Novacet). In cases of moderate to severe symptoms, an oral antibiotic such as tetracycline, 500 mg twice a day, erythromycin, 500 mg twice a day, or doxycycline, 50 mg twice a day, can be used in combination with a topical product. As lesions improve, the antibiotic can begin to be tapered after 2 months, with the goal of maintaining the patient on topical therapy.

Rhinophyma

Rhinophyma is a long-term sequela of rosacea. By controlling the symptoms of rosacea with avoidance of provocative factors and appropriate treatment, the development of rhinophyma may be prevented. Surgical interventions such as removal of redundant tissue with scalpel excision, carbon dioxide laser ablation, and dermabrasion have been utilized successfully in the treatment of rhinophyma.

Ocular Symptoms

Oral tetracycline (500 mg twice daily) and doxycycline (50 mg twice daily) are each very effective in treating the blepharoconjunctivitis associated with rosacea.

Alternative Therapeutic Options

Moderately severe rosacea can be treated with oral metronidazole or clindamycin. Isotretinoin (0.5 to 1.0 mg/kg/day) has been used to treat severe rosacea and its granulomatous varieties. Rosacea may respond to isotretinoin, but it often recurs with time. Owing to the side effect profile of these medications, they are not recommended as first-line agents in the treatment of rosacea.

PITFALLS AND PROBLEMS OF DIAGNOSIS AND THERAPY

Differential Diagnosis

Rosacea may appear similar to a variety of cutaneous disorders that affect the face (Table 42–1). Perioral dermatitis is characterized by erythema, scaling, and small papules and pustules occurring most commonly around the mouth and on the chin. Granulomatous rosacea can be distinguished from other cutaneous granulomatous processes such as sarcoid, tuberculosis, and leprosy on the basis of a skin biopsy.

Treatment Resistance

As previously mentioned, it is difficult to control the facial erythema associated with rosacea. It is therefore important to discuss this fact with patients in order to help them develop reasonable expectations.

Periodic exacerbations of rosacea may occur during maintenance therapy with topical antibiotics. These flares are characterized by the development of increased numbers of inflammatory lesions, and they can be effectively managed with reinstitution of an oral antibiotic regimen for 6 to 8 weeks.

TABLE 42–1

Differential Diagnosis of Rosacea

Systemic lupus erythematosus
Acne vulgaris
Perioral dermatitis
Seborrheic dermatitis
Cutaneous sarcoid
Cutaneous tuberculosis
Leprosy

Sensitive Skin

Many rosacea patients have sensitive skin that is easily irritated by harsh soaps, wind, sun, extremes of weather, and use of topical products including cosmetics and medications. Facial moisturizers (especially those containing a sunscreen) may often be beneficial in these patients.

Management of Steroid-Induced Rosacea

Steroid-induced rosacea is difficult to manage. Patients are often reluctant to stop using the implicated topical steroid because it may temporarily improve facial erythema through its vasoconstrictor action. It is difficult to convince many patients to break the cycle of topical steroid use. Patients must be cautioned that they will undergo a withdrawal period during which a temporary worsening of the condition will occur before improvement is achieved.

REFERRAL AND CONSULTATION GUIDELINES

Referral or consultation may be considered for:

1. Patients who fail to respond to standard treatment such as those with granulomatous rosacea, persistent facial edema, or steroid-induced rosacea
2. Patients with moderate to severe ocular symptoms including iritis and scleritis
3. Patients who are interested in surgical treatment of telangiectasia or rhinophyma

REFERENCES

1. Wilkin JK: Rosacea. Pathophysiology and treatment. Arch Dermatol 1994; 130:359–362.
2. Browning DJ, Proia AD: Ocular rosacea. Surv Ophthalmol 1986; 31:145–158.
3. Bonnar E, Eutace P, Powell FC: The *Demodex* mite population in rosacea. J Am Acad Dermatol 1993; 28:443–448.

CHAPTER 43

Scabies

James E. Rasmussen

CLINICAL APPEARANCE[1]

Scabies results from infestation with an eight-legged mite (*Sarcoptes scabiei*), 0.4 × 0.3 mm in size (Fig. 43–1). The usual clinical appearance varies tremendously with the age of the patient, the duration of infestation, poorly defined immunologic features, and prior attempts at therapy. In general, symptoms of the infestation begin insidiously as moderate pruritus with a characteristic distribution on the hands, genitalia, and axillary areas. Although it is stated that the pruritus is usually worse at night, this is a nonspecific finding, since most diseases itch more during this time. In children less than 3 to 6 years of age, lesions are widespread and may involve the scalp, face, trunk, extremities, palms, and soles. Older children and adults typically have a more restricted distribution, which usually spares the head and neck, and less involvement of the thickly keratinized palms and soles.

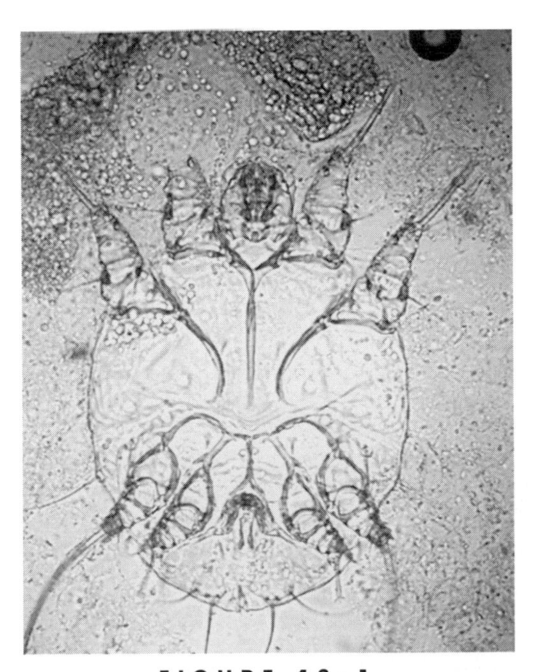

FIGURE 43–1
Sarcoptes scabiei mite.

More severe infections can produce cutaneous lesions that look like eczema, psoriasis, or impetigo. Erythema, scale, pyoderma, and nodular lesions are commonly seen over the extremities and the trunk. Nodular lesions are red-brown, 1 to 3 cm in diameter, and commonly occur around the genitalia and axilla (Fig. 43–2).

Patients with the most severe infestation usually have underlying diseases or conditions such as infection with the human immunodeficiency virus (HIV) or Down syndrome. In these individuals, the epidermal response to the massive infection is so remarkable that gross hyperkeratosis and psoriasiform thickening occur. The term *Norwegian scabies* is occasionally applied in this patient population.

DESCRIPTION OF DISEASE

Patients can be infested at any age. However, it usually takes 1 to 3 months following exposure for the mite population and the individual's immunity to reach a critical stage, so that lesions are usually not found in the first 2 to 3 months of life. The disease can be found in any part of the world and in any race, although it is

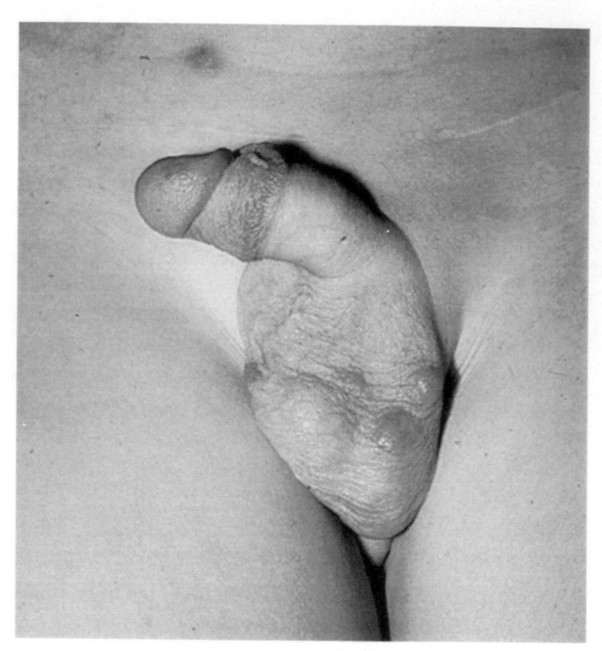

FIGURE 43-2
Nodules of scabies.

distinctly less common in blacks in the United States. It is much more common in warm, humid areas, since this probably facilitates transmission of the organism owing to increased survivability on fomites. Taplin and colleagues have reported from several countries in Central and South America where prevalence is near 100%.[2]

It is commonly stated that scabies occurs in epidemics with approximately 20-year cycles. Information for this is mostly anecdotal, since the disease is not reportable and is often misdiagnosed. Natural immunity may play some role in the spread of the disease, since it is uncommon to see patients infected with a second or third episode.

Left untreated, the disease can probably persist indefinitely and has given rise to such interesting nomenclature as the *7-year itch.*

Pathology

Female mites burrow vigorously in the outer portion of the epidermis, primarily in the stratum corneum. In severe cases, the stratum corneum may be thickened and honeycombed with burrows and eggs. Nodular lesions may contain mites or may represent a hypersensitivity reaction such as is seen with an insect bite granuloma.

Etiology/Pathogenesis

The disease is caused by *S. scabiei var. humanus,* which is probably host-specific and not transmitted from animals. Although animal scabies may occur, its clinical presentation is somewhat different from human scabies, as the organism probably cannot complete its life cycle in humans.

Female mites mate on the surface of the skin and live for a period of 30 to 60 days, during which time they burrow in the stratum corneum and lay several eggs per day. On hatching, the process is repeated and the mite population continues to expand. Melanby,[3] using painstaking microscopic examination of the entire skin surface of infected volunteers, determined that the number of adult mites was between 10 and 15 per infected individual. However, in cases of crusted scabies (Norwegian scabies) the number of mites probably ranges into the thousands and consequently makes these individuals more infectious.

It is believed that the itching is primarily an immunologic response to the presence of the mite eggs and feces. However, this has not been well established.

The disease is spread from direct person-to-person contact and through the use of fomites such as clothing and bedding. Live mites can be found in the living areas of many patients.[4] Because of the inability of the mite to travel any distance at room temperature and its very short viability off the human host (3 to 5 days), it usually takes pronounced and prolonged physical exposure to develop scabies. Many epidemics have been traced to hospitalized patients or those in nursing homes. Here the disease may spread to other patients and members of the health care team. It is common for only a few members of a family to be spared. Whether this is due to immunity is not known.

TREATMENT[1–5]

The number of agents available to treat scabies is quite extensive, although only a few are available in most countries of the world. Lindane 1% (cream or lotion) and permethrin 5% are the principal agents available in the United States. A variety of treatment protocols have been developed, but this author has had the greatest success treating all affected individuals from chin to toes overnight (approximately 8 hours) and washing the preparation off in the morning. This is followed at the end of 7 days with a second treatment. Infants should be treated from head to toes. It is important that all exposed individuals be treated, not just those who are symptomatic. Asymptomatic patients need be treated only once. In the interval between treatments, this author commonly uses antihistamines, topical antipruritics, and topical corticosteroids, since the symptoms and visible signs of the disease do not decline rapidly. This is probably due to the continued presence of the mite and its feces.

Both lindane and permethrin are absorbed (as is true of all active medications applied to the skin). The potential for toxic reactions, particularly neurologic, has been of increasing concern with the use of lindane.[4] Although this author has never seen a reaction to lindane, it is currently becoming much less popular to use this drug in infants and young children. Regardless of the product used, it is particularly important to emphasize that treatment should not be repeated on a daily basis and that the patient should be told the signs and symptoms will resolve slowly. This author insists that all patients be seen for follow-up examination in approximately 1 month's time unless they are completely free of signs and symptoms.

Crotamiton and precipitated sulfur are available but should be considered a second choice because of their low efficacy.[2]

Nodular lesions of scabies can be treated with injectable corticosteroids (once the acute infection has been treated) or with tar, topical steroids, or antipruritic agents.

Patients with severe scabies, such as those with concurrent HIV infections, frequently do not respond well to topical therapy with any modality. Multiple, repeat courses may be necessary, thereby exposing the patient to increased toxicity. Concomitant use of keratolytics to reduce the bulk of the scabies warren is sometimes successful, as is the use of a surgical scrub brush. Vigorous attention should be paid to keeping medication under the free edges of the nails, since this is often an untreated site and a common source of continued spreading of the disease.

Although some authors have been concerned about the development of resistance to scabies, this author believes this to be a very uncommon situation, where misdiagnosis has usually been confused with resistance to therapy. Few, if any, patients will fail to respond to two successive applications separated by a week, provided that all other exposed individuals are treated as well.

Meinking and associates have recently published on the systemic use of ivermectin.[5] A single dose of 200 μg/kg was 100% effective in patients with uncomplicated scabies. Patients with concurrent HIV infection and crusted scabies frequently required a second or, occasionally, a third dose.

In addition to specific therapy, it is important that all household articles in direct contact with the patient be thoroughly washed or disinfected, or both. It is not necessary, however, to routinely treat the entire house, since the organism cannot live for more than 2 to 3 days off a patient and is barely mobile.

Uncommonly in infants, the postscabetic syndrome occurs in which papules, vesicles, and pustules develop on the sides of the hands and feet. This syndrome may be confused with infantile acropustulosis and can occur in both blacks and whites. Topical steroids may be required for an extended period.

Diagnosis

The only diagnostic lesion of active scabetic infection is the burrow. Many texts and articles state that these lesions are uncommon. It is perhaps true that they are uncommonly found, but only because they are not carefully sought. In this author's experience, it is distinctly uncommon to see patients in whom the diagnosis of scabies is probable in the absence of burrows. These 3- to 9-mm, somewhat serpiginous, epidermal tracts are much more common on the webs of the fingers, sides of the hand, and in infants and children, the palms and soles (Fig. 43–3). The lateral and medial sides of the heel are also good places to evaluate for scabies. Often, a small gray-black dot (the female mite) can be seen at

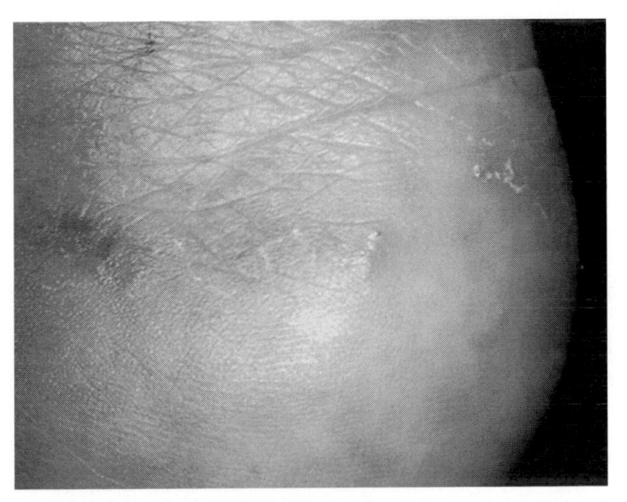

FIGURE 43–3
A scabies burrow.

the advancing end of the burrow. Good magnification and strong light are essential in searching for these lesions.

Once the diagnosis is suspected, a scraping of the burrow usually reveals the mature mite eggs or feces (scybala) (Fig. 43–4; see also 43–1). Remember, adults are easier to scrape than children.

For those who have difficulty in seeing the burrows, the ink test or topical tetracycline has been used. In these techniques, washable ink from a felt-tipped pen or topical tetracycline solution is spread over the suspected areas and then rinsed off. Burrows can then be sought by using the Wood lamp (for the tetracycline-treated) or regular light. In this author's experience, this has not been necessary. Skin biopsy is usually not necessary.

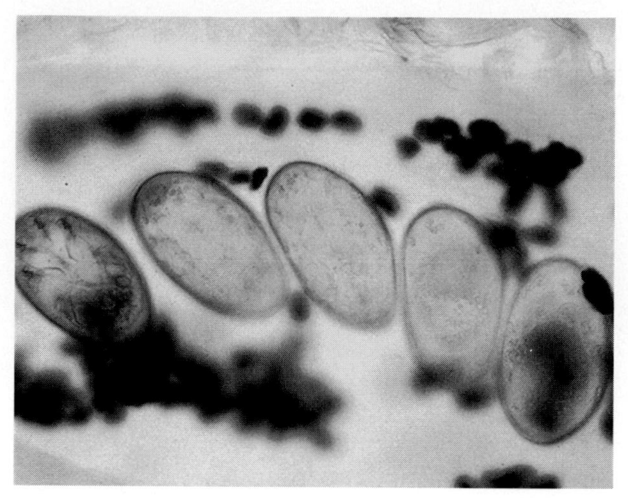

FIGURE 43–4
Eggs and scybala. (From Rasmussen JE: Body lice, head lice, pubic lice, and scabies. *In* Arndt KA, LeBoit PE, Robinson JK, Wintroub BU [eds]: Cutaneous Medicine and Surgery. Philadelphia: WB Saunders, 1996, p 1197.)

PITFALLS AND PROBLEMS

The most common error in misdiagnosing scabies is failure to consider it in any patient who complains of pruritus. Common misdiagnosis includes atopic eczema, insect bites, psoriasis, and xerosis. As many patients are overdiagnosed as are underdiagnosed in these situations. Only with consistent and persistent examination of the web spaces with strong light and magnification can the interested clinician be successful in correctly diagnosing the disease. It is not necessary to identify the mite if burrows are present. A history of spread among family members or nursing personnel is often the best historical clue. Patients who can feel mites crawling on the skin may have delusions of parasitosis. Mites move so slowly that their motion cannot usually be detected.

REFERRAL/CONSULTATION GUIDELINES

Patients with routine scabies can be treated by physicians in any branch of medicine. Those with crusted or HIV infections should be considered for referral, although with development of ivermectin therapy, this should be less common. Patients who continue to itch can be treated with topical corticosteroids and antipruritics and usually do not need retreatment with scabicides.

REFERENCES

1. Rasmussen JE: Scabies. Pediatr Rev 1994; 15:110–114.
2. Taplin D, Meinking TL, Chen JA, et al: Comparison of crotamiton 10% creme (Eurax) and permethrin 5% creme (Elimite) for the treatment of scabies in children. Pediatr Dermatol 1990; 7:67–73.
3. Melanby K: Scabies. Middlesex, Eng: EW Classey, 1972.
4. Arlian LG, Estes SA, Vyszenski-Moher DL: Prevalence of *Sarcoptes scabiei* in the homes and nursing homes of scabietic patients. J Am Acad Dermatol 1989; 19:806–811.
5. Meinking TL, Taplin D, Hermida JL, et al: The treatment of scabies with ivermectin. N Engl J Med 1995; 333:26–30.
6. Rasmussen JE: The problem of lindane. J Am Acad Dermatol 1981; 5:507–516.

CHAPTER 44

Seborrheic Dermatitis

Thomas G. Cropley and Bruce U. Wintroub

CLINICAL APPEARANCE

Definition

Seborrheic dermatitis is a subacute or chronic inflammatory disorder of unknown cause typically confined to the sebaceous gland–rich skin of the head and trunk and occasionally involving intertriginous areas. It is characterized by erythematous plaques exhibiting dry or oily scale. Seborrheic dermatitis occurs in adults and in early infancy, and the clinical morphology differs in these two groups.

Typical Lesions and Symptoms

Adults

Adults with seborrheic dermatitis usually have diffuse erythema and scaling of hair-bearing portions of the scalp. Commonly, but not invariably, well-defined pink plaques with powdery scale form in the eyebrows, nasolabial creases, and postauricular sulci. Seborrheic blepharoconjunctivitis is seen in persons with severe facial involvement. Patients with a mustache or beard commonly have involvement of those sites as well. Occasionally, the presternal, interscapular, or genital skin will also exhibit seborrheic changes. Truncal skin forms delicate arcuate plaques with crumbly or greasy scale that are referred to as *petaloid seborrhea,* whereas more diffuse involvement of the groin, particularly the hair-bearing skin, is typical of that site. Other intertriginous sites, especially the axillae, may also become involved.

Pruritus of the scalp is nearly universal in seborrheic dermatitis, but itching is more variable in other sites. Patients with facial seborrheic dermatitis may complain of an ''irritated'' or ''burning'' discomfort, rather than true pruritus.

Infants

Infantile seborrheic dermatitis typically involves the scalp, the flexural creases, and the diaper area. Skin exposed to saliva, such as perioral skin and the anterior neck crease, is often affected. Erythematous plaques with sharply defined borders and a glazed, or shiny, surface are characteristic. Small erythematous papules with fine scale may be scattered around and between larger plaques. In most flexural areas, scale may not be evident. On the other hand, seborrheic plaques on the scalp often develop thick, yellowish-white plates of scale colloquially termed *cradle cap.* Infants with seborrheic dermatitis are usually comfortable and seemingly oblivious to the rash, so one must conclude that pruritus is not an important feature of the infantile form of disease.

Atypical Presentation or Alternative Forms

Rarely, seborrheic dermatitis may become widespread, sometimes resembling pityriasis rosea, and can even eventuate in development of generalized exfoliative erythroderma. Seborrheic dermatitis in persons with the acquired immunodeficiency syndrome (AIDS) or with Parkinson's disease is distinguished more by greater severity and refractoriness to treatment (particularly in

AIDS) than by involvement of unusual sites or atypical morphologic features.[1]

DESCRIPTION OF DISEASE

Seborrheic dermatitis is a common disorder with a bimodal age distribution; it is seen in early infancy and in adulthood but only rarely in children older than 6 months of age. The incidence of seborrheic dermatitis in infants is not known.

Adult seborrheic dermatitis may begin at puberty but frequently does not appear until the third decade of life or later. The frequency of seborrheic dermatitis in adults is estimated to be 3 to 5%.[2] The condition usually continues throughout adult life. Seborrheic dermatitis is encountered in a large proportion of persons with human immunodeficiency virus (HIV) infection and in those with Parkinson's disease. The adult form is more common in men than in women. There does not appear to be any racial predilection.

The histopathology of both the adult and the infantile forms of seborrheic dermatitis is that of a spongiotic dermatitis and is not specific. Therefore, skin biopsy is rarely useful in patient management.

Although theories abound, the cause of seborrheic dermatitis remains unknown. Clinicians have long observed that the disorder preferentially involves sites rich in sebaceous glands, suggesting a direct or indirect role for sebum in its pathogenesis. This contention is supported by the age distribution of seborrheic dermatitis (i.e., early infancy and adulthood), which coincides with periods of sebaceous gland activity, and by the disorder's male predilection in adults. Further, sebum secretion rates in patients with Parkinson's disease correlate, albeit weakly, with activity of parkinsonian seborrheic dermatitis.[3]

The missing link between sebum and dermatitis may be *Pityrosporum ovale,* the lipophilic yeast that normally inhabits human skin. Two principal lines of reasoning suggest a role for this fungus in seborrheic dermatitis. First, the yeast is abundantly present in sebaceous skin and has been demonstrated to be even more evident in seborrheic scale.[4] Second, the dermatitis responds to a variety of medications that inhibit growth of *P. ovale,* including zinc pyrithione, selenium sulfide, nystatin, and ketoconazole.

TREATMENT

Therapeutic Expectations

Seborrheic dermatitis responds rapidly to topical therapy, and complete resolution of lesions should take 7 to 21 days. Less intense, long-term topical therapy is usually required to inhibit disease activity and prevent recurrence.

First-Line Therapy

Therapeutic efforts should focus on removal of scale and suppression of inflammation or treatment of the putative etiologic agent *P. ovale*. Initial therapy for scalp and body are described.

Scalp and Beard

A variety of shampoos are available and are highly effective for control of mild to moderate seborrheic dermatitis, including:

1. Ketoconazole (Nizoral) or selenium sulfide (Selsun) shampoos used daily for 7 to 10 days and then twice weekly
2. Shampoos containing 1 to 2% pyrithione zinc (DHS Zinc, Head & Shoulders, Zincon) used daily to twice weekly as needed
3. Coal tar shampoos (Pentrax, T/Gel, Zetar, DHS Tar, Ionil T) used daily to twice weekly as needed

In addition, moderate scalp disease with bothersome pruritus may require topical corticosteroids to achieve control. A steroid-containing solution (fluocinonide 0.05% [Lidex] or betamethasone valerate or diproprionate 0.05% [Valisone, Diprosone]) may be applied and massaged into the scalp before bed each night for 7 to 14 days and then as needed subsequently.

Body

Seborrheic dermatitis of nonscalp and beard skin is steroid-responsive and responds to desonide 0.5% (Tridesilon) or hydrocortisone 2.5% (Hytone) cream, lotion, or solution applied twice daily. In addition, ketoconazole (Nizoral) cream 2% may be used alone or with the mild topical corticosteroids.

Age Considerations

Infants require a different initial regimen:

1. Daily shampoo of scalp and face with baby shampoo. Keratolytic shampoos such as those containing sulfur and salicylic acid may be used for thick scales on the scalp, but more general use should be avoided because of the potential systemic toxicity of salicylic acid.

2. Mild topical corticosteroids (e.g., 1% hydrocortisone cream) may be used in short course when dermatitis is unresponsive to shampooing alone.

Alternative Therapeutic Options

1. Chloroxine (Capitrol) shampoo may be helpful.
2. A short hairstyle or close beard trim will decrease disease activity.
3. Seborrheic blepharitis will respond to either ophthalmic antibiotics or antimicrobials (erythromycin, sulfacetamide) applied bid or these agents used along with corticosteroids or vasoconstrictive agents (Blephamide, Vasocidin, Cetapred).
4. Phenol (P & S) lotion may be applied overnight to lessen adherent scaling.

PITFALLS AND PROBLEMS

1. Seborrheic dermatitis may appear similar to eruptions seen in serious systemic diseases (systemic lupus erythematosus, Langerhans' cell histiocytosis) or congenital diseases (complement deficiencies, Hailey-Hailey disease).
2. Chronic treatment is necessary to control seborrheic dermatitis. Continuing application of potent topical corticosteroids may lead to cutaneous atrophy and telangiectasia. The appearance of this adverse reaction resembles the original disorder, and the steroid side effects may gradually replace the seborrheic dermatitis without the patient's knowledge.
3. Seborrheic dermatitis is rare in children and adolescents. Dermatophyte infections must be considered in this age group, particularly in patients complaining of scalp scaling and itching.

REFERRAL AND CONSULTATION GUIDELINES

Lack of response to initial therapy may be caused by untreated accompanying bacterial impetiginization or improper diagnosis. The differential diagnosis (Table 44–1) is extensive and includes inflammatory, infectious, malignant, and inherited disorders, each of which requires specialized therapy appropriate to the proper diagnosis. Rarely, infantile seborrheic dermatitis will progress to generalized exfoliative erythroderma associated with severe diarrhea, recurrent bacterial infections including sepsis, and wasting. This severe seborrhea, known as *Leiner's disease,* is associated in some cases with familial C5 deficiency.

TABLE 44–1

Differential Diagnosis of Seborrheic Dermatitis

Infants	***Facial Dermatitis***
With Scalp/Face/Diaper Dermatitis	Seborrheic dermatitis
Seborrheic dermatitis	Perioral dermatitis
Psoriasis	Atopic dermatitis
Atopic dermatitis	Rosacea
Langerhans' cell histiocytosis	Alopecia mucinosa
Acrodermatitis enteropathica	Keratosis pilaris atrophicans faciei
Tinea (rare)	Darier's disease
Irritant diaper dermatitis	***Truncal or Intertriginous Dermatitis***
Candida albicans diaper dermatitis	Seborrheic dermatitis
With Exfoliative Erythroderma	Tinea
Seborrheic dermatitis	Candidiasis (groins, axillae)
Leiner's disease	Psoriasis
Atopic dermatitis (rare)	Reiter's Syndrome (Genitalia)
Psoriasis (rare)	Atopic dermatitis
Medication Reaction (Rare)	Contact dermatitis
Adults	Pityriasis rubra pilaris
Scalp Dermatitis	Parapsoriasis en plaques
Seborrheic dermatitis	
Psoriasis	
Tinea capitis	
Atopic dermatitis	
Pediculosis capitis	
Dandruff	
Darier's disease	

From Cropley TG: Seborrheic dermatitis. *In* Arndt KA, LeBoit PE, Robinson JK, Wintroub BU (eds): Cutaneous Medicine and Surgery. Philadelphia: WB Saunders, 1996, p 216.

REFERENCES

1. Mathes BM, Douglass MC: Seborrheic dermatitis in patients with acquired immunodeficiency syndrome. J Am Acad Dermatol 1985; 13:947–951.
2. Johnson M, Roberts J: Prevalence of Dermatological Diseases Among Persons 1–74 Years of Age. Publication No. 79. Washington, DC: Department of Health, Education and Welfare, 1977; p 1660.
3. Crowley NC, Farr PM, Shuster S: The permissive effect of sebum in seborrheic dermatitis: An explanation of the rash in neurological disorders. Br J Dermatol 1990; 122:1–6.
4. McGinley KJ, Leyden JJ, Marples RR, Kligman AM: Quantitative microbiology of the scalp in non-dandruff, dandruff, and seborrheic dermatitis. J Invest Dermatol 1975; 64:401.

CHAPTER 45

Seborrheic Keratosis

Clark C. Otley

CLINICAL APPEARANCE

Definition

Seborrheic keratoses are the most common benign, keratinocytic neoplasms of the epidermis, found on most adults over the age of 45 years. They are a problem only when irritated or cosmetically disfiguring or when they mimic malignant neoplasms. Whether the abrupt appearance of multiple seborrheic keratoses, the sign of Leser-Trélat, is a reliable indicator of an underlying internal malignancy is doubtful.[1]

Typical Lesions and Symptoms

There is considerable heterogeneity in the clinical appearance of seborrheic keratoses, both between individuals and on an individual patient.[2] Lesions range from slightly to markedly elevated, range in color from white, black, brown, tan, red, and yellow to skin-colored, and appear ''stuck on'' to the underlying skin (see Fig. 45–1 on Color Plate 17). The surface is more often rough than smooth, with a papillomatous texture and waxy or greasy character. Individual lesions range from 2 to 60 mm, and the number on an individual patient may range from one to hundreds. Horn cysts, 0.5 to 1 mm in size, can be visualized easily with magnification and can aid in differentiation from other neoplasms. Favored sites for seborrheic keratoses include the face and trunk, especially the back. Seborrheic keratoses are asymptomatic unless irritated.

Atypical or Alternative Forms

Erythema and crusting are indicative of an irritated seborrheic keratosis (see Fig. 45–2 on Color Plate 17), which also may appear normal with only symptomatic irritation. Two unique presentations of seborrheic keratoses include dermatosis papulosa nigra (see Fig. 45–3 on Color Plate 17), in which dozens of 1- to 2-mm pedunculated brown/black keratoses appear on the temples and cheeks, and stucco keratosis, in which dozens of barely elevated, white, adherent, 2- to 6-mm keratoses occur on the legs and dorsal hands.[3,4] Seborrheic keratoses can also form cutaneous horns.

DESCRIPTION OF DISEASE

Age/Population/Demographics

Seborrheic keratoses occur in men and women of all races over the age of 30 years and are very uncommon in patients under 20 years of age.[1] The majority of people over the age of 60 years have at least one seborrheic keratosis.

Natural History of Disease

The acquisition of seborrheic keratoses is usually progressive in predisposed individuals. Individual lesions enlarge over months and may remain stable for years. The loose scale of a seborrheic keratosis may shed periodically while the base remains intact. As mentioned previously, the abrupt appearance of multiple, pruritic keratoses, known as the *sign of Leser-Trélat,* is at best an uncommon and relatively nonspecific predictor of internal malignancy.[1]

Pathology

Benign hyperplasia of keratinocytes with horn cysts characterizes seborrheic keratoses.

Etiology/Pathogenesis

Given the familial occurrence of these benign neoplasms, the predisposition toward seborrheic keratoses may be an autosomal dominant trait. Although seborrheic keratoses may occur more often at sites of sun exposure and friction, a role for solar radiation and trauma in the pathogenesis of seborrheic keratoses has not been established.

Diagnosis

In the vast majority of cases, the diagnosis of seborrheic keratosis is made clinically. However, if uncertainty as to the identity of a lesion exists, dermatologic consultation or histologic confirmation should be obtained. The differential diagnosis of seborrheic keratosis includes wart, actinic keratosis, lentigo, melanoma, pigmented basal cell carcinoma, and squamous cell carcinoma.

TREATMENT

General Therapeutic Expectations

Only seborrheic keratoses that become irritated require treatment. Uncomplicated lesions are removable with minimal side effects by experienced practitioners. There is no effective topical medication for the treatment of these occasionally disfiguring growths.

First-Line Therapy

Cryotherapy with 3 to 8 seconds of liquid nitrogen spray or equivalent application with a cotton-tipped applicator, depending on the thickness of the lesion, is very effective. As with any benign neoplasm, undertreatment is preferable to permanent side effects. Biopsy is not usually necessary but should be performed if there is any question about the nature of a cutaneous neoplasm.

Age Considerations

Because seborrheic keratoses are usually confined to adults, the appearance of a similar lesion in a child or adolescent should raise the possibility of an alternate diagnosis.

Alternative Therapeutic Options

Curettage with or without electrodesiccation, chemical peels, and dermabrasion are among the destructive modalities employed in the treatment of extensive or recalcitrant seborrheic keratoses. Excision and radiation therapy are inappropriate modalities for seborrheic keratoses.

PITFALLS AND PROBLEMS

Patients should not be discouraged from having new cutaneous neoplasms evaluated regardless of prior history of typical seborrheic keratoses, especially if there is evidence of irritation, crusting, bleeding, or avulsion. Additionally, patients cannot be expected to evaluate the characteristics of their own neoplasms. Prompt evaluation of any suspicious cutaneous growth is in the interest of both patient and physician.

Malignant neoplasms may be associated with or mimic seborrheic keratoses.[5] Histologic examination of any atypical lesions is mandatory.[5] Horn cysts may occur in benign and malignant melanocytic neoplasms and should not be used as a sole predictor of benignity. Overly aggressive treatment of seborrheic keratoses may result in irreversible scarring or pigmentary changes.

REFERRAL AND CONSULTATION GUIDELINES

In the event of uncertainty about the nature of a cutaneous neoplasm or atypical response to treatment, consultative opinion or biopsy confirmation, or both, should be obtained. Evaluation by a dermatologist in difficult cases will increase diagnostic certainty and prevent unnecessary biopsies or procedures. Dermatologists can also be helpful in the treatment of seborrheic keratoses in cosmetically sensitive patients.

REFERENCES

1. Lindelof B, Sigurgeirsson B, Melander S: Seborrheic keratoses and cancer. J Am Acad Dermatol 1992; 26:947.
2. Berman A, Winkelmann RK: Seborrheic keratosis. Arch Dermatol 1982; 118:615.
3. Hairston MA, Reed RJ, Derbes VJ: Dermatosis papulosa nigra. Arch Dermatol 1964; 89:655.
4. Willoughby C, Soter NA: Stucco keratosis. Arch Dermatol 1972; 105:859.
5. Mikhail G, Mehregan A: Basal cell carcinoma in seborrheic keratosis. J Am Acad Dermatol 1982; 6:500.

CHAPTER 46

Stasis Dermatitis

Larisa C. Kelley

Primary care physicians frequently see elderly patients with red, swollen lower extremities. Many of these cases represent stasis dermatitis, the noninfectious cutaneous sequela of lower extremity venous insufficiency.

CLINICAL APPEARANCE

The clinical manifestations of stasis dermatitis are protean and dependent on the amount of venous congestion. Early signs of venous disease are calf edema or small arborizing veins and varicosities originating around the ankles.[1] As the disease process progresses, stasis dermatitis eventually ensues.

Stasis dermatitis usually alternates through acute and chronic phases. Acute stasis dermatitis presents as an erythematous, scaly, and occasionally weepy eruption that follows a rapid increase in static venous blood with subsequent calf edema (see Fig. 46–1 on Color Plate 17). The dermatitis typically originates around the medial malleolar area, with progression up the calf. Patients often complain of aching, itching, or burning sensations. During this phase, there is a high incidence of superinfection and ulceration resulting from small breaks in the skin. Chronic stasis dermatitis, the quiescent counterpart, clinically appears as thickened brownish-red plaques on atrophic calf skin (see Fig. 46–2 on Color Plate 17). There is less swelling during this phase, and the plaques are relatively asymptomatic. An acute flare can be precipitated by local infection, trauma, thrombophlebitis, or deep vein thrombosis.

Clinical Variants

Lipodermatosclerosis is a clinical manifestation of stasis dermatitis distinguished by remarkably tender, sclerotic erythematous or hyperpigmented plaques with loss of subcutaneous fat. The most impressive feature is the ''woody,'' indurated texture of the skin. Lipodermatosclerosis also starts around the medial malleoli (see Fig. 46–3 on Color Plate 17), with eventual progression up the lower calf, giving the leg an appearance of an inverted bottle.[2] Atrophie blanche is another variant of stasis dermatitis. It appears as circumscribed, ivory-white atrophic scars stippled with telangiectasia. These lesions commonly measure 2 to 4 cm and are surrounded by a halo of hyperpigmentation.

A common sequela of longstanding stasis dermatitis, despite meticulous care, is skin breakdown and ulceration. Skin ulceration adds significant morbidity to the clinical presentation and management of stasis dermatitis.

DESCRIPTION OF THE DISEASE

In a competent venous system, the direction of flow is from the superficial capillaries and veins through the perforating vessels to the deep veins, eventually emptying into the ileofemoral system.[3] The veins contain unidirectional valves. These valves as well as the calf muscle pump are integral parts of ensuring the direction of flow despite gravitational forces. In an incompetent network, the superficial venous or deep venous systems, or both, can be dysfunctional. The source of incompetence arises from either a defective calf muscle pump, valvular reflux, varicosities, arteriovenous fistulas, or thromboses, or any combination of these.[4] The end result is a reversal in the direction of venous flow, producing congested, static blood throughout the venous system. The cutaneous manifestations are a direct result of this congestion.

Edema, an early sign of venous disease, is produced by increased intravascular hydrostatic forces causing serous outflow from vessel walls.[1] Foreign exudate and proteins accumulate in the skin, and a sterile inflammatory (eczematous) reaction is produced in the epidermis. This gives the skin a red, weepy, scaly appearance seen in the acute phases of the disease. In this state, the skin defenses and healing capabilities are reduced, with a resulting increased incidence of contact dermatitis, infection, and ulceration.[1] As an acute flare resolves, hemosiderin and melanin pigment are deposited in the connective tissue, giving the skin the characteristic brownish-red color seen in chronic stasis dermatitis.[5] In longstanding disease, extravasated fibrinogen molecules form complexes around superficial dermal capillaries and in the dermal stroma. The fibrous stroma and pericapillary fibrin cuffs eventually form a barrier to diffusion of oxygen and other nutrients, which results in tissue fibrosis, ischemia, and ulceration.[5]

Histologically, the acute stage of the disease reveals edema and vesiculation in the epidermis. Chronic disease has a more thickened epidermis, with dilated vessels resting in a fibrotic dermis. Abundant dermal hemosiderin is found in both stages.

Predisposing circumstances to venous congestion are obesity, pregnancy, varicose veins, and long periods of immobility.[3] Venous disease and its cutaneous sequelae have a higher incidence in women.[2]

EVALUATION

Initial evaluation is clinical and therapeutic. In the absence of dramatic improvement with simple initial treatment, further evaluation may be required. Additional assessment of venous disease should focus on localizing the area of incompetence. Doppler ultrasonography is a noninvasive first-line screening maneuver that can determine the direction of venous flow but is not sensitive enough to discriminate between the superficial and the deep systems. Photoplethysonography is a more discriminating test that is based on the light absorption spectrum of hemoglobin and is able to differentiate deep versus superficial venous congestion. Air plethysonography is an equally sensitive test involving measurement of venous pressure by an external pressurized cuff. The advantage of air plethysonography is that an objective assessment can be made of the calf muscle pump by taking measurements during both exercise and rest. Most recently, duplex scanning has given excellent resolution of the flow of the venous system. It is important to properly evaluate the extent of venous incompetence and its etiology to determine the correct treatment.[4]

TREATMENT

Treatment of stasis dermatitis revolves around the basic premise of increasing lower extremity venous return.[1] The mainstay of treatment is elevation and compression. Elevating the legs above the level of the heart increases venous return by gravitational forces and is the most effective and simplest initial treatment of edematous legs.[4] Patients with considerable venous incompetence should be instructed not to stand idle for prolonged periods of time and, when sitting, to elevate the legs.

Compression therapy increases venous return by stabilizing incompetent vessel walls, increasing the tissue hydrostatic pressures, and enhancing the propulsive forces generated by the calf muscle pump. In addition to enhancing venous return, compression has been shown to induce fibrinolysis, therefore reducing tissue fibrosis and ischemia.[5] Graded elastic compression stockings are the most commonly used compression therapy. These are knee-high stockings fitted to provide 30 to 40 mmHg of compression. Ideally, measurements should be made during a time of minimal edema (i.e., morning). To obtain maximal benefit, they should be worn during all waking hours. Newer elastic stockings with zippers have been developed to promote easier use.[2, 5] An alternative to compression therapy is the use of rigid compression bandages. These are gauze wraps impregnated with zinc paste (i.e., Unna boot). Benefits of this type of compression therapy are dependent on the skill of the physician or nurse applying the dressing. One must be careful to apply even pressure without compromising the arterial system. Wrapping should always start at the forefoot and progress evenly up the calf, stopping at the knee.[1] Rigid compression bandages are most useful for patients who are unable to perform their own care or have broken down or ulcerated skin. It is recommended that these bandages be changed on a weekly basis or more frequently for more exudative eruptions. For severely edematous legs, pneumatic compression facilitates a faster reduction in edema.[5] Before starting compression therapy, it is important to evaluate the arterial system. Arterial competency can be easily assessed by comparing the ankle with the brachial systolic blood pressures. A ratio of less than 0.7 signifies arterial incompetence; therefore, compression therapy is contraindicated.[4]

Topical treatment is an important counterpart to elevation and compression. In most cases, hydration with a preservative-free ointment such as hydrated petrolatum is sufficient. Sixty to 80% of patients with stasis dermatitis have contact allergy induced by topical treatment;[1] therefore, ointments and creams with common sensitizers such as paraben, propylene glycol, lanolin, formaldehyde, ethylene diamine, cetyl stearyl alcohols, and neomycin should be avoided.[3] For acute eczematous flares, mild topical steroids (Classes VI to VII) can be applied twice daily for brief periods of time (1 to 2 weeks). Ointments (oil-based) rather than creams (water-based) are recommended because ointments contain fewer sensitizers and are better emollients.[5] Commercially available ointments such as hydrocortisone 2.5% (Hytone 2.5%) and desonide 0.05% (Tridesilon 0.05%) are recommended given their low potency and low concentration of vehicle sensitizers. One needs to be aware of the inactive ingredients of topical preparations prescribed to avoid sensitizing agents. Stronger topical steroids are usually not necessary and can increase the chances of ulceration by producing atrophy.

For patients with lipodermatosclerosis, who do not have improvement with compression or cannot tolerate the treatment owing to pain, stanozolol, 2 mg twice daily for 8 to 10 weeks, has been used to induce fibrinolysis.[2] Side effects to consider include abnormal liver and lipid profiles, hypertension, acne, and hirsutism.[2] These unfavorable side effects usually limit its use.

Small skin abrasions in an area of venous stasis dermatitis are at high risk of developing frank ulceration. These must be taken seriously and treated appropriately. Occlusive dressings such as hydrocolloids (e.g., DuoDerm) and hydrogels (e.g., Vigilion) facilitate quicker healing. These dressings are typically left in place until exudate has accumulated, resulting in loss of adherence of the dressing. The occlusive dressings protect the wound bed, prevent desiccation, and enhance epidermal growth factors.[5] A contraindication to an occlusive dressing is superinfection. In this case, saline dressings and topical antibiotics should be used until the ulcer bed is clear of infection. The least sensitizing topical antibiotics are erythromycin 2% in petrolatum base and mupirocin ointment (Bactroban).[5] Ulcers that do not heal with elevation, compression, and occlusive dressings may require skin grafting. Split-thickness skin grafts are the most commonly used; however, newer techniques such as autologous or allogenic grafting have gained popularity.

Patients with severe venous congestion should be evaluated for more invasive treatment such as sclerotherapy or surgical ligation. Indications for either treatment vary; however, varicosities of the larger saphenous veins and perforators usually need surgical ablation, whereas smaller reticular and arborizing varices are amenable to sclerotherapy.[1] The mechanism of these ablative procedures is to decrease the percentage of static venous flow, resulting in shunting of venous return through competent veins.

PITFALLS AND PROBLEMS

Allergic contact dermatitis to the active or inactive ingredients of topical medications is frequent. One should use bland topical agents, avoiding the common sensitizers mentioned previously.

Recurrent or chronic cellulitis is also a common problem and usually presents as markedly red, hot, and exquisitely tender plaques. It is often accompanied by lymphangitis, lymphadenopathy, and constitutional symptoms. Treatment should be directed toward the most common etiologic agents, staphylococci and streptococci. If there is no response to oral antibiotics, intravenous therapy should be considered.

Superficial thrombophlebitis is also seen in patients with lower extremity venous disease. It can be easily recognized as a red, tender, palpable cord and is the result of thrombotic venous occlusion with resulting inflammation of the venous wall. Treatment includes nonsteroidal anti-inflammatory medications, compression, and mobilization.

REFERRAL GUIDELINES

A consultation with a dermatologist or a leg ulcer/vascular clinic should be considered for patients with chronic, recalcitrant stasis dermatitis. In addition to recommending alternative noninvasive treatment options, these can help identify patients who would benefit from sclerotherapy or phlebectomy.

CONCLUSION

Physician awareness of the consequences of lower extremity venous disease is important for patient education and prevention. If calf edema is minimized, the cutaneous sequelae, dermatitis and ulceration, are less likely. Early treatment is essential.

REFERENCES

1. Braun-Falco O, Plewig G, Wolff HH, Winkelman RK: Diseases of the blood vessels. Dermatology. Berlin, Heidelberg: Springer-Verlag, 1991; pp 631–648.
2. Kirsner RS, Pardes JB, Eaglstern WH, Falanga V: The clinical spectrum of lipodermatosclerosis. J Am Acad Dermatol 1993; 28:623–627.
3. Ryan TJ, Burnand K: Diseases of the veins and arteries—Leg ulcers. *In* Rook A, Wilkinson DS, Ebling FJG (eds): Textbook in Dermatology. Oxford: Blackwell, 1992; pp 1963–2015.
4. Ongenae KC, Phillips TJ: Leg ulcers and wound healing. *In* Arndt KA, Robinson JK, LeBoit PE, Wintroub BU (eds): Cutaneous Medicine and Surgery. An Integrated Program in Dermatology. Philadelphia: WB Saunders, 1995; pp 558–571.
5. Phillips TJ, Dover JS: Leg ulcers. J Am Acad Dermatol 1991; 25:965–987.

CHAPTER 47

Sunburn

Charles R. Taylor

CLINICAL DESCRIPTION

Definition

Sunburn is a very common, acute, delayed skin injury resulting from overexposure to ultraviolet (UV) radiation, whether from sunlight or artificial sources, and appears as transient cutaneous inflammation in exposed areas, most commonly in fair-skinned individuals. Ordinary sunburn is the most common example of a first-degree burn, involving the epidermis. Occasionally, sunburns may present as second-degree injuries with blisters, representing injury down to the superficial dermis. Although ultraviolet B (UVB) radiation (290 to 320 nm) is largely responsible for sunburn, the large amount of ultraviolet A (UVA) radiation (320 to 400 nm) in terrestrial sunlight contributes up to 15% of the reaction.

Typical Lesions and Symptoms

With sharp lines of demarcation at sun-protected areas, acute sunburns do not show the type of eruption that occurs in abnormal responses to UV radiation, such as the papules or plaques seen in polymorphic light eruption or so-called sun poisoning. A mild sunburn is characterized by pink erythema, mild edema, and tenderness with a hot, dry, tight feeling. Pruritus is variable. Severe sunburns are characterized by bright erythema, intense edema, and blistering. The patient complains of intense pain and the inability to tolerate contact with clothing and linen. Constitutional symptoms and signs such as headache, nausea, malaise, tachycardia, chills, and fever often occur in the severely sunburned patient.

Typically, erythema begins within 2 to 6 hours of exposure and reaches a peak 24 to 48 hours later. Longer exposures cause a more rapid and persistent erythema. In the absence of further exposure, the erythema fades over 3 to 5 days as desquamation and tanning ensue.

DESCRIPTION OF DISEASE

Demographics

Most fair-skinned people experience sunburn in the first decade of life. Provided the exposure is long enough, individuals with dark complexions can, in fact, sunburn. A retrospective study analyzed 562 sun-related burns and found that females, mainly adults, represented 60.8% of all patients presenting with sunburn.[1] Occurring in all age groups and at all latitudes, sunburn is seen more often in beachgoers or those who take winter vacations in tropical areas and less often in populations indigenous to equatorial areas. Very young children and elderly persons appear to have a reduced capacity to sunburn.

Natural History of Disease

Complete recovery without scar formation or blemish is usual in sunburns. However, there can be permanent hypopigmentation, probably related to melanocytic destruction. Most sunburns resolve within a week, although the effects of severe ones may last longer.

Pathology

Microscopic changes become visible within 30 minutes of exposure in the form of dyskeratotic cells known as *sunburn cells,* which evolve from damaged keratinocytes and appear eosinophilic on routine histologic sections. Intercellular edema is seen along with lymphocyte exocytosis as well as melanocyte and Langerhans' cell vacuolization. The endothelial cells swell. The dermal infiltrate is superficial, perivascular, and mixed.

Etiology

The chromophores or molecules that absorb UV radiation and initiate the chemical pathways leading to UV-induced erythema have not been clearly identified. Whereas much evidence exists to suggest that DNA may be an important target, UV-induced injury to other cellular components probably also contributes to the response. Longer UV wavelengths penetrate the dermis, affecting the vessels, which gradually dilate. The mediators that cause erythema involve histamine for both UVB and UVA. Cytokines also appear to be involved, since UV radiation is a potent stimulus for their release by keratinocytes with local as well as systemic proinflammatory and immunomodulatory actions. Other known mediators include serotonin, lysosomal enzymes, and kinins. A detailed understanding of the precise mechanisms of UV-induced erythemogenesis is lacking.

TREATMENT

In general, sunburn is more easily prevented than treated. Certainly, prevention and avoidance of recurrent sunburns should be stressed. A history of "blistering" sunburns in youth is definitely a risk factor for the development of malignant melanoma in later years. Moreover, repeated sunburns result in photoaging changes or "dermatoheliosis" over time. Recommendations include sun avoidance whenever possible, especially during the hours from 10 A.M. to 3 P.M., and regular use of high (≥15) sun protection factor (SPF) sunscreens, which need to be reapplied after swimming or profuse sweating. Clothing such as wide-brimmed hats, long sleeves, and UV-protective sunglasses should be judiciously employed to avoid extensive sunburns.

When preventive techniques fail, accurate assessment of both the extent of the sunburn and the patient's general medical condition is essential for good management. For mild, localized sunburns, apply cool tap water or saline solution compresses for 20 minutes three or four times daily. If sunburn is more extensive, cool baths for 20 minutes three or four times a day should be used. A fluorinated topical corticosteroid ointment may be applied twice a day to reduce inflammation and sometimes pain. Bland emollients such as petroleum jelly or hydrated petrolatum should be used frequently to soothe and relieve dryness. All topical agents should be applied gently and can be diluted with equal parts of ice-cold water to minimize application pain. For analgesia, aspirin, when there is no contraindication, has been found to be effective. Synergistic beneficial effects of oral nonsteroidal anti-inflammatory drugs (NSAIDs) and topical steroids have been reported.[2] Other investigators have found that the early administration of NSAIDs alone, whether topical or oral, is effective, but the results are mixed.[3, 4] Local anesthetics are not very effective, with the exception of 20% benzocaine; moreover, they can sensitize the individual against related compounds. Systemic antihistamines may help to control pruritus.

For severe sunburns, bedrest is indicated and a short course of systemic steroids in the form of prednisone, 40 to 60 mg daily tapered over 7 to 10 days, may be useful. However, systemic steroid treatment has not been established to be efficacious by controlled studies. For children, systemic steroids are given in the dose of 1 mg/kg body weight. Such treatment should be instituted early—if possible, before erythema and symptoms are established—to abort the severe inflammation that will follow. Continuous cool compresses or frequent baths, topical fluorinated steroids, bland emollients, and analgesics should be added to systemic steroid therapy. Generally, the vesicles of a second-degree burn should not be opened, since they form a natural barrier against contamination with microorganisms. If blisters become tense and unduly painful, the fluid may be evacuated under aseptic conditions by puncturing the wall with a sterile needle, allowing the blister to collapse on the underlying wound. The wound is then covered with a topical antibiotic such as bacitracin or sulfadiazine. The patient must be observed for possible cutaneous bacterial superinfection.

PITFALLS AND PROBLEMS

Occasionally, an apparent sunburn may in fact be the result of a phototoxic reaction owing to a systemic or topical sensitizing medication. For example, patients on tetracyclines or thiazide diuretics may experience painful erythema on minimal sun exposure. Sulfonamides, phenothiazines, nalidixic acid, amiodarone, and psoralens are other common photosensitizing agents. Easy burning may also be seen in lupus or less often in erythropoietic protoporphyria. Rarely, exaggerated sunburns may be the presenting complaints of DNA repair disorders such as xeroderma pigmentosum or Cockayne's syndrome. Finally, many traditional local emollients, especially those containing fragrances and anesthetics, are potential sensitizers or irritants and may aggravate the sunburn.

REFERRAL AND CONSULTATION GUIDELINES

Patients with extensive burns, deep burns, or blistering burns involving the head, hands, feet, or perineum need to be closely monitored. Severely toxic patients are best managed in a specialized burn unit for fluid replacement and infection prophylaxis.

REFERENCES

1. Piccolo-Lobo MS, Piccolo NS, Piccolo-Daher MT, Cardoso VM: Sun tanning–related burns—A 3-year experience. Burns 1992; 18:103–106.
2. Hughes GS, Francom SF, Means LK, et al: Synergistic effects of oral nonsteroidal drugs and topical corticosteroids in the therapy of sunburn in humans. Dermatology 1992; 184:54–58.
3. Lichtenstein J, Flowers F, Sheretz EF: Nonsteroidal anti-inflammatory drugs. Int J Dermatol 1987; 26:80–87.
4. Schwartz T, Gschnait F, Greiter F: Photoprotective effect of topical indomethacin—An experimental study. Dermatologica 1985; 171:450–458.

CHAPTER 48

Tinea (Pityriasis) Versicolor

K. Robin Carder and Matthew J. Stiller

CLINICAL APPEARANCE

Tinea (pityriasis) versicolor is a noncontagious, chronically relapsing, superficial fungal infection characterized by scaling macules on the trunk (Fig. 48–1 on Color Plate 18). It is caused by the yeast *Malassezia furfur,* often synonymously referred to as *Pityrosporum ovale*, *Pityrosporum orbiculare*, or *Malassezia ovalis*. Tinea versicolor is most prevalent in warmer climates, often improving in the winter months, then flaring in the summer. Lesions become more noticeable in the summer, since affected areas often fail to tan normally. The color of the lesions varies from white to pink to light brown, according to the normal pigmentation of the patient; hence, the name *versicolor*. In general, darker-skinned individuals will develop macules that are hypopigmented and pale. The macules of fair-skinned individuals tend to be hyperpigmented. Lesions are typically small (about 1 cm) but can coalesce, becoming quite large. The scale, a characteristic feature of this condition, is not always readily apparent. Often, light scraping with a slide or fingernail is required for the scale to become evident. Distribution is greatest on the seborrheic regions of the body, with lesions most prominent on the upper chest and back, proximal extremities, abdomen, and neck. Patients are usually asymptomatic, although some may experience mild to moderate pruritus. The primary complaint is cosmetic.

Infection most commonly appears in the manner described previously, but alternate presentations exist. For example, in patients with the acquired immunodeficiency syndrome (AIDS), involvement can be more extensive, with distribution extending to the face, scalp, and genitalia. Infants, especially those with dark skin who live in warm climates, are prone to develop achromia parasitica. This condition is a severe form of *M. furfur* infection characterized by marked hypopigmentation of the diaper area that then spreads rapidly to other parts of the body.[1, 2] Involvement of the flexural surfaces is characteristic of another variant known as *inverse tinea versicolor*. Lastly, *M. furfur* overgrowth may occur in the hair follicles, resulting in a pruritic *Pityrosporum* folliculitis.

DESCRIPTION OF DISEASE

Tinea versicolor primarily affects adolescents and young adults, the age groups in which sebum production is highest, but any age group can be affected. The distribution is worldwide, with the greatest incidence in the tropics. In the United States, the incidence is estimated to be about 1%.[3] Studies vary as to the ratio of men and women, but overall the sexes appear to be affected equally. There is no racial predilection.[2]

Many predisposing factors exist for tinea versicolor infection. Humidity, warm climates, hyperhidrosis, pregnancy, and immunosuppression are known to increase frequency of infection. Less common factors include diabetes, Cushing's disease, adrenalectomy, malnutrition, use of oral contraceptives or parenteral steroids, striae, extensive burns, and ichthyosis.[3] There is also evidence to suggest an inherited predisposition. These factors are thought to trigger the conversion of *M. furfur* from the saprophytic yeast that is part of normal skin flora to the mycelial or hyphal form that is associated with development of clinical disease. Once infection occurs, depigmentation develops as a result of inhibition of tyrosinase (a key enzyme of melanin production) by C9–C11 dicarboxylic acids, products of *M. furfur*.[1]

Diagnosis of tinea versicolor can often be made clinically through recognition of the classic appearance and distribution. The diagnosis is confirmed by microscopic examination of scale using 10% potassium hydroxide. The classic finding on potassium hydroxide examination is the presence of both round budding blastospores and short septate hyphae, often described as ''spaghetti and meatballs'' (see Fig. 48–1 on Color Plate X). Wood's lamp examination is also helpful in diagnosis and reveals golden-yellow fluorescence. Biopsy, rarely necessary for diagnosis, shows organisms (yeast) in the stratum corneum.[2]

TREATMENT

Many topical agents have been used successfully to treat tinea versicolor. Antifungal preparations are often the first line of therapy. One of the more widely used preparations is selenium sulfide (Selsun) 2.5% lotion or shampoo applied for 10 minutes once a day for 2 weeks, then once every 2 to 4 weeks as prophylaxis. The topical imidazoles (miconazole 2% cream, clotrimazole 1% cream/lotion, ketoconazole 2% cream/shampoo, econazole 1% cream, sulconazole 1% cream/solution) are effective treatment options. Other useful antifungal agents are haloprogin 1% cream, tolnaftate 1% cream, terbinafine 1% cream, naftifine 1% cream/gel, and ciclopirox 1% cream/lotion (applied twice daily for 2 to 3 weeks); zinc pyrithione 1% shampoo (once daily for 10 minutes for 1 to 2 weeks); 2% sulfur in an ointment base; and sodium hyposulfite (20% aqueous solution). Sodium thiosulfate 25% (Tinver lotion), used twice daily for 2 to 4 weeks, is one of the more successful therapies.

Keratolytic agents such as 50% propylene glycol in water (applied twice daily for 2 weeks), salicylic acid, sulfur and salicylic acid (Sebulex) soap or shampoo, and Whitfield's ointment (benzoic acid 12%, salicylic acid 6%—half strength may be used if irritation develops) provide additional topical treatment options. Retinoic acid 0.005% lotion/cream has been used in refractory cases.[2]

The primary disadvantage of topical therapy is inconvenience. Elimination of infection requires frequent and regular applications of medication to the entire trunk, neck, arms, and thighs even though only a portion of these areas may be affected.[4] This is not only time-consuming but also can be cosmetically objectionable, since some topical therapies have unpleasant (sulfur) odors. Clearance, if achieved, can take weeks to months.

Oral medications provide an appealing alternative with shorter durations of treatment, greater convenience, and more rapid results. Oral ketoconazole has been shown to be effective as a single dose of 400 mg (or 200 mg/day for 5 days) with greater than 95% of patients cleared within 4 weeks. Efficacy can be further enhanced with exercise, as sweating increases drug delivery to the skin surface. Following single-dose therapy, patients remain clear for an average of 8 months.[3]

Ketoconazole is not without problems, however, and 1 to 3% of patients develop nausea, vomiting, headaches, malaise, diarrhea, pruritus, or abdominal pain. The most common side effect has been a transient elevation in liver enzymes. In 1 of 12,000 patients, symptomatic hepatitis may develop. Hepatitis is typically seen after a few weeks to a month of therapy, especially in patients having a history of prior idiosyncratic drug reactions, hepatitis, or prior treatment with griseofulvin. Hepatotoxicity rarely occurs in patients receiving treatment for less than a week.[5] Other effective oral agents are fluconazole (a single 400-mg dose) and itraconazole (200 mg/day for 1 week). Griseofulvin is not effective in tinea versicolor. Because of the potential risks, oral therapy should be reserved for those patients who fail topical therapy, have extensive involvement with frequent recurrences, or are immunocompromised. Once the infection has been cleared, repigmentation can be stimulated with sunlight or phototherapy but may still take months to achieve.

Despite adequate treatment, recurrences of tinea versicolor are common: 60% within 1 year of therapy and 80% within 2 years.[4] Prophylaxis is crucial for control of the disease. Prophylaxis can be topical, with application of the medication every 2 to 4 weeks, or oral, with ketoconazole (400 mg) once a month or at the first sign of reinfection. Prophylaxis is most necessary in immunocompromised patients who experience more frequent relapses.

DIFFERENTIAL DIAGNOSIS

Many conditions can mimic tinea versicolor. Vitiligo and postinflammatory hypopigmentation resemble the hypopigmented form. The former can be distinguished (with the aid of a Wood lamp) by its progressive and complete loss of pigmentation and lack of scale. Nevus depigmentosus and nevus anemicus can also appear similar, but these are typically localized and do not progress. Pityriasis rosea, seborrheic dermatitis, pityriasis alba, dermatophyte infections, and psoriasis are scaling conditions that must be included in the differential diagnosis. They can usually be differentiated from tinea versicolor by history, appearance, distribution, and potassium hydroxide examination.

REFERRAL/CONSULTATION GUIDELINES

Tinea versicolor is a chronic condition that is difficult and frustrating to treat. It has a high recurrence rate and is often slow to respond to topical therapy. Nevertheless, temporary clearing can be achieved in most patients. Because of the resemblance of tinea versicolor to other dermatologic conditions, complete failure to respond to proven therapies should warrant reconsideration of the diagnosis. Immunodeficiency should be suspected in cases that are unusually extensive, resistant to treatment, or more frequently relapsing.

REFERENCES

1. Martin AG, Kobayashi GS: Yeast infections: Candidiasis, pityriasis (tinea) versicolor. *In* Fitzpatrick TB, Eisen AZ, Wolff K, et al (eds): Dermatology in General Medicine. 4th ed. New York: McGraw-Hill, 1993; pp 2452–2467.
2. Rippon JW: Medical Mycology: The Pathogenic Fungi and the Pathogenic Actinomycetes. 3rd ed. Philadelphia: WB Saunders, 1988.
3. Borelli D, Jacobs PH, Nall L: Tinea versicolor: Epidemiologic, clinical, and therapeutic aspects. J Am Acad Dermatol 1991; 25:300–305.
4. Faergemann J: *Pityrosporum* infections. J Am Acad Dermatol 1994; 31:S18–S20.
5. Goodless DR, Ramos-Caro FA, Flowers FP: Ketoconazole in the treatment of pityriasis versicolor: International review of clinical trials. DICP 1991; 25:395–398.

CHAPTER 49

Urticaria

Michael D. Tharp

CLINICAL APPEARANCE AND DESCRIPTION

Urticaria or angioedema occurs in up to 20 to 25% of all individuals at some time during their lives, and it is seen in all age groups. Whereas acute urticaria is more common in children and young adults, chronic urticaria is more prevalent in adults, with a greater incidence in women than in men.[1] In one retrospective study of patients with urticaria/angioedema, 49% had both types of lesions, 40% had urticaria alone, and 11% had angioedema alone.[2] Fifty percent of patients experiencing chronic urticaria will be free of their hives after 1 year, whereas 20% continue to experience their eruption for more than 20 years. In contrast, 50 to 75% of patients with combined urticaria and angioedema can have active disease for up to 5 years, and 20% for more than 20 years.[2, 3]

Urticaria (hives) consists of pale to red, well-demarcated, transient, pruritic swellings involving the dermis, and the swellings can vary from a few millimeters to many centimeters in size. They are often round or oval, but they may coalesce into plaques with irregular borders or evolve into annular, arcuate, or serpiginous lesions. Urticarial lesions do not scale or demonstrate pigmentary changes, but they may be surrounded by an area of pallor or erythema. Individual lesions of urticaria typically have an abrupt onset and last less than 24 hours, which differentiates them from other cutaneous disorders that present with a hivelike morphology (Fig. 49–1). Urticaria lasting up to 6 weeks has been empirically classified as acute disease, whereas recurrent attacks of hives lasting more than 6 weeks are arbitrarily defined as chronic urticaria. Although urticaria represents a cutaneous reaction pattern for which there are multiple potential causes (Table 49–1), many patients with chronic urticaria (80% or more) have idiopathic disease. Patients with chronic urticaria may also have an associated physical urticarial reaction. In one series of 96 chronic urticaria patients, 37% experienced delayed pressure urticaria, 22% dermatographism, and 11% cholinergic urticaria.[3, 4]

Angioedema is the term used to describe deeper swellings of the skin and subcutis, and it may be acute or chronic. These lesions have poorly defined borders and often retain their normal skin color. They may be asymmetric and slightly painful or pruritic. Angioedema most often involves the eyelids, lips, tongue, genitalia, hands, and feet, with the larynx, gastrointestinal tract, and urinary bladder being less commonly affected. Angioedema, like urticaria, is an acute or chronic reaction pattern for which there are multiple potential causes or associated disorders (see Table 49–1), and it can occur without urticaria.[2, 5–7] Most cases are idiopathic; however, angioedema has been associated with physical and contact urticarias as well as recurrent attacks consisting

TABLE 49–1

Common Causes of Urticaria and Angioedema

Infections
Medications
Contactants
Physical agents (heat, cold, vibration, pressure, light, and water)
Foods and food additives
Insect bites

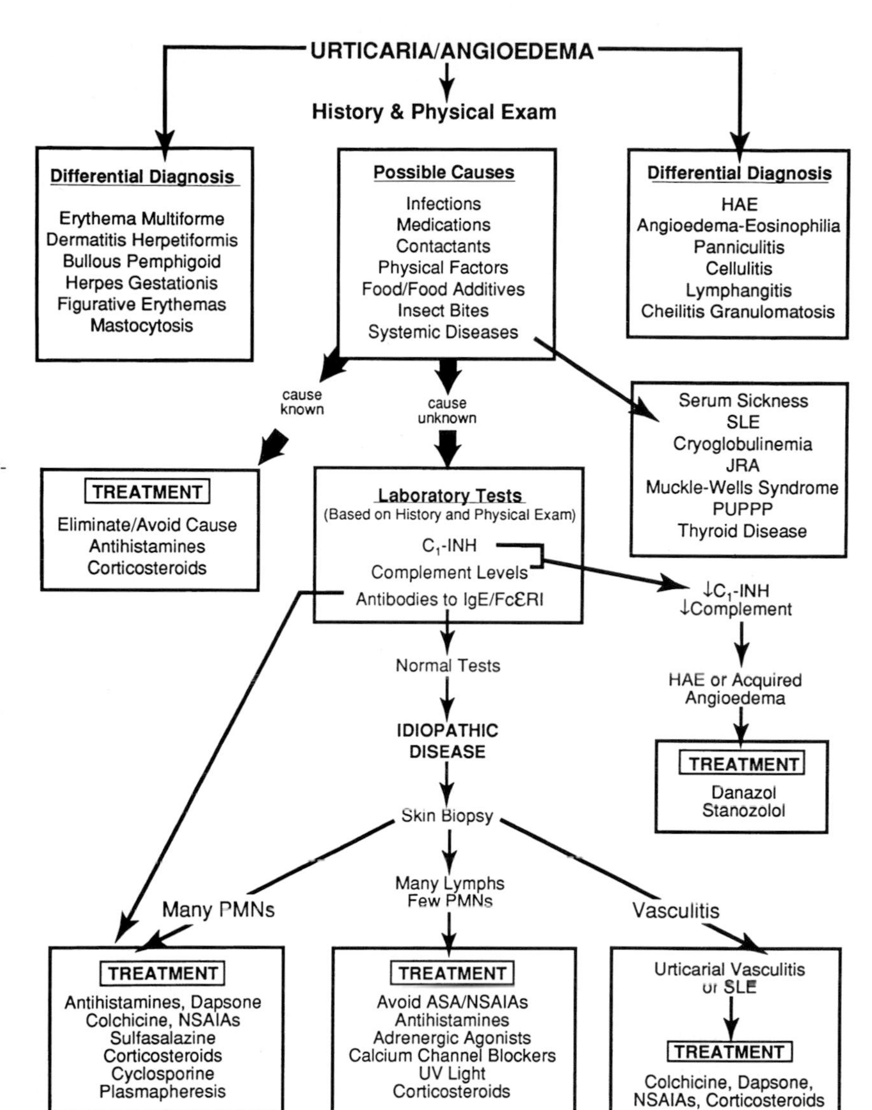

FIGURE 49-1

Approach to the diagnosis and treatment of urticaria and angioedema. *Abbreviations:* Exam, examination; HAE, hereditary angioedema; C_1-INH, C1-esterase inhibitor; IgE/FcεRI, immunoglobulin E/high-affinity IgE receptor; SLE, systemic lupus erythematosus; JRA, juvenile rheumatoid arthritis; PUPPP, pruritic urticarial papules and plaques of pregnancy; PMNs, polymorphonuclear neutrophils; Lymphs, lymphocytes; NSAIAs, nonsteroidal anti-inflammatory analgesics; ASA, acetylsalicylic acid; UV, ultraviolet.

of eosinophilia, fever, and acute weight gain.[5, 8] Hereditary forms of angioedema are well characterized. Lesions in patients with hereditary angioedema (HAE) appear as deep swellings that last up to 2 to 4 days.[9, 10] Urticaria does not occur in conjunction with HAE. The clinical course of HAE is characterized by recurrent attacks of painful angioedema of the skin and mucosa of the upper respiratory and gastrointestinal tracts. Death from laryngeal edema can occur in as many as 26% of affected, untreated persons.[10] Many factors initiate attacks of HAE, including minor trauma, emotional upset, infections, and exposure to sudden temperature changes. HAE is most often due to an autosomal dominant, genetically determined deficiency of the C1-esterase inhibitor (type I HAE).[11] Less commonly, impaired activity of this enzyme underlies HAE (type II).[12] Without C1-esterase inhibitor, the complement cascade is activated, resulting in the generation of the anaphylatoxins C3a and C5a as well as other pharmacologically active chemical mediators. Acquired forms of angioedema associated with the C1-esterase inhibitor have been described and include angioedema associated with autoantibodies that bind to the C1-esterase inhibitor, thereby blocking its activity.[13] Patients with lymphoproliferative disorders may develop angioedema that results from anti-idiotypic antibody formation and complement activation leading to C1-esterase inhibitor consumption.[14, 15]

DIAGNOSIS

The diagnosis of urticaria and angioedema is usually made on the physical examination; however, a thorough history is important not only for establishing the diagnosis but also for elucidating possible causes. General screening laboratory tests and skin testing are neither helpful nor cost-effective for these disorders; however, specific tests based on information gained from the history and physical examination may be of value. Although routine skin biopsies are not indicated for most patients with chronic urticaria or angioedema, they may prove useful in identifying a subset of patients who have predominance of polymorphonuclear neutrophils (PMNs) in lesional skin. It is noteworthy that these patients can often be identified clinically by their resistance to antihistamine therapy.[16–18]

Testing for the presence of physical urticarias can be useful if indicated by the history. Although the diagnosis of cholinergic urticaria is often made from the history, patients may be challenged by exercising or by immersing an extremity in warm (42° C) water for 15 minutes. Wheals generally appear within 2 to 20 minutes and last from 30 to 60 minutes. Injection of 10 mg of methacholine in 100 ml of normal saline solution will also reproduce the tiny wheals of cholingeric urticaria in approximately 30% of these patients. Dermatographism may be diagnosed by firm *stroking* of the skin using a retracted pen or blunt instrument (lesion appears within minutes). Pressure urticaria may be induced by hanging a *strap* with 15 pounds of weight on the shoulders or thigh for 20 minutes (lesion appears within hours). Approximately 33% of patients with pressure urticaria will have a mildly elevated sedimentation rate, and 20% will have a peripheral blood leukocytosis; however, these tests are not particularly useful for diagnosis.[4, 5] Patients suspected of having solar urticaria should be tested to ultraviolet A (UVA), ultraviolet B (UVB), and visible light using appropriate light sources. Heat-induced urticaria can be diagnosed by a challenge of 40° to 43° C water in a conductive flask for 1 to 5 minutes. Vibratory urticaria often is induced within minutes after the use of a vortex apparatus, which is available in most clinical laboratories. An ice-cube test is the classic provocation test for cold urticaria. An ice cube or a glass filled with ice is placed on the forearm for 5 to 20 minutes. Urticarial lesions typically appear as the site rewarms. A 20-minute challenge is required before the test is considered negative, and as many as 5% of patients with cold urticaria will not react to this challenge. In this patient group, immersion of an extremity in cold water or total-body exposure to a cold room is required to provoke an urticarial response.[5] The diagnosis of aquagenic urticaria is confirmed by application to the skin of a gauze pad soaked in 37° C water for several minutes.[19] Identifying patients with contact urticaria requires open or closed patch-testing, but patches must be read within 15 to 30 minutes.[20]

Among the patients with angioedema, it is most important to establish the diagnosis of HAE. A history of recurrent attacks of swelling, beginning in childhood, that often follow trauma is characteristic. Approximately 80% of patients have a positive family history for this disorder. The complement component C4 is diminished in the serum of HAE patients during asymptomatic periods and usually undetectable during an episode of angioedema. The level of C2 is usually normal during asymptomatic periods but diminished during attacks. Determination of C1-esterase inhibitor is the most specific test for HAE; however, up to 15% of patients with HAE have type II disease, in which levels of this protein are normal but its activity is impaired. Therefore, a functional assay is required to establish the diagnosis of type II HAE.[10–12] Patients with acquired forms of angioedema associated with decreased concentrations of C1-esterase inhibitor have been reported. These patients have low levels of C1, which is not seen in HAE.[10, 14] Episodic angioedema with eosinophilia is a rare cause of angioedema. Four patients have been described who experienced attacks of recurrent angioedema, urticaria, and fever associated with increased body weight, leukocytosis, and peripheral eosinophilia.[8]

TREATMENT

The most effective treatment of urticaria and angioedema is the identification and elimination of the cause. Patients with a physical urticaria often benefit from a thorough explanation of their disease that enables them to reduce the number and severity of symptomatic episodes by altering their lifestyle. Those patients with cold-induced urticaria, for example, should be advised to wear warm gloves and socks as well as to protect their face from cold air in order to minimize the frequency of attacks. In addition, these patients need to be cautioned about diving into a swimming pool filled with cool water, since anaphylaxis is possible. For patients with UVB-induced solar urticaria, sun avoidance and the use of sunscreens may be adequate treatment; however, sunscreens are often unsatisfactory for urticaria patients who are sensitive to UVA and visible light. Interestingly, some patients with solar urticaria will improve by gradually increasing their exposure to natural or artificial light. Unfortunately, the number of patients who have a detectable cause for their chronic urticaria and angioedema is relatively small. Nevertheless, a number of pharmacologic agents are effective for the treatment of urticaria and angioedema, and these medications are discussed in the following sections.

Antihistamines

Antihistamines are the only available specific inhibitors of a mast cell mediator and, therefore, are the first line of therapy. They are most effective in acute urticaria, cholinergic urticaria, and dermatographism; somewhat effective in solar, cold, aquagenic, and chronic idiopathic urticaria; and rarely useful in delayed pressure urticaria.[5, 19, 21–24] There are six classes of first-generation antihistamines, with the ethanolamines (diphenhydramine), ethylenediamines (tripelennamine), and phenothiazines (promethazine) causing the most sedation. Piperidines (cyproheptadine) are especially effective for cholinergic and cold-induced urticaria. Alkylamines (chlorpheniramine, dexchlorpheniramine, brompheniramine, and hydroxyzine) appear to be the most useful agents in initial therapy because of efficacy, tolerance, and cost. Dosing should be continuous and is generally increased in strength every 5 to 7 days to tolerance.[25–27] It has been suggested that dosing with hydroxyzine once nightly may decrease the objective signs but not the subjective symptom of sedation while still being effective.[28] This is probably due to the longer half-life of the active metabolite of hydroxyzine, which is cetirizine. Dosing of antihistamines in the elderly may need to be decreased, owing to a reduction in renal excretion.[29] Most of the antihistamines may lead to weight gain, and the anticholinergic effects of traditional antihistamines can rarely lead to movement disorders after chronic use.[30] All antihistamines, except cetirizine, undergo significant metabolism in the liver.[31]

Over the last several years second-generation antihistamines (terfenadine, astemizole, loratadine, and cetirizine), which are less sedating, have been developed. These agents have limited access to the central nervous system and tend to be more specific for H_1 receptors as well as less active at serotonin and muscarinic receptors. Thus, many of the side effects associated with first-generation H_1 antihistamines, including impaired motor and cognitive skills, do not occur with second-generation H_1 blockers.[32–35] This antihistamine group is best for patients who cannot tolerate, or are not helped by, first-generation antihistamines. The combination of two different H_1 antihistamines may prove effective in some urticarial/angioedema patients who are unresponsive to a single agent. In this case, a sedating antihistamine can be taken at night, and a second-generation antihistamine can be used during the day. Both terfenadine and astemizole have been reported to cause cardiac tachyarrhythmias and prolongation of the Q-T interval as a result of accumulation of unmetabolized parent drug in patients with liver disease or those taking ketoconazole, erythromycin, and related antibiotics and antimycotics, as well as quinine.[36–38] The recommended dosage for second-generation antihistamines should not be exceeded for these medications, and loading doses should not be prescribed. H_2 antihistamines also may be effective in the treatment of some patients with chronic urticaria and angioedema. Although early studies documented an additive effect of cimetidine and chlorpheniramine only in dermatographism, several studies have suggested an additive effect of H_1 and H_2 blockers in some chronic urticaria patients.[39, 40] The tricyclic antidepressant doxepin has potent anti–H_1- and anti–H_2-receptor activity and can be effective for the treatment of urticaria.[41, 42] Because of its extended half-life, doxepin can be used in doses of 10 to 20 mg twice a day; however, its sedating effects may limit its use to 25 to 30 mg each night. This drug should be used with caution in patients with a history of cardiac arrhythmias, and its anticholinergic side effects may limit its use in the elderly.

Other Treatments

ADRENERGIC AGENTS. Subcutaneous epinephrine (1:1000 aqueous epinephrine) at a dose of 0.2 to 0.4 ml in adults or 0.01 mg/kg of body weight for children is useful for treating acute episodes of urticaria and angioedema. The clinical effects of epinephrine last for only a few hours; therefore, another medication, such as a H_1 antihistamine, must be given in conjunction with subcutaneous epinephrine. Oral terbutaline at doses ranging from 1.25 to 2.5 mg three times per day in combination with antihistamines has proved helpful for the treatment of chronic urticaria.[43] Ephedrine also may be used at doses from 25 to 50 mg every 6 hours in adults, and at 2 to 3 mg/kg of body weight per 24 hours, divided into four doses in children.

CALCIUM CHANNEL BLOCKERS. Nifedipine has been reported to control symptoms in some urticaria patients. A double-blind, placebo-controlled crossover trial of nifedipine at 10 to 20 mg three times per day in 10 patients with chronic idiopathic urticaria who continued their antihistamines throughout the study found a significant improvement in pruritus and hives after 2 weeks of treatment.[44] However, in a double-blind crossover trial on symptomatic dermatographism, no beneficial effect of nifedipine at 10 mg orally three times per day was found.[45] Thus, it appears that nifedipine is most effective as an adjunctive agent rather than as a primary medication for the treatment of urticaria and angioedema.

CORTICOSTEROIDS. The use of systemic corticosteroids in patients with chronic idiopathic urticaria or angioedema should be reserved for those who are unresponsive to other therapies, and there are clearly isolated cases in which corticosteroids are indicated. Owing to their numerous side effects, however, daily systemic corticosteroids are to be avoided. Most patients with chronic idiopathic urticaria and angioedema respond to oral daily doses of 30 to 40 mg of prednisone within 4 to 5 days. During this time, different combinations of antihistamines or new medications such as calcium channel blockers or adrenergic agents can be introduced. Changes in the treatment regimen often permit the discontinuation of oral corticosteroids after 4 to 5 days. Systemic corticosteroids are also effective in the management of patients with delayed pressure urticaria and angioedema due to C1-esterase inhibitor antibodies; however, they frequently are needed on a chronic basis.[4, 5]

NONSTEROIDAL AGENTS. Nonsteroidal anti-inflammatory agents may be useful in some patients with pressure urticaria, and occasionally in patients with chronic urticaria.[46] However, these agents appear to worsen urticaria and angioedema in approximately 50% of patients.[1, 2]

COLCHICINE AND DAPSONE. These medications may be useful in conjunction with antihistamines for the treatment of patients who have a predominance of PMNs in their urticarial lesions.[16, 17, 47] A serum glucose-6-phosphate dehydrogenase level must be obtained prior to the use of dapsone. Therapeutic doses of dapsone range from 100 to 200 mg per day. Colchicine is best tolerated at a dose of 0.6 mg twice to three times a day.

SULFASALAZINE. This agent in doses of 2 to 3 g per day has been reported to be effective in a few patients with chronic urticaria who had a PMN–rich infiltrate on skin biopsy and required systemic corticosteroids for control.[48]

CYCLOSPORINE. Cyclosporine has been demonstrated to inhibit immunoglobulin E (IgE)–mediated human skin mast cell histamine release and to suppress chronic urticaria.[49] Symptoms promptly recur after discontinuation of the drug. The side effects and cost make cyclosporine unacceptable for the treatment of urticaria and angioedema except in cases of life-threatening disease unresponsive to all other treatments.

ANDROGENS. Androgens have been used in patients who have systemic corticosteroid–dependent urticaria. Danazol (200 mg twice per day) and stanozolol (1 to 2 mg twice per day) have induced a therapeutic response within days, allowing for the tapering of systemic corticosteroids.[50] These agents, at similar doses, are also effective for preventing episodes of angioedema in patients with HAE. Once attacks of angioedema have been controlled, dosages may be decreased.[10–12]

ULTRAVIOLET LIGHT. A controlled study of UVA light versus psoralens and UVA light (PUVA) reported an approximately 25% reduction (for both therapies) of symptom scores in patients with chronic urticaria over 16 weeks.[51] UVA light desensitization in solar urticaria also may be useful and appears most efficacious with PUVA therapy, although some patients have been treated with UVA light alone. Pretreatment with antihistamines or systemic steroids may be required. One study demonstrated a therapeutic response after 13 to 27 treatments of UVB light alone in patients with dermatographism, cholinergic urticaria, and cold urticaria. No positive effect was seen in patients with idiopathic urticaria.[46]

PLASMAPHERESIS. Urticaria patients with circulating antibodies to the high-affinity immunoglobulin E receptor have been treated with plasmapheresis three times over a 5-day period. Remissions of 4 to 8 weeks or significant improvement was observed in six of these eight patients.[52] Plasmapheresis has also been suggested in the management of solar urticaria.[52]

PITFALLS

Clinical pitfalls are most commonly related to therapy and diagnosis. First-line treatment almost always requires use of antihistamines, and for this reason, sedation, particularly in older individuals with decreased renal function, is problematic and may require use of the more expensive second-generation antihistamines. When using the latter agents, cardiac toxicity—associated with terfenadine and astemizole in patients with liver disease and in those also taking ketoconazole, erythromycin, and related antibiotics, and antimycotics and quinine—is a potential pitfall. To date, neither loratadine nor cetirizine is known to cause this problem.

Lack of expected therapeutic response to antihistamines is the best indication of a diagnostic error. In this setting, diagnoses other than routine urticaria must be considered and include neutrophil-rich urticaria, urticarial vasculitis, collagen vascular disease, chronic drug reaction, and other difficult-to-diagnose conditions.

REFERRAL/CONSULTATION GUIDELINES

The absence of expected response to antihistamines is excellent evidence that referral to a clinician with special expertise in management and diagnosis of urticarial disorders is appropriate.

REFERENCES

1. Juhlin L: Recurrent urticaria: Clinical investigation of 330 patients. Br J Dermatol 1981; 104:369–381.
2. Champion RH, Roberts SOB, Carpenter RG, et al: Urticaria and angio-oedema: A review of 554 patients. Br J Dermatol 1969; 81:588–597.
3. Margolis CF, Nisi R: Urticaria in a family practice. J Fam Pract 1985; 20:57–64.
4. Greaves MW: The physical urticarias. Clin Exp Allergy 1991; 1:284–289.
5. Barlow RJ, Warburton F, Watson K, et al: Diagnosis and incidence of delayed pressure urticaria in patients with chronic urticaria. J Am Acad Dermatol 1993; 29:954–1005.
6. Lawrence C: Cholinergic urticaria with associated angiooedema. Br J Dermatol 1981; 105:543–550.
7. Kivity S: The effect of food and exercise on the skin response to compound 48/80 in patients with food-associated exercise-induced urticaria-angioedema. J Allergy Clin Immunol 1988; 81:1155–1158.
8. Gleich GJ, Schroeter AL, Marcoux JP, et al: Episodic angioedema associated with eosinophilia. N Engl J Med 1984; 310:1621–1626.
9. Warin RP: The role of trauma in the spreading wheals of hereditary angiooedema. Br J Dermatol 1983; 108:189–194.
10. Landerman NA: Hereditary angioneurotic edema. J Allergy Clin Immunol 1962; 33:316–329.
11. Donaldson VH, Evans RR: A biochemical abnormality in hereditary angioneurotic edema: Absence of serum inhibitor of C1 esterase. Am J Med 1963; 35:37–44.
12. Rosen FS: Genetically determined heterogeneity of the C1-esterase inhibitor in patients with hereditary angioedema. J Clin Invest 1971; 50:2143–2147.
13. Gelfand JA: Acquired C1-esterase inhibitor deficiency and angioedema: A review. Medicine 1979; 58:321–328.
14. Alsenz J: Autoantibody mediated acquired deficiency of C1-inhibitor. N Engl J Med 1987; 316:1360–1363.
15. Jackson J: An IgG autoantibody which inactivates C1 inhibitor. Nature 1986; 323:722–724.
16. Jones RR, Bhogal B, Dash A, et al: Urticaria and vasculitis: A continuum of histological and immunopathological changes. Br J Dermatol 1983; 108:695–703.
17. Winkelmann RK, Reizner GT: Diffuse dermal neutrophilia in urticaria. Hum Pathol 1988; 19:389–393.
18. Zvadak D, Tharp M: Chronic urticaria as a manifestation of the late phase reaction. Immunol Allergy Clin North Am 15:4, 745–760, 1995.
19. Shelley WB, Rawnsley HM: Aquagenic urticaria: Contact sensitivity reaction to water. Arch Dermatol 1964; 189:895–898.
20. Kanerva L: Contact urticaria. *In* Lenfant C (ed): Dermatology Progress and Perspectives. The Proceedings of the 18th World Congress of Dermatology. New York: Parthenon Publishing, 1993; pp 745–749.
21. Neittaanmaki H: Cold urticaria: Clinical findings in 220 patients. J Am Acad Dermatol 1985; 13:635–644.
22. Champion RH: Urticaria, then and now. Br J Dermatol 1988; 119:427–436.
23. Kalz F, Bower CM, Pritchard H, et al: Delayed and persistent dermographia. Arch Dermatol Syphilol 1950; 61:772–780.
24. Baughman RD, Jillson DE: Seven specific types of urticaria: With special reference to delayed persistent dermatographism. Ann Allergy 1963; 21:248–255.
25. Soter NA: Acute and chronic urticaria and angioedema. J Am Acad Dermatol 1991; 25:146–154.
26. Kennard CD, Ellis CN: Pharmacologic therapy for urticaria. J Am Acad Dermatol 1991; 25:176–187.
27. Monroe EW: Urticaria. Int J Dermatol 1981; 20:32–41.
28. Goetz DW, Jacobson JM, Apaliski SJ, et al: Objective antihistamine side effects are mitigated by evening dosing of hydroxyzine. Ann Allergy 1991; 67:448–454.
29. Simons KJ, Watson WT, Chen XY, et al: Pharmacokinetic and pharmacodynamic studies of the H_1-receptor antagonist hydroxyzine in the elderly. Clin Pharmacol Ther 1989; 45:9–14.
30. Samie MR, Ashton AK: Choreoathetosis induced by cyproheptadine. Mov Disord 1989; 4:81–84.
31. Drouin MA: H1 antihistamine: Perspectives on the use of the conventional and new agents. Ann Allergy 1985; 55:747–752.
32. Monroe EW: Chronic urticaria: Review of nonsedative H_1 antihistamines in treatment. J Am Acad Dermatol 1988; 19:842–849.
33. Kalvis J, Breneman D, Tharp M, et al: Urticaria: Clinical efficacy of cetirizine in comparison with hydroxyzine and placebo. J Allergy Clin Immunol 1990; 86:1014–1018.
34. Paul E, Bodcher R-H: Comparative study of astemizole and terfenadine in the treatment of chronic idiopathic urticaria: A randomized double-blind study of 40 patients. Ann Allergy 1989; 62;318–320.
35. Simons FER: New H_1-receptor antagonists: Clinical pharmacology. Clin Exp Allergy 1990; 10(Suppl 2):19–24.
36. Wilen JF II, Gelber ML, Henreteg FM, et al: Clinical laboratory observations: Cardiotoxic effects of astemizole oxidase in children. J Pediatr 1992; 120:799–802.
37. Homig PK, Woosley RL, Zamani K, et al: Changes in the pharmacokinetics and electrocardiographic pharmacodynamics of terfenadine with concomitant administration of erythromycin. Clin Pharmacol Ther 1992; 52:231–238.
38. Monahan BP, Ferguson CL, Killeary ES, et al: Torsades de pointes occurring in association with terfenadine use. JAMA 1990; 264:2788–2790.
39. Singh G: H_2 blockers in chronic urticaria. Int J Dermatol 1984; 23:627–628.
40. Monroe EW, Cohen SH, Kalsfleisch J, et al: Combined H_1 and H_2 antihistamine therapy in chronic urticaria. Arch Dermatol 1981; 117:404–407.
41. Sullivan TJ, Parker KL, Stenson W, et al: Pharmacologic modulation of the whealing response to histamine in human skin: Identification of doxepin as a potent in vivo inhibitor. J Allergy Clin Immunol 1982; 69:260–267.
42. Greene SL, Reed CE, Schroeter AC: Double-blind crossover study comparing doxepin with diphenhydramine for the treatment of chronic urticaria. J Am Acad Dermatol 1985; 12:669–675.
43. Kennes B, De Maubeuge J, Delespesse S: Treatment of chronic urticaria with beta$_2$-adrenergic stimulant. Clin Allergy 1977; 7:35–39.
44. Bressler RB, Sowell K, Huston DP: Therapy of chronic idiopathic

urticaria with nifedipine: Demonstration of beneficial effect in a double-blind, placebo-controlled, crossover trial. J Allergy Clin Immunol 1989; 83:756–763.
45. Lawlor F, Ormerod AD, Greaves MW: Calcium antagonist in the treatment of symptomatic dermatographism: Low-dose and high-dose studies with nifedipine. Dermatologica 1988; 177:287–291.
46. Sussman GL, Harvey RP, Schocket AL: Delayed pressure urticaria. J Allergy Clin Immunol 1982; 70:337–342.
47. Lawlor F, Kobza-Black A, Ward AM, et al: Delayed pressure urticaria: Objective evaluation of a variable disease using a dermatographometer and assessment of treatment using colchicine. Br J Dermatol 1989; 120:403–408.
48. Jaffer AM: Sulfasalazine in the treatment of corticosteroid-dependent chronic idiopathic urticaria. J Allergy Clin Immunol 1991; 88:964–965.
49. Fradin MS, Ellis CN, Goldfarb MT, et al: Oral cyclosporine for severe chronic idiopathic urticaria and angioedema. J Am Acad Dermatol 1991; 25:1065–1067.
50. Brestel EP, Thrush LB: The treatment of glucocorticosteroid-dependent chronic urticaria and stanozolol. J Allergy Clin Immunol 1988; 82:265–269.
51. Olafsson JH, Larko O, Roupe G, et al: Treatment of chronic urticaria with PUVA or UVA plus placebo: A double-blind study. Arch Dermatol Res 1986; 278:228–231.
52. Grattan CE, Francis DM, Slater NG, et al: Plasmapheresis for severe, unremitting chronic urticaria. Lancet 1992; 339:1078–1080.

Viral Rashes (Those With Consequences and Those Without)

Neil S. Prose and Richard J. Antaya

Many viral and bacterial infections are accompanied by generalized rashes (exanthems) and mucous membrane eruptions (enanthems). These result either from direct invasion by the organism or by host immune response. Because of limited patterns of response, different organisms or drugs may elicit a similar response; and conversely, because of differences in immunity, the same virus may produce dissimilar eruptions. Owing to this fact, the approach to diagnosis of viral exanthems should include consideration of other physical and laboratory findings (toxicity, lymphadenopathy, complete blood count), epidemiologic data (age, season, exposures), and historical data (prodrome, evolution of rash, immune status of host).

MEASLES (RUBEOLA)

CLINICAL APPEARANCE

Definition

Measles is a self-limited, highly contagious systemic illness caused by a paramyxovirus. It has only one antigenic strain, and humans are the natural hosts and only reservoir of the infection. Prior to the introduction of vaccine in the 1960s, it was the most common childhood exanthem. It still is a problem owing to incomplete immunization in children and waning immunity in adults.

Typical Lesions and Symptoms

The typical lesions and symptoms of measles occur in three stages:

1. There is an incubation period of 9 to 14 days with few or mild symptoms and, rarely, a transitory macular or urticarial rash.
2. The prodromal stage, lasting 2 to 4 days, is characterized by a brassy cough, coryza, and conjunctivitis accompanied by fever (high at times), photophobia, and constitutional symptoms. Koplik's spots, the enanthem, first observed after prodromal symptoms have begun, are 1- to 3-mm, grayish or bluish-white elevations speckling an erythematous, granular base. These spots begin on the buccal mucosa opposite the lower molars and spread throughout the oropharynx. Koplik's spots may be transient, lasting only a few hours, but they generally precede the rash by 2 days.
3. The final stage is heralded by an erythematous

macular exanthem, which begins along the hairline and becomes increasingly confluent and papular as it spreads downward from head to foot by day 2 or 3. It is generally nonpruritic and fades in the same sequence as it appeared over the following 3 to 6 days, sometimes leaving areas of fine desquamation. The fever and constitutional symptoms peak with the progression of the rash, and most patients are quite ill appearing.

Atypical Presentations

Atypical measles is due to a wild-type measles infection in persons immunized with the "killed" measles vaccine that was available in the 1960s. It is characterized by high fever, severe respiratory symptoms, peripheral edema, and a macular, vesicular or petechial rash, primarily involving the distal extremities. It must be differentiated from Rocky Mountain spotted fever.[1]

TREATMENT

Therapeutic Expectations

Measles is self-limited, and no effective antiviral agent is available.

First-Line Therapy

Symptomatic treatment with antipyretics, analgesics, and hydration is helpful but does not alter the course of the disease.

Alternative Therapeutic Options

Vitamin A appears to reduce morbidity and mortality of measles in vitamin A–deficient patients. The American Academy of Pediatrics Committee on Infectious Diseases recommends the use of vitamin A for select cases, such as children hospitalized with complications of measles and patients with immunodeficiencies or with underlying conditions predisposing to malabsorption.

PITFALLS AND PROBLEMS

The most common complications are otitis media, pneumonia (interstitial and secondary bacterial), and encephalitis; less commonly seen are myocarditis and laryngotracheobronchitis. Hemorrhagic measles (black measles), resembling disseminated intravascular coagulation (DIC), is extremely rare.

Neurologic complications are more common in measles than in any other viral exanthem, with an incidence of 1 to 2 per 1000 cases of measles reported.

REFERRAL AND CONSULTATION GUIDELINES

All cases of rubeola should be reported to the local health department, and isolation precautions should be observed for all hospitalized patients.

RUBELLA (GERMAN MEASLES, 3-DAY MEASLES)

CLINICAL APPEARANCE

Definition

Rubella is a mild, self-limited, highly communicable illness of childhood or early adulthood. It has few significant sequelae, except congenital rubella syndrome when the infection is transmitted in utero.

Typical Lesions and Symptoms

Subclinical infection is common and may represent up to 80% of infections. Systemic illness is generally mild.

After exposure from an infected person by droplet spray, an incubation period of 14 to 21 days is followed by a prodromal stage with mild upper respiratory and constitutional symptoms, the most distressing of which is pain on lateral and upward eye movement.

The exanthem, which can be variable and mild, consisting of discrete pink macules and papules, begins on the face and progresses to the trunk and lower extremities. The face is usually clear by the second day, and the remainder of the rash disappears by the third day. Its most distinctive characteristics are its rapid change in appearance, frequently over a few hours, and its pink-red lesions, which distinguish it from the purplish-red lesions of measles.

The enanthem (Forchheimer's sign), observed early in the course, consists of petechiae on the soft palate.

Tender retroauricular and suboccipital adenopathy is a characteristic, although nondiagnostic, finding.

TREATMENT

There is no specific treatment, but live vaccine is now widely administered to prevent disease.

PITFALLS AND PROBLEMS

The risk of congenital rubella infection is highest when women contract rubella early in the first trimester of pregnancy. Exposed pregnant women who have an unknown rubella status should have their rubella titer checked emergently. The routine use of immune globulin for postexposure rubella prophylaxis in early pregnancy is not recommended, and this should be considered only if termination of the pregnancy is not an option.[2]

Other complications include arthritis, especially in older women, neuritis, and rarely, encephalitis.

REFERRAL AND CONSULTATION GUIDELINES

All cases of rubella should be reported to the local health department.

VARICELLA (CHICKENPOX)

See Chapter 14.

ROSEOLA INFANTUM (EXANTHEM SUBITUM)

CLINICAL APPEARANCE

Definition

Roseola, caused by human herpesvirus 6 (HHV6), is a common, self-limited illness and the most common viral exanthem of children under age 3 years (mostly between 6 and 18 months of age).[3]

Typical Lesions and Symptoms

The disease is characterized by 3 to 5 days of high fever (≥40° C), usually of sudden onset, accompanied by mild constitutional symptoms and febrile seizures in about 10% of patients.

Pharyngitis may be present, and some patients appear well.

The rash, characterized by discrete 2- to 5-mm, rose-pink macules and papules, occurs mainly on the trunk and neck. The most distinguishing feature is the development of this rash after defervescence and accompanying clinical improvement, either on the same day or 1 to 2 days later. It fades without desquamation in hours to days.

Atypical Presentations

HHV6 infection may occur as an undifferentiated febrile illness without rash, a rash without preceding fever, or an asymptomatic infection.

TREATMENT

Treatment is supportive, mostly limited to antipyretics, even for patients predisposed to febrile seizures.

PITFALLS AND PROBLEMS

The diagnosis is made clinically by its characteristic progression of defervescence followed by rash. However, during the febrile phase of the illness, common infections of the affected age group must be ruled out: otitis media, urinary tract infection, meningitis, and most importantly, occult bacteremia. A relative leukopenia after day 2 of illness may be helpful in differentiating roseola from the others.

FIFTH DISEASE (ERYTHEMA INFECTIOSUM)

CLINICAL APPEARANCE

Definition

Erythema infectiosum is a self-limited, moderately contagious disease that affects mainly children (usually 3 to 12 years old). It is caused by human parvovirus B19.

Typical Lesions and Symptoms

The incubation period is generally around 2 weeks. There are few, if any, prodromal symptoms. The rash evolves in three clinical stages:

1. Sudden onset of an intense macular erythema of the cheeks suggests a ''slapped cheek'' or ''sunburn'' appearance.
2. Over the following days, the facial rash fades as an erythematous maculopapular eruption begins over the extensor aspects of the proximal extremities and, to a lesser extent, the trunk and buttocks.
3. On or about the sixth day, fading of the rash begins, with areas of central clearing. This creates a distinctive and characteristic reticulated or marbled appearance, especially of the proximal extremities (see Fig. 50–1 on Color Plate 18). This rash may last 1 to several weeks or may subside only to recur intermittently over a 4- to 8-week period, usually intensified by heat, friction, exercise, or emotional outbursts.

TREATMENT

There are usually no symptoms requiring treatment for erythema infectiosum. Children should be allowed to attend school, as patients are no longer contagious after the onset of rash.[4]

PITFALLS AND PROBLEMS

The most troublesome, albeit rare, complications from parvovirus B19 are aplastic crises in patients with underlying hemolytic anemias (such as sickle cell disease and hereditary spherocytosis) and hydrops fetalis. Exposed pregnant women with positive serologic testing may require ultrasound evaluation.

The most common complication in adults, but rare in children, is arthritis. Adults also manifest more constitutional symptoms.

ENTEROVIRAL INFECTION

CLINICAL APPEARANCE

Definition

Enteroviruses of the echovirus and coxsackievirus groups are responsible for the majority of viral exanthems in the late summer and early fall. Spread mostly by a fecal-oral route, they can cause virtually any type of exanthem, but the hand-foot-and-mouth syndrome, caused by coxsackievirus A16, is the most distinctive. Rash is more common in children.

Typical Lesions and Symptoms

In most cases of enteroviral infection, an incubation period of 3 to 7 days is followed by the sudden onset of fever, often associated with some combination of pharyngitis, cervical adenopathy, myalgia, abdominal pain, or gastrointestinal symptoms. The exanthem usually begins on the face and, within hours, spreads to involve the trunk and limbs. The lesions, which may persist for 2 to 7 days, may be erythematous macular, papular, urticarial, or rubelliform. Rarely, the rash may be petechial, suggestive of meningococcal infection, or may even resemble roseola. Some echoviruses produce small papules characterized by a dilated, blanchable vessel centrally and surrounded by a white halo.

Hand-foot-and-mouth disease presents—after 1 to 2 days of low-grade fever and malaise—with the development of small red 1- to 3-mm macules that vesiculate and ulcerate on the soft palate, buccal mucosa, tongue, and uvula, usually sparing the lips. Pain occasionally interferes with eating. One to 2 days later, cutaneous lesions appear as multiple, 3- to 7-mm, round or oval, asymptomatic vesicles, favoring the lateral aspects of the palms and soles. The dorsal and, less commonly, volar aspects of the hands and feet may be involved. The vesicles resolve in 7 to 10 days in most cases.

TREATMENT

There is no specific antiviral therapy for enteroviral infections. Supportive treatment with antipyretics, analgesics, cool dairy products for mouth discomfort, and fluids to prevent dehydration is helpful.

PITFALLS AND PROBLEMS

Enteroviruses may also produce complications such as aseptic meningitis and, rarely, myocarditis. When clinical presentations are suggestive, it is crucial to rule out life-threatening bacterial infections such as meningitis or sepsis.

EPSTEIN-BARR VIRUS INFECTIONS

CLINICAL APPEARANCE

Definition

Epstein-Barr virus (EBV) is a herpesvirus. Its clinical manifestations vary depending on the age of the host. It presents as infectious mononucleosis in the adolescent and young adult and as an upper respiratory infection with rash in young children.[5]

Typical Lesions and Symptoms

Infectious mononucleosis presents as an acute illness with fever, exudative tonsillopharyngitis, fatigue, adenopathy (particularly posterior cervical), and occasionally, hepatosplenomegaly and jaundice. Often, there is a petechial enanthem on the anterior soft palate. Rash is rarely seen, except when patients are treated with ampicillin or amoxicillin. The exanthem, occurring 1 to 2 days after beginning the antibiotic, presents as erythematous or copper-colored macules and papules on the trunk and then disseminates, often becoming confluent, particularly on the extensor surfaces of the extremities. The rash fades in 4 to 5 days and does not represent a true drug allergy.

In young children, EBV may present with signs and symptoms similar to those of infectious mononucleosis, except rash is more frequent in this age group. This exanthem is usually maculopapular; however, petechial, papulovesicular, urticarial, erythema multiforme–like eruptions have been observed.

Some less frequently observed cutaneous manifestations associated with primary EBV infection are infantile papular acrodermatitis (Gianotti-Crosti syndrome), acute urticaria, erythema multiforme, and erythema nodosum.[6]

Diagnosis is usually based on clinical presentation and confirmed by hematologic and serologic tests. The widely used monospot test is unreliable in young children.

TREATMENT

Treatment is supportive (see ''Pitfalls and Problems'' below).

PITFALLS AND PROBLEMS

Patients with splenomegaly should avoid athletics. The rare deaths from EBV are often from splenic rupture.

Corticosteroids are occasionally indicated for upper airway obstruction due to enlarged lymphoid tissue.

Antibiotics should be reserved for culture-proven infections, such as secondary streptococcal pharyngitis. Avoid the use of ampicillin and amoxicillin during EBV infections.

REFERENCES

1. Frieden IJ, Resnick SD: Childhood exanthems: Old and new. Pediatr Clin North Am 1991; 8(4):859–887.
2. American Academy of Pediatrics: Parvovirus B19. *In* Peter G (ed): 1994 Red Book: Report of the Committee on Infectious Diseases. 23rd ed. Elk Grove, IL: American Academy of Pediatrics, 1994; pp 345–347.
3. Yamanishi K, Okuno T, Shiraki K, et al: Identification of human herpesvirus-6 as a causal agent for exanthem subitum. Lancet 1988; 1:1065–1067.
4. Prose NS, Resnick SD: Cutaneous manifestations of systemic infection in children. Curr Probl Dermatol 1993; 5:81–112.
5. Sumaya CV, Ench Y: Epstein-Barr virus infectious mononucleosis in children: I. Clinical and general laboratory findings. Pediatrics 1985; 75:1003–1010.
6. Baldari U, Cancellieri C, Celli B, et al: Skin disorders and Epstein-Barr virus primary infection: Results of a 31-month survey. J Eur Acad Dermatol Venereol 1995; 4:239–247.

CHAPTER 51

Vitiligo

Pearl E. Grimes

Vitiligo is a common acquired disease characterized by patches of depigmented skin. The disease occurs in a generalized, acral, acrofacial, localized, or segmental distribution. Lesions are typically asymptomatic without clinical signs of inflammation. Hypopigmented lesions may coexist with depigmented areas. The white patches usually begin on sun-exposed sites with eventual dissemination to other areas. Areas of depigmentation vary from a few millimeters to many centimeters in size (see Fig. 51–1 on Color Plate 18). The borders of lesions are often distinct. Vitiliginous patches may slowly progress or remain stable for years. A small minority of patients undergo almost complete spontaneous depigmentation in a few years.

DESCRIPTION

In light of the stark contrast between depigmented and normal skin, vitiligo is probably the most psychologically devastating of all pigmentary disorders, particularly in darker-complexioned individuals. It affects approximately 1 to 2% of the population. The disease may begin at any age, but has its peak incidence in the second and third decades of life. Vitiligo affects females more often than males, and there is a familial incidence in 25 to 30% of patients. The disorder is often precipitated by factors such as emotional stress, sunburn, trauma, or physical illness.

The precise pathogenesis of vitiligo is unknown. However, advances in pigmentation research suggest that vitiligo is probably a heterogeneous disease with multiple etiologies. Potential pathogenic mechanisms include the classic autoimmune, self-destruction, and neural hypotheses, whereas newer theories suggest that melanocytes are destroyed in vitiliginous patches because of an intrinsic genetic defect of melanocytes, local growth factor defects, cytomegalovirus infection, aberrant catecholamine responses, or excessive local accumulation of free radicals.[1] Histopathologic studies document an absence of melanocytes, basilar vacuolopathy, and in some cases, lymphohistiocytic infiltrates.

Despite advances in our knowledge of the epidemiology, genetics, clinical spectrum, and treatment of vitiligo, many clinicians still regard the disease as a trivial cosmetic malady and continue to perpetuate the myth of vitiligo as an ''untreatable'' disease.

TREATMENT

General Expectations

Although no panacea for repigmentation of vitiliginous lesions has been identified, a variety of effective medical and surgical treatments have been used.[2, 3] The most consistent results have been obtained with psoralen plus ultraviolet A (PUVA) (see Fig. 51–2 on Color Plate 18) and corticosteroids. Mean repigmentation of at least 50% can be achieved using these therapeutic modalities. Efficacious surgical therapies include autologous minigrafting, suction blister grafting, and autologous transplantation of melanocyte cultures. Depigmentation is a viable alternative in patients with extensive disease. Maximal repigmentation occurs on the face and neck, the areas of greatest cosmetic concern to the patient. Intermediate responses occur on the trunk, arms, and legs. The hands and feet are difficult to repigment regardless of the therapeutic modality employed.

First-Line Medical Therapies

Steroid Therapy

Topical, intralesional, intramuscular, and oral steroids have been used to treat vitiliginous skin lesions. Partial or complete repigmentation has been reported in 10 to 80% of cases treated with midpotency to high-potency topical steroids. Topical steroids should be considered in the initial treatment phases of individuals with limited (less than 10%) vitiligo. These preparations can also be used in children less than 2 years of age, who are too young for PUVA therapy. Low-potency to midpotency topical steroids are used in young children. High-potency topical steroids can be used in older children and adults. Class I steroids are applied once or twice daily for the first month or two, then tapered to lower-potency preparations. They should be applied to very limited or localized areas of involvement. Patients must be monitored closely to avoid steroid-induced side effects, including atrophy, striae, and telangiectasia. Because of case reports of steroid-induced glaucoma, midpotency to high-potency topical steroids should be used with caution when treating periorbital areas of depigmentation. Short courses of systemic steroids may be indicated in patients with rapidly progressive vitiligo. This should be done only by physicians experienced in treating this disease.

Topical Photochemotherapy

Topical photochemotherapy is also an option for patients with limited involvement (less than 20% of the body surface). It avoids many of the systemic side effects associated with oral psoralens. A thin coat of 0.1% methoxalen ointment is routinely used for in-office topical PUVA. Oxsoralen solution 1% (ICN Pharmaceuticals, Costa Mesa, CA) is diluted to a concentration of 0.1% in Aquaphor or petrolatum. A thin coat of this preparation is applied to vitiliginous areas 30 minutes prior to UVA exposure. The initial UVA dose is 0.12 to 0.25 joules and is increased by increments of 0.12 to 0.25 joules weekly according to the patient's skin type. Initial lower UVA doses may be necessary for patients with skin types I and II. After moderate asymptomatic erythema is achieved, the UVA dosage should be maintained at a dosage sufficient to retain erythema. The treated areas should be washed with soap and water immediately after UVA exposure, followed by application of a broad-spectrum sunscreen. Treatments are administered in the office weekly. The major side effect of topical photochemotherapy using this regimen is a severe phototoxic or blistering reaction and perilesional hyperpigmentation. Patients should be made cognizant of these side effects prior to initiating therapy. Oxsoralen ointment 0.1% with sunlight as a UVA source should be avoided because of the increased potential of developing severe phototoxic reactions. The major advantages of in-office topical photochemotherapy include its lower cumulative UVA dose and its lack of systemic and ocular toxicity when compared with oral PUVA.

In light of the difficulties of in-office PUVA for many patients and their families (time and cost), we recently modified our topical PUVA protocol to allow for daily sunlight exposure as the UVA light source, using a very dilute (0.001%) concentration of Oxsoralen. It is recommended for patients with less than 10% cutaneous surface involvement. A thin coat of 0.001% Oxsoralen ointment is applied to lesional skin 30 minutes prior to sun exposure. The affected areas are exposed to sunlight for 15 to 30 minutes between 10:00 A.M. and 4:00 P.M. After 2 weeks, exposure time can be increased to 45 minutes to 1 hour if mild erythema has not occurred. Following sun exposure, the treated areas are washed with soap and water, followed by application of a broad-spectrum sunscreen. This treatment approach minimizes the adverse reactions routinely associated with in-office topical photochemotherapy. Costs are minimal, and it provides increased therapeutic accessibility to larger segments of the vitiligo population.

Oral Photochemotherapy

Oral photochemotherapy is reserved for patients with more extensive involvement and for individuals recalcitrant to topical photochemotherapy. A dosage of 0.3 to 0.4 mg/kg of 8-methoxypsoralen (8-MOP) (Oxsoralen-Ultra, ICN Pharmaceuticals) is ingested with food 1.5 hours prior to UVA exposure. The initial UVA dose should be in a range of 1 to 2 joules, with increments of 1 joule on every other visit until moderate asymptomatic erythema is achieved. The UVA dosage can then be maintained at a level necessary to retain 1+ or 2+ erythema of vitiliginous lesions. As with the topical protocols, a broad-spectrum sunscreen should be applied to exposed areas prior to leaving the treating facility. Protective UVA sunglasses should be worn indoors and outdoors for 18 to 24 hours after ingestion of 8-MOP.

Treatments are given twice weekly and never on two consecutive days. Oral psoralens should not be used in children younger than 9 years. Ocular defects, including cataracts, and abnormal liver function tests are contraindications for oral PUVA, and in general, photosensitivity disorders contraindicate the use of oral or topical PUVA. Trisoralen, which is less phototoxic and associated with fewer gastrointestinal side effects, may be used as an alternative drug. Clinical trials suggest that 5-MOP is comparable with 8-MOP in efficacy, but 5-MOP is associated with fewer side effects. The U.S. Food and Drug Administration has not approved 5-MOP for use in the United States.

If the patient is unable to come to the physician's office for oral photochemotherapy, trisoralen and sunlight can be prescribed in a dose of 0.6 to 0.8 mg/kg. Following ingestion of trisoralen, the initial sun exposure should be 5 minutes between 10:00 A.M. and 4:00 P.M., and subsequent sun exposure is increased by 5 minutes until erythema is achieved. Treatments are given three times weekly. Because of the increased susceptibility of male genital skin to PUVA-induced skin cancer and the poor response of vitiliginous genital skin to PUVA therapy, these areas should either be shielded from PUVA exposure or be treated on every third visit.

Side effects of oral photochemotherapy include nausea and vomiting, pruritus, erythema and edema, hypertrichosis, diffuse hyperpigmentation, xerosis, premature aging, skin cancer, cataracts, and immunologic defects. In contrast to psoriasis, studies have not documented a PUVA-induced increase in skin cancer in vitiligo. Compared with topical PUVA, the major advantages of oral PUVA therapy include its effectiveness in limiting the progression of actively spreading vitiligo, its lower frequency of blistering reactions, and its superiority as a repigmenting agent in patients with skin types I and II.

Depigmentation Therapy

Depigmentation, or removal of pigmentation from the remaining pigmented skin areas, can be considered in patients with greater than 50% cutaneous involvement who have demonstrated recalcitrance to repigmentation. Furthermore, it is a therapeutic option in patients with extensive disease who have no desire to undergo repigmentation. The depigmentation agent is monobenzylether of hydroquinone. It irreversibly destroys melanocytes and therefore must never be used as a hypopigmenting agent for other disorders. Monobenzylether of hyroquinone 20% should be diluted to a 10% concentration for the first month of application to avoid acute irritation. After 4 to 6 weeks, the full-strength product may be applied twice daily. The major side effect of this treatment is contact or irritant dermatitis, which usually responds to topical or systemic steroid therapy.

Other less common side effects include pruritus, xerosis, conjunctival melanosis, and corneal pigment deposition.

First-Line Surgical Therapies

Surgical approaches for repigmenting vitiliginous lesions should be considered when medical therapies fail. These approaches can also be used in combination with medical therapies. The most practical in-office surgical therapy utilizes 2-mm autologous minigrafts.[2, 4] Melanocyte cultures offer efficacious results; however, the technique is expensive and requires special laboratory culture expertise.[5] Although efficacious, suction blister graft procedures are cumbersome as they often necessitate special office equipment.

Micropigmentation should be reserved for treatment of mucosal sites such as the lips. When treating cutaneous sites with micropigmentation, several problems are common and include koebnerization of the treated lesion, progressive fading of the implanted pigment, and further discoloration of the pigment by the Tyndall effect. Surgical therapies should be considered for patients with rather localized, stable vitiliginous lesions unresponsive to medical treatment. A history of hypertrophic scarring or keloid formation contraindicates surgical intervention. The major advantage of grafting procedures is the transfer of a reservoir of viable melanocytes to vitiliginous skin to undergo proliferation and migration into areas of depigmentation.

Age Considerations

Children make up a unique subgroup of vitiligo patients. In general, they demonstrate an enhanced repigmentation response compared with that of adults.

Children less than 2 years of age can be given a trial of low-potency topical steroids. Children greater than 2 years of age with limited involvement can be treated with higher-potency topical steroids or topical PUVA. Children older than 9 years of age having extensive disease (greater than 20%) should be treated with oral PUVA.

Alternative/Adjunctive Therapeutic Options

Alternative Medical Therapies

Alternative therapies include tar emulsions, phenylalanine, khellin, immunomodulators such as isoprinosine, cyclosporine, and levamisole, UVB phototherapy, and nutritional approaches using vitamins such as folic acid, vitamin E, vitamin B_{12}, and ascorbic acid.[1, 2]

Adjunctive Therapies

Broad-spectrum sunscreens can be an extremely effective therapeutic approach in persons with skin types I and II. These agents minimize tanning, thereby limiting the contrast between vitiliginous and normal skin.

Cosmetic camouflage with stains and makeup or self-tanning preparations is also used as an alternative to permanent repigmentation or in conjunction with efforts to induce repigmentation. Makeups such as Dermablend may be useful. Stains provide a longer-lasting camouflage and include Vitadye, Chromelin, and a variety of self-tanning products. The active ingredient in staining products is dihydroxyacetone.

PITFALLS

Other disorders characterized by depigmentation may occasionally mimic vitiligo clinically. These include piebaldism, nevus depigmentosus, nevus anemicus, postinflammatory depigmentation/hypopigmentation, pityriasis alba, tinea versicolor, discoid lupus erythematosus, scleroderma, hypopigmented cutaneous T-cell lymphoma, and sarcoidosis. Therefore, in certain instances, a skin biopsy may be necessary to substantiate the diagnosis of vitiligo.

REFERENCES

1. Grimes PE: Diseases of hypopigmentation. *In* Sams WM Lynch PJ (eds): Principles and Practice of Dermatology. 2nd ed. New York: Churchill Livingstone, 1996; pp 843–853.
2. Grimes PE: Vitiligo: An overview of therapeutic approaches. Dermatol Clin 1993; 11:325–338.
3. Nordlund JJ, Halder RM, Grimes PE: Management of vitiligo. Dermatol Clin 1993; 11:27–33.
4. Falabella R: Treatment of localized vitiligo by autologous minigrafting. Arch Dermatol 1988; 124:1649–1655.
5. Olson MJ, Juhlin L: Transplantation of autologous cultured melanocytes in vitiligo. Br J Dermatol 1995; 132:587–591.

CHAPTER 52

Warts

Suzanne Grevelink

CLINICAL APPEARANCE

Definition

Warts, or verrucae, are benign, slow-growing proliferations of the epidermis due to infection with one of a family of double-stranded DNA viruses known as *papillomavirus.* The clinical presentation of warts varies according to the specific type of papillomavirus causing infection, as well as the location of infection. The appearance of lesions ranges from flesh-colored to slightly erythematous, in morphology from papules to coalescing plaques, and in surface texture from smooth to rough or filiform (see Figs. 52–1 through 52–3 on Color Plate 19). Warts are in general asymptomatic, but they may occasionally be associated with varying degrees of tenderness or discomfort, especially with warts on the plantar surfaces.

The various types of warts, along with their most common location and morphology, are defined in Table 52–1. Many of the less common wart types deserve further definition here. Butcher's warts, for example, consist of multiple verrucous papules on the dorsal, periungual, or plantar aspect of the hands of meat cutters. Bowenoid papulosis presents as multiple soft papules on the external genitalia that histologically reveal cellular atypia resembling squamous cell carcinoma in situ. Although these lesions are often infected with human papillomavirus (HPV) types associated with malignancy including HPV-16, the rate of malignant degeneration is lower for bowenoid papulosis than for HPV-16 infection of the cervix. Lesions of bowenoid papulosis may serve as a reservoir for transmission of potentially oncogenic HPV types, and female patients as well as the female partners of male patients should be examined for cervical cancer.

Verrucous carcinoma is a low-grade form of squamous cell carcinoma that presents clinically in three different forms. *Verrucous carcinoma of the anogenital area,* also known as *giant condylomata acuminata of Buschke and Löwenstein,* consists of multiple cauliflower–like proliferations commonly located on the glans penis, foreskin, vulva, and anus. *Verrucous carcinoma of the oral cavity* is also known as *oral florid papillomatosis* and consists of white, soft papules on the oral mucosa. *Verrucous carcinoma of the plantar surface,* also called *epithelioma cuniculatum,* presents as an exophytic mass that slowly penetrates deeply into the underlying skin, forming deep crypts. The name *cuniculatum* is used because these crypts resemble the burrows of rabbits.

Focal epithelial hyperplasia, also called *Heck's disease,* is characterized by soft pink papules on the oral mucosa. Respiratory (laryngeal) papillomatosis is usually seen in infants and presents as multiple papules on the larynx, oropharynx, and bronchopulmonary epithelium. The lesions are thought to be transmitted during delivery from virus present in maternal cervical papillomas or condyloma acuminatum. Respiratory papillomatosis is benign and often resolves spontaneously, but recurrences are common.

Atypical Presentation: Epidermodysplasia Verruciformis

Epidermodysplasia verruciformis (EV) is a rare, lifelong, autosomal recessive disease associated with

TABLE 52-1

Types of Warts

Type of Wart	Location	Morphology
Common (verruca vulgaris)	Hands	1-mm–4-mm rough, verrucous papules Single or grouped
Flat warts (verruca plana)	Face, hands, legs	2-mm–4-mm flat-topped papules
Plantar/palmar (verruca plantaris)	Plantar/palmar surfaces	Painful, endophytic papules
Mosaic	Plantar/palmar surfaces	Coalescence of plantar or palmar warts into large plaques
Filiform	Face, mucous membranes	Pedunculated papules with multiple projections on a narrow stalk
Butcher's	Hands, fingers	Verrucous papules, often multiple
Anogenital (venereal warts) (condylomata acuminata)	Anogenital area, oropharynx	Small to large "cauliflower-like" papules and plaques
Bowenoid papulosis	Genitalia	2-mm–3-mm papules, often multiple
Buschke-Löwenstein tumor	Anogenital area	Giant condyloma acuminatum Form of verrucous carcinoma
Oral florid papillomatosis	Oral cavity	Multiple verrucous papules; form of verrucous carcinoma
Epithelioma cuniculatum	Plantar surface	Form of verrucous carcinoma
Focal epithelial hyperplasia	Buccal, gingival, or labial mucosa or hard palate	1-mm–3-mm soft pink to white papules
Respiratory (laryngeal) papillomatosis	Larnyx, oropharynx, bronchopulmonary area	Multiple verrucous papules
Epidermodysplasia verruciformis	Face, neck, chest, extremitics	Variable: flat papules, red macules, thin pink/brown plaques with scale

chronic infection with HPV. Cutaneous lesions vary from red macules to flat-topped papules to tinea versicolor–like plaques (see Fig. 52–4 on Color Plate 19). Lesions present during early childhood and are often disseminated over the face and extremities. The oral and genital mucosa are, in general, spared. Approximately a third of patients will develop actinic keratoses and malignant tumors, primarily on the sun-exposed areas during the third and fourth decades of life. Patients with EV are often infected with more than one HPV, with the most frequently encountered HPVs including HPV-5, -8, -17, and -20. HPV-5 and -8 appear to have the highest oncogenic potential and are most often associated with malignant lesions in patients with EV.

DESCRIPTION OF DISEASE

Demographics

Nongenital warts occur in approximately 10% of children and young adults, with a peak incidence from ages 12 to 16 years. Anogenital warts are uncommon in children and are found most often in adults where the incidence is between 1 and 10%. Since the mid-1950s, there has been a dramatic increase in the number of office visits for anogenital warts. In adults, anogenital warts are almost always sexually transmitted, whereas genital warts in children may result from inoculation at birth from an infected mother (vertical transmission), inoculation from cutaneous warts of a caregiver, or sexual abuse.

Etiology/Pathogenesis

HPV is a double-stranded DNA virus of the family Papovaviridae, which is trophic to human squamous epithelial cells. Over 70 different types of papillomavirus have been identified, and most of these types are associated with a preferred clinical presentation and site of infectivity (Table 52–2). The various HPV types may be classified as follows: (1) nongenital types (e.g., HPV types 1, 2, 3), (2) anogenital (e.g., HPV types 6, 11, 16, 18), and (3) EV, a rare, autosomal recessive disorder characterized by chronic infection with HPV types 5, 8, and others.

After gaining access to the superficial epithelium, HPV resides in the basal cell layer and replicates within

TABLE 52-2

Human Papillomavirus Types and Clinical Presentation

Clinical Lesion	Types
Common warts	1, 2, 4, 26–29
Plantar warts	1, 4, 63
Flat warts	3, 10, 26–29, 41
Epidermodysplasia verruciformis	5, 8, 9, 12, 14, 15, 17, 19–25, 36–38, 46, 47, 49, 50
Genital warts	6, 11, 16, 18, 30–32, 42–44, 51–55
Laryngeal papillomas	6, 11, 55
Butcher's wart	7
Keratoacanthomas	9, 37
Focal epithelial hyperplasia (oral)	13
Bowenoid papulosis	16, 18, 31–32, 34, 39, 42, 48, 51–54
Bowen's disease	34, 48
Cervical dysplasia	16, 18, 31–32, 35, 42, 51–54
Cervical carcinoma	16, 18, 31–33, 35, 39, 42, 51–54

the upper level, differentiated cells of the epidermis. The virus-induced excessive epidermal proliferation and the retention of stratum corneum result in epidermal acanthosis, producing the clinical morphology of a papule. Histopathology reveals epidermal acanthosis with papillomatosis, hyperkeratosis, and parakeratosis. Koilocytes, large keratinocytes with a pyknotic nucleus surrounded by a perinuclear halo, are commonly seen in the stratum malpighii of HPV-infected tissue. The dermis is characterized by dilated vessels and occasionally a mononuclear cell infiltrate.

Transmission of HPV is apparently via direct contact with inoculation of virus into the skin through small epidermal defects. New warts may develop around the original lesion owing to the initial exposure or from autoinoculation. The reservoir of infection with HPV is thought to be individuals with clinical or subclinical infection and, possibly, infectious viral particles on inanimate objects in the environment. The incidence and extent of subclinical infection in clinically normal tissue are unknown. HPV DNA has been recovered from the laryngeal mucosa of patients with respiratory papillomatosis who were in clinical remission and in clinically normal skin surrounding treatment sites of genital warts. It is unknown whether this DNA is infectious or represents a ''latency'' state of noninfectious, nonreplicating virus.

Warts frequently resolve spontaneously with an incidence thought to be as high as 66%. Warts that are present in an immunocompromised host and warts associated with EV do not tend to resolve spontaneously and are often refractory to treatment.

Papillomavirus and Oncogenesis

Infection with papillomavirus is most often associated with biologically benign lesions; however, certain types of papillomavirus have oncogenic potential. As mentioned previously, HPV-5 and -8 are often found in the squamous cell carcinomas arising in sun-exposed warts of patients with EV. HPV-6 and -11 are also often seen in verrucous carcinoma, a low-grade, well-differentiated squamous cell carcinoma. HPV-6 and -11 are also commonly found in cervical papillomas and early dysplasia, whereas HPV-16, -18, -31, and -33 are found in cervical cancers. Carcinoma of the penis, vulva, and anus has also been associated with HPV infection. In summary, infection with certain HPV types appears to be associated with oncogenesis, but most likely other cofactors are necessary for the development of a malignant phenotype.

TREATMENT

Overview

The management of warts depends on several important variables, including the patient's age, the type of wart, the duration and extent of the lesions, the patient's immunologic status, and the patient's motivation for therapy. The rate of spontaneous remission is estimated at 67% within 2 years, but many new warts may appear during this time period.

Current treatment modalities all involve either physical destruction of infected tissue or induction of an immune response, or both. Several investigational treatments are designed to be specifically ''antiviral'' and inhibit the synthesis of new virus (e.g., antisense oligonucleotides), but these are not yet available for clinical use. The degree of pain, cost, inconvenience, risk of scarring, and other side effects should all be carefully considered when deciding on a management approach. Patients with anogenital warts or bowenoid papulosis should be informed about the risk of sexual transmission, and all sexual partners should be examined. In addition, owing to the association of these wart types with cervical cancer, female patients and the female partners of male patients should have an examination of the uterine cervix.

Table 52–3 provides a list of the therapeutic options for the management of warts. Several forms of treatment are considered conventional or first-line, including benign neglect, salicylic acid, cantharidin, and cryotherapy. Podophyllin resin, podophyllotoxin, and cryotherapy are all conventional first-line treatment options for anogenital warts. Many of the other therapies listed are second-line and are used most often for refractory warts.

Treatment Protocols

Protocols of the different forms of therapy vary. Tape occlusion or ''adhesiotherapy'' involves application of various types of tape to the wart for 1 to 6 days at a time, with a quarter to half a day off between applications. The hyperthermia protocol consists of immersion of the affected area into a 45° C water bath for 30 minutes three times a week.

Treatment with salicylic acid is done with a variety of over-the-counter preparations ranging in concentration from 5 to 40%. Salicylic acid in collodion and nitrocellulose-based preparations may be painted on the wart with a 1- to 2-mm margin and allowed to dry. Salicylic acid may also be present in plasters that may be cut to fit the wart. The medication is typically applied after soaking the affected area. After 24 hours, the area is gently débrided with an emory board or pumice stone before the medication is reapplied. Daily applications should continue for approximately 1 week after clinical clearing.

Cryosurgery is done most often with liquid nitrogen (−196° C); less commonly used cryogens include carbon dioxide snow (dry ice, −79° C), freon-12 (−30° to −90° C), and chlorodifluoromethane (−30° to −90° C). Liquid nitrogen is applied to the wart with a cotton swab or via a cryospray delivery system with two rapid-freeze, slow-thaw cycles. Patient response may vary from minimal erythema to hemorrhagic bullae with lo-

TABLE 52–3

Treatment of Warts

Therapy	?Painful	Cost	Frequency	Comment
Benign neglect	No	None	—	Rate of spontaneous remission approximately 67%
Tape occlusion	No	Inexpensive	Change qd-qwk	Anecdotal reports only
Hyperthermia	Yes	None	3 times qwk	Immersion in 45° C for 30 minutes Anecdotal reports only
Cryotherapy	Yes	Moderate	q 2–4 wks	40–80% effective following multiple treatments May develop painful hemorrhagic blisters, ring wart
Salicylic acid	No*	Low	qd	Reported success as high as 84%
Cantharidin	No*	Low	q 2–4 wks	May develop painful hemorrhagic blisters, ring wart
Podophyllum resin (20–25%)	No*	Low	q 2–4 wks	Potency of preparations vary; cytotoxic, possible toxicity with systemic absorption
Podophyllotoxin (0.5%)	No*	Low	qd	The most active component of podophyllin, reproducible activity
Electrodessication and curettage	No†	Moderate	Once	High risk of scarring; useful for warts that are small and few in number
Bichloroacetic and trichloroacetic acid	Yes	Low	q 2–4 wks	Causes immediate superficial tissue necrosis
Dinitrochlorobenzene	No	Low	qwk	90% efficacy has been reported
5-Fluorouracil	No	Moderate	qd	Primarily for flat warts
Tretinoin	No	Moderate	qd	Primarily for flat warts
Excision	No†	Expensive	Once	High risk of scarring; success rate is not higher than with other treatment modalities
Carbon dioxide laser	No†	Expensive	Once–several	Risk of scarring, prolonged healing time
Pulsed dye laser	Yes	Expensive	q 4 wks	72–99% clearing reported; success rate likely lower
Bleomycin	Yes	Expensive	q 2–4 wks	60–100% success rate; given intralesionally systemic toxicity
Cimetidine	No	Moderate	qd for 2 mos	Recent placebo-controlled trial showed no difference between cimetidine and placebo
Interferon	Yes	Expensive	2 times a wk	Case reports of resolution of common warts; flu-like symptoms, fever, transient leukopenia
Hypnosis	No	Expensive	q 2–4 wks	Several reports of success

Abbreviations: qd, every day; qwk, every week; q, every; mos, months.
*Not painful during application, but subsequent reaction may be painful.
†Local anesthesia prevents discomfort during removal; may be somewhat painful afterward.

calized pain and tenderness. Tense bullae may be decompressed by allowing the fluid to dry, after which the site may be covered with antibiotic ointment and a bandage.

Cantharidin is a chemical extract from the blister beetle *Coleopteres heteromeres* that induces focal destruction of the epidermis with vesicle formation. The liquid is carefully applied to each wart with a 1- to 2-mm margin and allowed to dry. The treated areas may be occluded with tape or a bandage for 4 to 6 hours, after which the medication should be thoroughly washed off. As with liquid nitrogen treatment described previously, patients may experience a range of effects from mild redness to large painful bullae. Patients should follow the same wound care instructions as for liquid nitrogen treatment.

Podophyllin is a crude extract from the may apple plant that is provided in a resin ranging in concentration from 20 to 25%. The potency of podophyllin preparations may be highly variable. Prior to applying podophyllin, the surrounding area should be protected with a bland emollient or barrier cream. One to 2 drops of podophyllin liquid extract is then carefully applied with the blunt end of a cotton-tipped swab. The treated area should be thoroughly washed 3 to 4 hours after application. The most active component of podophyllin is podophyllotoxin, which has very reproducible activity, unlike the crude preparation. Podophyllotoxin is available in the prescription product Condylox, which is applied twice-daily 3 consecutive days a week for a month or until clinical clearing is achieved. Podophyllin should not be used in pregnant women.

Electrodessication and curettage is associated with a high risk of scarring, but it may be useful for a limited number of small warts in cosmetically unimportant areas. The area to be treated should first be anesthetized with lidocaine (Xylocaine). The warts are then removed with a curet, and the base of the wound is cauterized by electrodessication or electrocautery. Small warts respond very well to this treatment; however, patients should be aware that it is possible for the wart to recur within and adjacent to the treated area. In addition, the vapor produced by electrodessication or by electrocautery has been shown to contain intact papillomavirus DNA. All personnel including the patient should wear masks designed to inhibit the passage of viral particles, and a vacuum plume evacuator should be used during the procedure.

Bichloroacetic acid and trichloroacetic acids in concentrations up to 80% are available for the treatment of warts in the office. The acid should be meticulously applied to the wart, followed by thorough rinsing of the area after the desired time interval. The acid causes an immediate painful localized skin necrosis, the depth of which is dependent on the concentration and duration of application.

Dintrochlorobenzene (DNCB) causes sensitization in most people after topical application and is used to treat warts by causing a localized allergic contact dermatitis. Although DNCB has been used to treat warts since the mid-1970s, its use is controversial since it is mutagenic by the Ames test of mutagenicity. Patients are instructed to apply the DNCB each day to the warts until the area becomes mildly erythematous and pruritic. Some protocols call for an initial sensitization by applying DNCB to the medial forearm in increasingly concentrated solutions until a reaction occurs. After sensitization, a diluted solution of DNCB is then applied to the warts daily. If tolerated, the concentration of DNCB is increased every 2 weeks until clinical clearing is achieved.

Topical tretinoin (Retin-A) cream and 5-fluorouracil (Efudex) creams have been used primarily in the treatment of verruca plana. These creams may be used separately or together on a daily basis with or without occlusion until the area becomes irritated and erythematous. 5-Fluorouracil cream has been reported to produce hyperpigmentation and erosions on the treated areas and, when applied periungually, may cause onycholysis.

Removal of warts by excision has an increased risk of scarring and, contrary to popular belief, is no more effective than some of the more conventional therapies. It may be difficult to justify the presence of a symptomatic scar on a weight-bearing area or a disfiguring scar in a cosmetically sensitive area, since most warts should spontaneously resolve. For these reasons, removal of warts by excision is rarely, if ever, a reasonable treatment option.

Treatment of warts with the carbon dioxide laser is similar to surgical removal, with similar risks of scarring and anesthesia requirements. The newer ''pulsed'' carbon dioxide lasers emit a series of high-energy short duration pulses that allow the depth of tissue destruction to be precisely controlled, limiting scarring. As with electrosurgery, it is important to be aware that the vapor produced by the carbon dioxide laser during treatment of warts has been shown to contain intact papillomavirus DNA. A vacuum plume evacuator should be used during the procedure, and all personnel including the patient should wear masks designed to inhibit the passage of viral particles.

The pulsed tunable-dye laser at 585 nm has been used

in the treatment of warts. The laser energy is specifically absorbed by oxyhemoglobin and, theoretically, should be effective in destroying the abundant blood supply of the wart. A preliminary study in 1993 showed 72% clearing of recalcitrant warts after just 1 to 2 treatments, and a more recent study in 1995 reported an overall response rate of 99% for body, limb, and anogenital warts, 95% for hand warts, and 84% for plantar warts. Despite the very optimistic data from these two studies, many practitioners feel that the success rate of this modality is probably lower than what has been reported.

Bleomycin, a glycoprotein with cytotoxic properties, may be administered intralesionally every 2 to 4 weeks at a concentration of 0.5 to 1.0 U/ml. Success rates of 60 to 100% have been reported, but the treatment is limited by side effects including pain, edema, and erythema up to 1 week after injection. In addition, because plasma concentrations may be close to what is seen with slow-infusion cancer chemotherapy, patients receiving bleomycin therapy for warts should also be monitored for possible systemic effects.

Cimetidine, an H_2-receptor antagonist, has been used in the recent past to treat recalcitrant warts in children and adults. Treatment is based on the fact that H_2 receptors are present on T-suppressor cells, and blockage of these receptors may induce an increase in cell-mediated immunity. In experimental studies, cimetidine has been shown to inhibit suppressor T-cell function and to increase delayed-type hypersensitivity responses. Initial clinical studies reported 81% clearing of widespread recalcitrant warts in children receiving cimetidine in doses of 25 to 40 mg/kg/day for 2 months in an uncontrolled prospective trial. A second uncontrolled study revealed 84% clearing or dramatic improvement of recalcitrant warts in adults receiving 30 to 40 mg/kg/day for 3 months. However, a recent randomized, placebo-controlled, double-blind study in children and adults reported no significant difference in the efficacy of cimetidine and placebo in the treatment of warts.

Interferons, a family of glycoproteins produced by various cell types, have been utilized in the treatment of warts owing to their ability to inhibit viral replication. All three types of interferon have been tried in the treatment of warts including: (1) interferon-alfa produced primarily from leukocytes, (2) interferon-beta produced by epithelial cells and fibroblasts, and (3) interferon-gamma produced by lymphocytes. Interferons are generally used in the treatment of genital warts, where success rates of up to 70% have been reported. Interferon-alfa and -beta are generally administered intralesionally once to three times weekly, and interferon-gamma may be given by intramuscular injection. Interferon is used most frequently in the treatment of genital warts; however, common warts, flat warts, and lesions of EV have been treated as well. Patients commonly experience side effects from the treatment, including flulike symptoms, fever, and transient leukopenia.

As mentioned previously, in general adult patients with warts are treated initially with one of the conventional or first-line treatments, including cryotherapy or salicylic acid. In patients with anogenital warts, the first-line treatments include podophyllin resin, podophyllotoxin, and cryotherapy. If the warts are refractory to the conventional treatments, the second-line therapies may be tried or the patient may be referred to a practitioner who specializes in the treatment of refractory warts.

Age Considerations

The treatment of warts in children should be modified according to a few guidelines. First, benign neglect is a safe, cost-effective treatment for warts that are asymptomatic and present for less than 2 years. For children whose warts are extensive, spreading, painful, or present for more than 2 years, the clinician should carefully inform the child and parents about the variety of treatment alternatives. Convenient, minimally painful, inexpensive treatments should be tried first, and painful treatments should be reserved only for motivated children with symptomatic, disfiguring, or widespread warts present for over 2 years. Treatment modalities with a high risk of scarring should be avoided in children, especially in cosmetically sensitive areas. Finally, since treatment often involves multiple visits and may involve pain either during or after administration, children may become increasingly anxious, making subsequent visits more difficult.

PITFALLS AND PROBLEMS

The presence of anogenital warts raises two separate issues including sexual abuse and oncogenesis. Anogenital warts in children raises the question of sexual abuse, but warts in this location may also result from inoculation at birth from an infected mother or from inoculation from a caregiver. A careful history should be obtained from the child and parents in these cases, and the child should be examined for other signs of abuse. Although most anogenital warts are caused by infection with HPV-6 and -11 with low oncogenic potential, similar lesions may be produced by HPV-16 and -18, which carry a higher risk of malignancy.

When the treatment of a wart results in a bulla, there is an increased risk of a resultant ''ring-wart'' phenomenon. This phenomenon involves the appearance of a new annular or ring-shaped wart at the perimeter of the treatment site of the original wart. This new ring-wart is larger and therefore more difficult to treat than the original wart and is thought to arise from the presence of live, infectious HPV that somehow escapes the destructive forces of the treatment modality as well as the immunologic response associated with that treatment.

Prior to initiating any treatment for a wart, the clinician should be convinced that the diagnosis is correct. The differential diagnosis of a common wart may include molluscum contagiosum, seborrheic keratosis, nevus, acrochordon, clavus, and squamous cell carcinoma. It is especially important not to miss a squamous cell carcinoma, and when suspected, a punch biopsy should be performed to rule out this possibility. Multiple verruca plana may resemble an epidermal nevus, lichen nitidus, and lichen planus. Lesions of condyloma acuminatum may mimic condyloma lata, a manifestation of secondary syphilis, or pseudoverrucous papules and nodules, an inflammatory condition in the perianal area associated with chronic fecal incontinence. Finally, plantar warts are clinically similar to clavi, corns, and punctate palmar and plantar keratoses. Gentle paring of the stratum corneum over a wart reveals tiny red to brown hemorrhagic punctata, representing the multiple superficial capillaries present in a wart.

REFERRAL/CONSULTATION GUIDELINES

When warts are unresponsive after a reasonable therapeutic trial, the clinician should reconsider the differential diagnosis before turning to an alternative treatment option. Alternative treatments, including the use of laser surgery, bleomycin, interferon, and hypnosis, require referral to a practitioner with expertise in the technique.

BIBLIOGRAPHY

Cobb MW: Human papillomavirus infection. J Am Acad Dermatol 1990; 22:547–566.

Committee on Guidelines of Care: Guidelines of care for warts: Human papillomavirus. J Am Acad Dermatol 1995; 32(1):98–103.

Frasier LD: Human papillomavirus infections in children. Pediatr Ann 1994; 23:354–360.

Siegfried EC: Warts on Children—An Approach to Therapy. Annual Meeting of the American Academy of Dermatology, Washington, DC: February 1996.

Yilmaz E, Alpsoy E, Basaran E: Cimetidine therapy for warts: A placebo-controlled, double-blind study. J Am Acad Dermatol 1996; 34:1005–1007.

SECTION

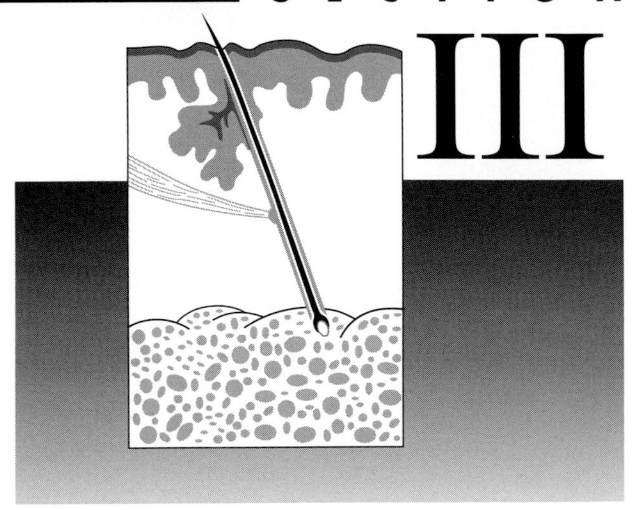

III

Dermatologic Emergencies and Critical Problems

CHAPTER 53

Bullous Pemphigoid and Other Immunologically Mediated Blistering Diseases

Neil J. Korman

Blisters in the skin may be caused by infections (including bacterial, viral, and fungal etiologies), allergic hypersensitivity reactions (including erythema multiforme and allergic contact dermatitis), metabolic disorders (including porphyria cutanea tarda), inherited genetic defects (including the epidermolysis bullosa group of diseases), and immunologically mediated blistering skin diseases. In this chapter, we focus on the immunologically mediated blistering diseases, which are among the most intriguing, well-characterized, and sometimes, serious skin diseases known.

Immunologically mediated blistering diseases are not frequently encountered in a general medical practice. Diagnosis is aided by determining the nature of the lesions, their clinical distribution, and their patterns (Table 53–1). However, in all cases, definitive diagnosis of these diseases can be made only after histologic and immunopathologic studies are performed. A routine skin biopsy for histology interpreted by an experienced dermatopathologist should be the first diagnostic test. The most accurate diagnostic features are obtained from skin biopsies that sample early lesions including inflamed skin or small vesicles. Older lesions including ruptured blisters or healing erosions rarely reveal any useful information and should not be biopsied. In all cases, a second biopsy should be obtained from perilesional unaffected skin or from perilesional erythematous nonblistered skin, processed for direct immunofluorescence (IF) studies, and interpreted by an experienced immunodermatologist. Direct IF is a technique that allows a determination of whether there are antibodies bound in the skin and, if so, what pattern and specificity they have. In addition, indirect IF studies, which probe for the presence of circulating antibodies directed against molecules found in the skin, are indicated in the diagnostic evaluation of many of these conditions. The importance of accurate diagnosis cannot be overemphasized because several of these diseases may have similar or overlapping histologic and immunopathologic features (see Table 53–1), and treatment plans for management can differ significantly from disease to disease.

Once an immunologically mediated blistering disease has been properly diagnosed, the physician is faced with management issues. Most of these diseases tend to be chronic and require treatment with potent medications, including systemic glucocorticosteroids, immunosuppressive agents, such as cyclophosphamide and azathioprine, dapsone, gold, and hydroxychloroquine (Plaquenil). As primary care physicians are likely to encounter bullous pemphigoid, this chapter discusses this disorder in detail and considers the other immunologically mediated blistering diseases in an abbreviated format.

TABLE 53–1

Differential Diagnosis of Immunologically Mediated Blistering Disease

Disease	Clinical Appearance	Histology	Immunopathology
Bullous pemphigoid	Urticarial plaques and tense blisters on skin of elderly	Subepidermal blisters with eosinophils	Linear basement membrane zone deposits of IgG and C3
Cicatricial pemphigoid	Blisters and erosions of mucous membranes with scarring	Subepithelial blisters with inflammatory infiltrate	Linear basement membrane zone deposits of IgG and C3
Herpes gestationis	Urticarial plaques and tense blisters in pregnancy	Subepidermal blisters with eosinophils	Linear basement membrane zone deposits of C3
Epidermolysis bullosa acquisita	Mechanobullous trauma-induced blisters or tense inflammatory blisters	Subepidermal blisters with or without neutrophilic infiltrate	Linear basement membrane zone deposits of IgG
Dermatitis herpetiformis	Symmetrically distributed pruritic vesicles of elbows/knees	Dermal papillary neutrophilic microabscesses	Granular deposits of IgA in the dermal papillae
Linear IgA bullous dermatosis	Papulovesicles and blisters of skin	Subepidermal blisters with neutrophils	Linear basement membrane zone deposits of IgA
Bullous systemic lupus erythematosus	Urticarial papules, plaques, and tense blisters	Dermal papillary neutrophilic microabscesses	Linear/granular basement membrane deposits of IgG, IgM, IgA, and C3
Pemphigus vulgaris	Flaccid blisters on skin and mucous membranes	Blisters in suprabasilar epidermis	Keratinocyte cell surface deposits of IgG
Pemphigus foliaceus	Scaly, crusted lesions of scalp, face, chest, and back	Blisters in superficial layer of epidermis	Keratinocyte cell surface deposits of IgG
Paraneoplastic pemphigus	Mucous membrane blisters and erosions with erythema multiforme–like skin lesions in the setting of a lymphoreticular neoplasm	Blisters in suprabasilar epidermis along with keratinocyte necrosis	Keratinocyte cell surface deposits of IgG along with basement membrane zone deposits of IgG

Abbreviations: IgG, immunoglobulin G; IgA, immunoglobulin A; IgM, immunoglobulin M.

BULLOUS PEMPHIGOID

CLINICAL APPEARANCE

Bullous pemphigoid is an acquired blistering disease that is most commonly seen in the elderly. The lesions of bullous pemphigoid are tense blisters that occur on normal-appearing skin or on an erythematous base (see Fig. 53–1 on Color Plate 20). The blisters most commonly occur on the flexor surfaces of the arms and legs, axilla, groin, and abdomen. Oral disease may be seen in a minority of patients, but the lesions are usually transient and of minimal importance. At disease onset, patients may have only urticarial or hivelike plaques. This urticarial phase of bullous pemphigoid may be sustained for long periods of time, or the urticarial lesions may evolve into blisters. The lesions of bullous pemphigoid can be very pruritic, and occasional patients may present with only pruritus without any skin lesions. Therefore, bullous pemphigoid should enter into the differential diagnosis of elderly patients presenting with pruritus in the absence of any skin lesions. When the blisters break, the patient is left with erosions that may become crusted and subsequently heal. Some patients have disease localized to the legs, hands, or other sites. Laboratory abnormalities are not commonly recognized, but many patients will have a peripheral blood eosinophilia. Notwithstanding earlier misconceptions, patients with bullous pemphigoid do not have any increased risk of internal malignancy when compared with appropriately matched controls.

DESCRIPTION

Bullous pemphigoid most commonly presents in the elderly population, with the majority of patients over age 60 years at the onset of disease. There is no definitive sexual or racial predilection, and bullous pemphigoid occurs throughout the world. The incidence of bullous pemphigoid is approximately 10 cases per 1 million population per year. It tends to be a relatively benign disease, and if untreated, patients will have disease that may persist from months up to 5 to 7 years. The mortality rate in bullous pemphigoid is low, even in the absence of treatment, but deaths do occur in elderly or debilitated patients.

The major histologic feature of bullous pemphigoid is a subepidermal blister with an inflammatory infiltrate that is often eosinophil-rich but may also contain lymphocytes, histiocytes, or neutrophils. Since these histologic findings are seen in several other related conditions, further diagnostic testing is necessary. Direct IF studies performed on normal-appearing or erythematous nonbullous perilesional skin will reveal linear basement membrane zone deposits of immunoglobulin G (IgG) and the third component of complement (C3) in the majority of patients, but similar findings can be observed in epidermolysis bullosa acquisita, cicatricial pemphigoid, herpes gestationis, and bullous eruption of systemic lupus erythematosus. The sera of approximately 70% of patients with bullous pemphigoid will have circulating IgG antibodies that bind to the basement membrane. Similar findings may also be observed in patients with epidermolysis bullosa acquisita. The level of these circulating antibodies has no correlation with the degree of disease activity.

Although the reasons that patients develop circulating antibodies directed against bullous pemphigoid antigens are not well understood, it is known that these antibodies are directed against two distinct molecules, of 230,000 and 180,000 molecular weight, that are both part of the hemidesmosome found in all stratified squamous epithelia. These hemidesmosomes are thought to play an important role in the attachment of keratinocytes to the basement membrane. Once the IgG antibodies form in the circulation, they become deposited in situ in the skin, where they are very strong activators of the complement cascade. This leads to the accumulation and activation of leukocytes and mast cells. Activation of the leukocytes and mast cells leads to the generation of multiple soluble factors whose net effect is the destruction of the epidermal basement membrane with blister formation.

TREATMENT

Patients with localized disease can often be successfully treated with high-potency topical steroids. Patients with mild generalized disease are usually successfully treated with low-dose prednisone (approximately 0.5 mg/kg/day, in a single morning dose). Patients with more severe disease should be treated with moderate-dose prednisone (0.75 to 1.25 mg/kg/day, in a single morning dose). As the disease comes under control, prednisone should be tapered to an alternate-day regimen to minimize steroid side effects. The dosage should be decreased in 10-mg increments every other day on an every 2-week basis until the patient is on alternate-day therapy. The alternate-day dosage is then tapered in 10-mg increments every 2 weeks until the dosage is 20 mg of prednisone every other day, assuming that there is no major disease flare during this taper. The taper is continued in 5-mg increments until the patient is off therapy. Patients with contraindications to systemic steroid therapy may be treated with dapsone, a combination of tetracycline and nicotinamide, or immunosuppressive agents, particularly azathioprine. The combination of tetracycline and nicotinamide has been used with great success in younger patients with strong contraindications to systemic corticosteroids. Older patients with generalized disease, who have strong contraindications to systemic corticosteroids, may be treated with azathioprine alone (1.0 to 1.5 mg/kg/day) with excellent results. These patients generally respond within 2 to 6 months of treatment initiation. Subsequent flares of disease respond well to reinstitution of azathioprine. Older patients with bullous pemphigoid who have severe disease can often be successfully managed with the combination of moderate-dose prednisone along with azathioprine. As the disease comes under control, the prednisone is tapered to alternate days, as described previously. After the patient is off prednisone, treatment is continued with azathioprine for another few months until the disease is suppressed and then the azathioprine is discontinued. Other options to be considered in patients with the most progressive disease that is uncontrollable with this combination therapy include the combination of moderate-dose prednisone with cyclophosphamide or chlorambucil, pulse steroids, and plasmapheresis.

PITFALLS AND PROBLEMS

In order to distinguish bullous pemphigoid from conditions such as epidermolysis bullosa acquisita, special studies, such as indirect IF studies utilizing salt-split skin, are necessary. In this technique, which currently is available only in immunodermatology laboratories, normal human skin is treated with 1.0-M sodium chloride solution for 3 days. This treatment causes a split to occur within the epidermal basement membrane such that most bullous pemphigoid antibodies will bind only to the epidermal side, while all epidermolysis bullosa acquisita antibodies will bind solely to the dermal side of split skin.

The treatment of bullous pemphigoid is fraught with many problems, particularly in patients treated with systemic steroids or immunosuppressive agents. Systemic glucocorticosteroids may lead to numerous complications, some of which are life-threatening, such as sepsis and gastrointestinal bleeding. Other major morbidities of systemic corticosteroids include diabetes mellitus, osteoporosis, myopathy, cataracts, and central nervous system toxicity. The elderly may be particularly at risk for adverse effects of glucocorticosteroids, since treatment with these agents will exacerbate many conditions such as diabetes mellitus, hypertension, osteoporosis, diminished wound healing, and decreased host response to infection, which already occur with increased frequency in the elderly. It is therefore suggested that when elderly patients are treated with glucocorticosteroids, all attempts should be made to keep the dosage to a minimum and patients should be carefully monitored for toxicities.

When treating patients with azathioprine, the complete blood count is carefully monitored to ensure that bone marrow suppression, particularly leukopenia, does not occur. Liver function tests are also followed, since hepatitis can occur with azathioprine treatment. Other side effects of azathioprine include a gastrointestinal hypersensitivity reaction characterized by nausea, vomiting, or diarrhea that typically occurs in the first few weeks of therapy and a possible increased long-term risk of malignancy. This potential risk is the reason to reserve azathioprine therapy for elderly patients, who may not outlive the latency period for these malignancies.

REFERRAL/CONSULTATION GUIDELINES

Bullous pemphigoid may present in a localized form that will usually respond very nicely to potent topical steroid preparations. Patients with more generalized disease who require treatment with systemic glucocorticosteroids for longer than 2 months or with other immunosuppressive agents should be seen and managed jointly by a dermatologist and the primary care provider.

CICATRICIAL PEMPHIGOID

Cicatricial pemphigoid is a chronic subepidermal blistering disease of the middle to older age group that shares several features with bullous pemphigoid. Bullous pemphigoid generally involves the skin, but some patients also have mucous membrane lesions. Cicatricial pemphigoid almost always involves the mucous membranes, with occasional concurrent skin involvement. The mucous membrane lesions in cicatricial pemphigoid are typically small blisters that rapidly rupture, leaving painful erosions. Although disease of the oropharynx is the most common manifestation, patients may also have involvement of the conjunctiva, larynx, nasopharynx, and esophagus, as well as the genitalia and rectal mucosa. Patients with cicatricial pemphigoid have prominent scarring at the site of blister formation, whereas patients with bullous pemphigoid do not scar. Scarring, caused by injury to the dermis, with collagen damage and subsequent repair, is a permanent process. Pigmentary changes (hyperpigmentation or hypopigmentation), which occur owing to injury of the epidermal melanocytes, tend to resolve over 1 to 2 years. Since patients with both bullous pemphigoid and cicatricial pemphigoid may have lesions that leave temporary pigmentary alterations and patients with only cicatricial pemphigoid have scarring, this distinction is important in the classification of these diseases. The histologic and immunopathologic features of cicatricial pemphigoid are very similar to those of bullous pemphigoid, such that clinical features generally must be used to distinguish these two entities. Occasional patients with cicatricial pemphigoid may show a predominance of plasma cells on their biopsies, but that is because mucosal lesions tend to accumulate plasma cells when there is inflammation. In addition to circulating IgG antibodies, some patients with cicatricial pemphigoid may have circulating immunoglobulin A (IgA) antibodies.

Cicatricial pemphigoid patients may present to the dentist, ophthalmologist, gastroenterologist, or otolaryngologist for evaluation of mouth sores, sore throat, difficulty swallowing, dry eyes, or ocular complaints. The disease is a chronic one with periods of exacerbations and remissions. Treatment of cicatricial pemphigoid is dictated by the organs involved. For patients with disease limited to the nasopharynx or oropharynx, treatment with topical steroids, intralesional steroids, or dapsone is indicated. For those patients with involvement of the eyes, esophagus, or larynx, the morbidity can be very severe and includes blindness, dysphagia, and laryngeal stenosis. Aggressive treatment with systemic glucocorticosteroids and immunosuppressive agents is indicated for these patients.

HERPES GESTATIONIS

Herpes gestationis is a subepidermal blistering disease that occurs during or shortly after pregnancy and shares several features with bullous pemphigoid. This disease has absolutely no relationship to infection with the herpesvirus. It was given this name in the late 1800s when the term *herpes* was applied to any eruptions having grouped lesions. Many experts have proposed that this disorder be renamed *pemphigoid gestationis* to emphasize its similarities to bullous pemphigoid and to eradicate any confusion regarding its possible relationship to herpesvirus infection. Herpes gestationis is a rare disease with an incidence of approximately 1 case in every 50,000 pregnancies. The disease usually occurs in the second and third trimesters and is characterized by urticarial papules and plaques on the trunk and extremities that evolve into blisters. Lesions often start within or immediately adjacent to the umbilicus. Herpes gestationis resolves within a few weeks after delivery but often recurs in subsequent pregnancies and, occasionally, in a milder form, after ingestion of oral contraceptives or with the menses.

The histologic and immunopathologic features are very similar to those of bullous pemphigoid, but patients with herpes gestationis have a unique circulating IgG1 antibody that avidly fixes complement. The circulating antibodies in herpes gestationis bind to the same 180,000-molecular-weight protein that is recognized in some patients with bullous pemphigoid. The pathogenesis of herpes gestationis is thought to be very similar to that of bullous pemphigoid. Although the etiology is not fully understood, there is evidence demonstrating an increased incidence of the human leukocyte antigen (HLA)–DR3 and HLA-DR4 genotypes, suggesting a genetic predisposition to the disease. The majority of patients with herpes gestationis will require treatment with systemic glucocorticosteroids. There is debate whether there is any risk of fetal morbidity or mortality in babies born to mothers with herpes gestationis. It is therefore reasonable to have the mother followed by an obstetrician who has the facilities and expertise to handle a potentially high-risk infant. Rarely, infants born to mothers with herpes gestationis will have transient skin blisters that spontaneously resolve.

EPIDERMOLYSIS BULLOSA ACQUISITA

The term *epidermolysis bullosa* refers to a group of more than 20 distinct inherited blistering diseases characterized by the development of blisters secondary to the presence of mechanically fragile skin. The various subtypes differ in their modes of inheritance, distribution and types of lesions, presence of extracutaneous disease, and specific immunohistochemical or ultrastructural changes. Recent advances in molecular biology have allowed us to pinpoint the exact defects responsible for several of these subtypes of inherited epidermolysis bullosa. We focus our attention in this chapter on epidermolysis bullosa acquisita, a disease first recognized as a chronic blistering disease that has many features reminiscent of inherited epidermolysis bullosa but is acquired in adults having no personal or family history of a blistering disorder. Patients with epidermolysis bullosa acquisita may have mechanobullous, noninflammatory, trauma-induced blisters similar to those in inherited epidermolysis bullosa, but they may also present with inflammatory blisters of the skin and mucous membrane involvement that can be clinically indistinguishable from bullous pemphigoid (see Fig. 53–2 on Color Plate 20). Both types of epidermolysis bullosa acquisita lesions will heal with scarring. Some patients may present with inflammatory lesions that later evolve into noninflammatory lesions. Epidermolysis bullosa acquisita tends to be a chronic condition. It most commonly occurs in middle life and has been reported to occasionally occur in association with inflammatory bowel disease.

The histologic findings reveal a subepidermal blister containing only few inflammatory cells when mechanobullous lesions are sampled or a neutrophil-rich leukocyte infiltrate when inflammatory blisters are sampled. Direct IF studies obtained from normal-appearing perilesional skin reveal linear deposits of IgG and occasionally C3 at the epidermal basement membrane. Circulating IgG autoantibodies that bind to the epidermal basement membrane are found in about 50% of patients with epidermolysis bullosa acquisita. When assayed on 1.0-M sodium split human skin, antibodies from epidermolysis bullosa acquisita patients bind to the dermal side of the split. The antigen recognized by these circulating antibodies is a 290,000-molecular-weight protein that is a part of the carboxy terminal domain of type VII collagen. The pathogenesis of epidermolysis bullosa acquisita is not known but is thought to involve antibody binding to the basement membrane zone followed by complement activation. Neutrophils are recruited into the area and activated, leading to proteolytic enzyme release that causes blister formation.

The course of the disease is chronic, and it tends to be very difficult to treat successfully. Patients with noninflammatory lesions are largely resistant to therapy. Patients with inflammatory lesions are also difficult to treat, but some will respond to systemic glucocorticosteroids alone or with immunosuppressive agents (such as cyclophosphamide, azathioprine, or particularly, cyclosporine). Some patients with neutrophil-rich inflammatory lesions may respond to dapsone therapy.

DERMATITIS HERPETIFORMIS

Dermatitis herpetiformis is an intensely pruritic, chronic blistering disease of the skin that occurs most commonly in the second to fourth decades of life. The primary lesions are small, tense vesicles that tend to be symmetrically distributed over the elbows, knees, buttocks, and nuchal areas. Owing to the extreme pruritus, it is uncommon to see patients with intact vesicles because they have usually been scratched off prior to presentation, leaving only excoriations. Sometimes, the pruritus precedes the onset of new lesions by several hours, allowing the patient to predict where new lesions may occur. Oral mucous membrane involvement is quite rare.

Skin biopsy of an early lesion of dermatitis herpetiformis will reveal small subepidermal clefts with accumulation of neutrophils in the neighboring dermal papillae. If the skin biopsy is not performed until the lesion is more developed, it may be very difficult to distinguish dermatitis herpetiformis from other subepidermal blistering diseases such as bullous pemphigoid, epidermolysis bullosa acquisita, and linear IgA bullous disease. Biopsy of normal-appearing perilesional skin for direct IF will reveal granular deposits of IgA at the epidermal basement membrane zone concentrated at the dermal papillary tips. Whereas these cutaneous deposits of IgA are thought to be important in the pathogenesis of dermatitis herpetiformis, their exact role is not completely understood.

The large majority of patients with dermatitis herpetiformis will have an associated subclinical gluten-sensitive enteropathy, and most express the HLA-B8/DRW3 haplotype. Associated abnormalities in patients with dermatitis herpetiformis include thyroid disease (both hyperthyroidism and hypothyroidism), achlorhydria, atrophic gastritis, and antigastric parietal cell antibodies. Most patients do not manifest overt gastrointestinal symptoms, but if a biopsy of the small bowel is performed, it will reveal blunting of the intestinal villi with a lymphocytic infiltrate in the lamina propria. These gastrointestinal changes are potentially reversible if the patient is placed on a gluten-free diet. In fact, if the patient stays on the gluten-free diet for a long period of time, the skin disease may also improve or sometimes even be fully controlled.

The most effective therapy is dapsone, which will be beneficial in almost all patients. The major toxicities of dapsone include hemolysis, methemoglobinemia, and agranulocytosis. Patients should be screened for glucose-6-phosphate dehydrogenase deficiency because use of dapsone in such a patient will lead to severe hemolysis. Patients need to be followed with regular blood counts. Dapsone requirements may be decreased by following a gluten-free diet, but this diet must be truly gluten-free in order to be beneficial. A gluten-free diet must be maintained for many months before benefit may be realized. Since this diet can be very difficult to follow, it is important that patients be properly counseled by an experienced dietician. As dermatitis herpetiformis is a chronic disease, patients must remain on dapsone or their gluten-free diet indefinitely if they are to remain under control.

LINEAR IgA BULLOUS DERMATOSIS

Linear IgA bullous dermatosis is a subepidermal blistering disease that until recently was considered a variant type of dermatitis herpetiformis. Clinical lesions consist of papulovesicles or blisters along with urticarial plaques, and sometimes, the patients may have an arcuate pattern with a "cluster of jewels" grouping of blisters (see Fig. 53–3 on Color Plate 20). The lesions tend to be more generalized than those in dermatitis herpetiformis and are not usually symmetric. Lesions of the oral mucous membranes are frequently seen. Occasionally, ocular involvement with subsequent scarring may occur similar to that found in cicatricial pemphigoid. Patients with linear IgA bullous dermatosis do not have any gastrointestinal disease, do not have an increased frequency of the HLA-B8/DRW3 phenotype, and will not show any benefit from a gluten-free diet.

Linear IgA bullous dermatosis may occur with increased frequency in patients over 60 years of age, but it may be seen throughout adulthood. A blistering disease found in children, known as *chronic bullous disease of childhood,* appears to be the childhood counterpart of linear IgA bullous dermatosis.

The histology of linear IgA bullous disease can be indistinguishable from that seen in dermatitis herpetiformis, or some patients may show neutrophils along the entire epidermal basement membrane zone, unlike in dermatitis herpetiformis where the neutrophils tend to be limited to the dermal papillae. Direct IF studies obtained from normal-appearing perilesional skin will reveal linear basement membrane zone deposits of IgA. Indirect IF studies performed on salt-split skin will often reveal a low-titer circulating IgA antibody that almost always binds to the epidermal side of salt-split skin. The majority of patients with linear IgA disease will respond to dapsone. Some patients may require the addition of systemic glucocorticosteroids in order to control their disease. Rare patients who have ocular disease must be treated aggressively with systemic glucocorticosteroids and cyclophosphamide to control the disease and prevent ocular scarring.

BULLOUS SYSTEMIC LUPUS ERYTHEMATOSUS

This eruption is characterized by the presence of a blistering skin disease occurring in the setting of a patient with systemic lupus erythematosus. It occurs in a small minority of patients with systemic lupus erythematosus and is characterized by tense blisters, urticarial papules, and plaques that may resemble either bullous pemphigoid or dermatitis herpetiformis. The histology of these lesions is very characteristic, showing features similar to those of dermatitis herpetiformis with dermal papillary microabscesses of neutrophils. Routine direct IF testing reveals the presence of linear or granular deposits of IgG, IgA, immunoglobulin M (IgM), and C3 at the epidermal basement membrane zone. Indirect IF studies reveal the presence of circulating IgG antibodies that bind to the dermal side of salt-split skin in a pattern indistinguishable from that of epidermolysis bullosa acquisita antibodies. The antigen recognized by these circulating antibodies appears to be identical to the 290,000-dalton type VII collagen that is recognized by circulating antibodies in epidermolysis bullosa acquisita. Bullous eruption of systemic lupus erythematosus is usually treated with dapsone with very good results, and most patients will eventually be able to discontinue therapy without recurrence of the disease.

PEMPHIGUS

The term *pemphigus* refers to a group of autoimmune blistering skin diseases characterized by blister formation within the epidermis due to a process known as *acantholysis.* Acantholysis is defined as the loss of cohesion between epidermal cells. Pemphigus vulgaris and pemphigus foliaceus are the two major types of pemphigus. In pemphigus vulgaris, the more common type, the blister occurs in the suprabasilar region (an area just above the basal keratinocytes), whereas in pemphigus foliaceus, the blister occurs in a subcorneal location (an area just below the stratum corneum).

The lesions of pemphigus vulgaris consist of flaccid blisters on either normal-appearing or erythematous skin. The lesions usually start in the oropharynx and then spread to involve the trunk, the head and neck, and intertriginous areas including the axilla and groin. Almost all patients have oropharyngeal involvement at some point in their course. Patients with severe disease may have involvement of other mucosal surfaces including laryngeal, esophageal, conjunctival, vulval, and rectal surfaces. Since the blisters are flaccid, they tend to break easily, leaving denuded areas of skin that may crust and then enlarge from the periphery (see Fig. 53–4 on Color Plate 20). The lesions do not heal without appropriate therapeutic intervention. With the onset of new skin lesions, patients may experience some burning, local discomfort, or itching, but after the blisters break, pain becomes the major complaint. Patients with pemphigus vulgaris may often present to the dentist or otolaryngologist with complaints of sore throat or sores in the mouth. The involvement of the oral cavity can become extensive, and in these patients, the pain of denuded mucous membranes can be very severe, causing poor oral intake of solids and liquids that may even lead to malnutrition if left untreated. The lesions of pemphigus vulgaris generally heal without scarring, except for sites that may have become secondarily infected. Postinflammatory hyperpigmentation or hypopigmentation at the site of old lesions commonly occurs and usually resolves within 1 to 2 years.

Pemphigus may occur in association with myasthenia gravis or thymoma or, rarely, with other autoimmune disorders. Although pemphigus is generally considered to be idiopathic, certain medications, including penicillamine and captopril, may occasionally induce pemphigus.

Pemphigus foliaceus presents clinically with erythema, scaling, and crusting localized to the face, scalp, and upper trunk. Since the lesions are histologically more superficial, intact blisters are rarely observed, and patients usually present with shallow erosions. Patients with pemphigus foliaceus, unlike those with pemphigus vulgaris, rarely have mucous membrane involvement. This is an important distinguishing feature between these two variants of pemphigus.

Pemphigus is a relatively rare disease, with an incidence of 1 to 2 cases per 1 million population per year. It affects both sexes and is most common in middle age, with occasional onset in children or in the older population. Although it is found in all ethnic groups, there is an increased incidence of pemphigus vulgaris in the Ashkenazi Jewish population, and it is associated with the HLA-DR4/HLA-DR6 phenotype.

Routine skin biopsies in pemphigus should be performed from early skin lesions in order to demonstrate the characteristic histology of acantholysis. Direct IF biopsy should be performed on normal-appearing or erythematous nonbullous perilesional skin and will reveal cell surface deposits of IgG (in all patients) and C3 (in up to 50% of patients). The IgG deposits in the skin occur because of the presence of a circulating IgG antibody that is targeted to keratinocyte cell surface antigens. These circulating IgG antibodies are found in the large majority of patients with pemphigus and are detected by the indirect IF technique. The amount of antibody (as measured by the titer) tends to correlate roughly with the degree of disease activity. Pemphigus vulgaris and pemphigus foliaceus show identical findings by direct IF testing, but subtle differences can be distinguished by indirect IF studies. The autoantibodies in pemphigus vulgaris target a 130,000-molecular-weight protein known as *desmoglein III,* which is a member of the cell adhesion family of molecules called *cadherins.* The autoantibodies in pemphigus foliaceus target a 160,000-molecular-weight protein, *desmoglein I,* another member of the cadherin family, that is closely related to desmoglein III. Compelling evidence from animal studies clearly demonstrates that the autoantibodies in both major types of pemphigus are pathogenic, meaning that they are capable of reproducing the clinical, histologic, and immunopathologic features of pemphigus.

Before glucocorticosteroids became available in the 1950s, the mortality rate from pemphigus ranged from 60 to 90%. After glucocorticosteriods became available, the mortality rate diminished to the 15 to 45% range. More recently, with the use of adjuvant therapy including the immunosuppressive agents, the mortality rate has further decreased to the 5 to 10% range. The most common cause of death in patients with pemphigus now is from side effects of the therapy. Poor prognostic factors include extensive disease, old age at presentation, and extensive disease progression prior to the initiation of therapy. All patients with pemphigus vulgaris will require systemic therapy with glucocorticosteroids to clear the circulating antibodies. Pemphigus foliaceus patients tend to have a more benign course, can often be treated with lower dosages of glucocorticosteroids, and occasionally respond to topical steroid therapy alone.

Patients with pemphigus are generally treated with prednisone at 1 to 2 mg/kg, depending on disease severity, with tapering toward an alternate-day dosage within a 1- to 3-month time period, as the disease allows. Short-term and long-term toxicities of prednisone are numerous and include gastrointestinal bleeding, diabetes mellitus, cataracts, osteoporosis, increased risk of infection, and central nervous system changes. Every effort should therefore be made to minimize the dosage of systemic glucocorticosteroids and to switch to alternate-day dosing as soon as is feasible. Immunosuppressive agents, most commonly cyclophosphamide and azathioprine, are used, particularly in pemphigus vulgaris, for their steroid-sparing effects. Cyclophosphamide appears to be the more effective of the two, but it has numerous toxicities, including bone marrow suppression, hemorrhagic cystitis, bladder fibrosis, sterility, alopecia, and an increased risk of malignancy. The major toxicities of azathioprine include bone marrow suppression, hepatotoxicity, and increased risk of malignancy. Monitoring of patients treated with these immunosuppressive agents should include frequent blood counts, urinalyses, and liver function testing. Other therapies, used in specific settings but with lower success rates as steroid-sparing agents in pemphigus, include dapsone, the combination of tetracycline and niacinamide, hydroxychloroquine, gold, and cyclosporine. Patients with the most severe disease may be treated with the combination of systemic glucocorticosteroids and immunosuppressive agents along with plasmapheresis.

PARANEOPLASTIC PEMPHIGUS

Paraneoplastic pemphigus is a relatively recently recognized autoimmune syndrome that has features of both pemphigus vulgaris and erythema multiforme. Patients with this disease have an underlying malignancy, usually lymphoreticular in origin. The disease is characterized by numerous ocular and oral blisters and erosions along with generalized skin lesions that may resemble toxic epidermal necrolysis, lichen planus, bullous pemphigoid, or erythema multiforme. The disease is rapidly progressive, leading to death in most patients who have an associated malignant neoplasm (such as lymphoma) but may resolve in patients who have an associated benign neoplasm (such as thymoma) that is surgically removed. Histologic features of both pemphigus vulgaris (suprabasilar acantholysis) and erythema multiforme (basal keratinocyte necrosis and lymphocyte infiltrate) may be present. IF studies show the presence of circulating and tissue-bound IgG antibodies in paraneoplastic pemphigus that bind to the cell surface of stratified squamous epithelia in a pattern indistinguishable from pemphigus antibodies. These same circulating IgG antibodies also recognize the cell surface of simple epithelia such as liver and heart, in contrast to pemphigus IgG antibodies, which recognize only the cell surface of stratified squamous epithelia. In addition, there may be IgG antibodies, which bind to the basement membrane. The circulating antibodies in paraneoplastic pemphigus recognize a complex of epidermal proteins that include 250- and 210-kd proteins (desmoplakin I and II), the 230-kd bullous pemphigoid antigen, and as yet uncharacterized 190- and 170-kd proteins. Although the etiology of this severe mucocutaneous disease is poorly understood, it is thought that it may result from the combination of both a cellular and a humoral immune response to tumor antigens but also may have overlapping reactivity to normal components of skin and other epithelia.

The syndrome of paraneoplastic pemphigus must be considered in patients with severe mucocutaneous disease reminiscent of pemphigus who present with atypical features. These patients may not have a known neoplasm at the time of presentation. If there is sufficient suspicion for the diagnosis of paraneoplastic pemphigus, then a search for an occult neoplasm is warranted. This will often entail extensive laboratory and diagnostic investigation because these patients may have associated tumors that are difficult to diagnose including rare entities such as retroperitoneal sarcoma, thymoma, or Waldenström's macroglobulinemia, along with more commonly recognized tumors such as Hodgkin's lymphoma and chronic lymphocytic leukemia. Most patients must be treated very aggressively with high-dose glucocorticosteroids along with immunosuppressive agents, often with less than outstanding results. The best treatment for patients who have an associated benign tumor is surgical removal of the tumor. Unfortunately, the majority of patients with paraneoplastic pemphigus have associated malignant tumors, and there are no known effective therapies. These patients present exceedingly difficult management problems and will require coordination of care between the experienced immunodermatologist and the primary care physician.

BIBLIOGRAPHY

Anhalt GJ, Kim SC, Stanley JR, et al: Paraneoplastic pemphigus: An autoimmune mucocutaneous disease associated with neoplasia. N Engl J Med 1990; 323:1729–1735.

Hall RP: The pathogenesis of dermatitis herpetiformis: Recent advances. J Am Acad Dermatol 1987; 16:1129–1144.

Korman NJ: Bullous pemphigoid. Dermatol Clin 1993; 11:483–498.

Korman NJ: Pemphigus. J Am Acad Dermatol 1988; 18:1219–1238.

Woodley DJ: Epidermolysis bullosa acquisita. Prog Dermatol 1988; 22:1–13.

CHAPTER 54

Erysipelas

Julie S. Prendiville

CLINICAL APPEARANCE

Definition

Erysipelas is a bacterial infection of the dermis and adjacent subcutaneous tissue. It is considered a superficial variant of bacterial cellulitis. Group A β-hemolytic streptococcus is the most common infecting organism. Other streptococci (groups G, C, and B) may also cause erysipelas.[1] *Staphylococcus aureus* has been isolated from occasional cases, although its role as a primary pathogen is questioned.[1, 2]

Typical Lesions and Symptoms

Erysipelas is characterized by sudden onset of a painful, erythematous, warm, swollen plaque with a well-defined, rapidly advancing margin. Sites of predilection are the face and lower extremities (see Fig. 54–1 on Color Plate 20). Lesions on the face may extend over both malar areas and the bridge of the nose in a "butterfly" distribution.

Peau d'orange induration is seen in some patients and is attributed to involvement of cutaneous lymphatics. Intense edema of the skin may result in vesicles or large surface bullae within 2 to 3 days of onset. Systemic manifestations include fever and chills, malaise, nausea, headache, myalgia, and a polymorphonuclear leukocytosis. Lymphangitis and regional lymphadenopathy are sometimes observed. Resolution of inflammation is accompanied by desquamation.

Atypical Presentation or Alternative Forms

Erysipelas and cellulitis may be difficult to distinguish and are generally considered to be variants of the same disease process. Classic erysipelas is a superficial infection of the dermis and subcutaneous tissues and has a distinct border, whereas cellulitis involves deeper tissues and is less well defined. In practice, the two conditions show considerable overlap and the distinction is not always clear-cut.

Erysipelas may present in the immunocompromised host with atypical features such as absence of fever or less intense local inflammation. Cases of recurrent erysipelas may also develop in a less florid or atypical manner.

Group B streptococcus has been associated with erysipelas in the perineal area in adults. This organism may also be responsible for skin and soft tissue infections in newborn infants.

DESCRIPTION OF DISEASE

Erysipelas is seen in all age groups but is most common in the elderly. Predisposing factors include diabetes, alcoholism, venous insufficiency, and lymphedema.[2] The portal of entry for the infecting organism is usually a break in the skin.[3] Surgical wounds, ulcers, trauma, insect bites, excoriated dermatoses, and interdigital tinea pedis are commonly described sources of infection. In many cases, particularly those involving the face, no entry site is apparent.

Laboratory confirmation of infection is difficult. Bacteriologic diagnosis by needle aspiration of the advancing edge or culture of skin biopsy material is often unrewarding because of the small number of bacteria present.[4] Culture of surface blisters or portal of entry sites is sometimes useful but may be misleading. Blood cultures are positive in only a small percentage of cases. Serologic testing of paired serum samples does not invariably show evidence of streptococcal infection despite an adequate response to penicillin therapy. Direct immunofluorescence of lesional skin biopsy specimens, using antistreptococcal antibodies, has confirmed group A streptococcus to be the predominant infecting organism.[5]

Complications of erysipelas are uncommon. These include septic shock, cavernous sinus thrombosis, abscess formation, gangrene, osteomyelitis, and glomerulonephritis. Airway obstruction has been described in a patient with infection involving the soft tissues of the neck.

Repeated recurrence of erysipelas in the same location is a well-recognized problem. This may be more common in patients with preexisting venous insufficiency or lymphedema. Damage to the local lymphatic system as a result of infection is believed to contribute to recurrent disease.[1]

TREATMENT

Therapeutic Expectations

The aim of treatment is to eradicate infection and minimize the risk of recurrence. Patients respond rapidly to appropriate therapy and should clearly improve within 24 to 48 hours after treatment begins.

First-Line Therapy

Penicillin is the treatment of choice. This may be given intravenously (penicillin G 2.4 to 8 million units per day in divided doses), intramuscularly (procaine penicillin G 1.2 million units daily in divided doses), or orally (penicillin V 250 to 500 mg four times daily). Parenteral administration is indicated in patients with severe disease, and may be indicated with young children, elderly debilitated patients, and the immunocompromised. Treatment should be continued for at least 10 days.

Potential portal of entry sites, for example, skin ulcers or tinea pedis, should be treated appropriately to lessen the risk of recurrence.

Age Considerations

The treatment of children is identical to that of adults. Young children with erysipelas are at greater risk for bacteremia. Hospitalization is warranted if they are very ill, but it is not necessary in all cases.

Hemophilus influenzae cellulitis must be considered in the differential diagnosis of facial lesions in children.

Alternative Therapeutic Options

Cephalexin (500 mg four times daily) and erythromycin (500 mg four times daily) are acceptable alternatives to oral penicillin.

PITFALLS AND PROBLEMS

The differential diagnosis of erysipelas includes allergic contact dermatitis, thrombophlebitis, and erysipeloid. Allergic contact dermatitis is characterized by erythema, swelling, and pruritus without evidence of systemic toxicity. In superficial thrombophlebitis, tenderness and erythema occur in a linear or oval distribution overlying the inflamed vessel. Erysipeloid is an infection of butchers and meat handlers caused by the organism *Erysipelothrix rhusiopathiae;* skin lesions are usually localized to the hand and lack the acute onset and systemic toxicity of erysipelas.

Erysipelas must not be confused with necrotizing fasciitis, a deeper and much more virulent infection of the subcutaneous tissues. Necrotizing fasciitis should be considered in any patient not responding to parenteral penicillin within 48 hours of initiating treatment.

Whereas penicillin alone is appropriate therapy for classic erysipelas, an antistaphylococcal antibiotic should be initiated when cellulitis of the deeper subcutaneous tissues is present. Intravenous ampicillin is the treatment of choice for facial cellulitis due to *H. influenzae* in children.

Long-term antibiotic prophylaxis with oral penicillin or a macrolide may be necessary in patients with a high frequency of recurrent erysipelas.

REFERRAL AND CONSULTATION GUIDELINES

Referral is recommended for cases in which the diagnosis is uncertain or when response to antibiotic therapy is not seen within 24 to 48 hours.

REFERENCES

1. Chartier C, Grosshans E. Erysipelas. Int J Dermatol 1990; 29:459–467.

2. Jorup-Ronstrum C: Epidemiologic, bacteriological and complicating features of erysipelas. Scand J Infect Dis 1986; 18:519–524.
3. Ronnen M, Suster S, Schewach-Millet M, Modan M: Erysipelas: Changing faces. Int J Dermatol 1985; 24:169–172.
4. Leppard BJ, Seal DV, Colman G, Hallas G: The value of bacteriology and serology in the diagnosis of cellulitis and erysipelas. Br J Dermatol 1985; 112:559–567.
5. Bernard P, Bedane C, Mounier M, et al: Streptococcal cause of erysipelas and cellulitis in adults: A microbiologic study using a direct immunofluorescence technique. Arch Dermatol 1989; 125:779–782.

CHAPTER 55

Erythroderma

John Q. Binhlam and Lloyd E. King, Jr.

CLINICAL APPEARANCE

Exfoliative dermatitis or erythroderma is a clinical syndrome characterized by widespread erythema, fine or large scales, and desquamation of a significant portion of the body surface. The clinical presentation of a patient with erythroderma can vary depending on the severity of the underlying process and its complications. Cutaneous manifestations include erythema (100%) followed by scaling (100%), alopecia (17 to 25%), dystrophic nails (up to 78% in erythrodermic psoriasis), and areas of hyperpigmentation or hypopigmentation.[1–5] Scales are usually larger in acute processes and smaller in chronic or longstanding erythrodermas. The palms and soles are typically involved (keratoderma), whereas the mucous membranes are spared (see Figs. 55–1 through 55–3 on Color Plate 21).

Symptoms typically occurring in these patients include chills, malaise, and pruritus. Systemic manifestations due to erythrodermas are variable and may include tachycardia, hyperthermia or hypothermia, lymphadenopathy, hepatomegaly, splenomegaly, and edema. Laboratory evaluations are also variable and may show leukocytosis (41 to 51%), anemia (19 to 64%), peripheral eosinophilia (32 to 48%), elevated sedimentation rate (36 to 50%), hypoalbuminemia (17 to 44%), hypocalcemia, or azotemia.[1, 2, 4, 5] Serum protein electrophoresis may be abnormal, with a nonspecific polyclonal elevation of immunoglobulin G (IgG) or immunoglobulin E (IgE). Sézary's cells, which are mononuclear cells with large hyperchromatic cerebriform nuclei, can be seen on peripheral blood smears in erythrodermas due to benign or malignant lymphoproliferative causes.

DESCRIPTION OF DISEASE

Estimates of the incidence of exfoliative dermatitis range from 2 to 71 per 1000. Men are more frequently affected than women with a male-to-female ratio of approximately 2.3:1. Although erythroderma has been reported in both the neonate and the elderly, the patient population affected tends to be older, with an average age of 55 years.[1] Physiologic studies have shown that approximately 0.5 to 1.0 g of exfoliated material is lost from the surface of normal hair-bearing human skin each day. There is also wide regional variation in the amount that is lost, with skin from the scalp, forehead, and palms showing the greatest loss and skin from the chest, forearm, and lower legs showing the least. In exfoliative dermatitis, 20 to 30 g of exfoliated material can be lost each day. Skin biopsies in patients with chronic exfoliative dermatitis are mandatory and show a spectrum of histologic patterns ranging from acute to chronic dermatitis. Histologic features in erythrodermic patients vary from characteristic or pathognomonic to nonspecific findings. Over half of the cases of erythrodermas are due to aggravation of a preexisting skin disease that often has diagnostic findings (see later in this chapter).

Just as the histology of the erythroderma syndrome is variable, the underlying etiology of exfoliative dermatitis is variable but can be categorized into the following five groups: (1) erythrodermas due to preexisting dermatoses, (2) erythrodermas induced by drugs, (3) erythrodermas induced by malignancies, (4) miscellaneous conditions associated with erythroderma, and (5) idiopathic erythrodermas.

TABLE 55–1

Dermatoses Associated With Erythroderma

Actinic reticuloid	Leiner's syndrome	Psoriasis
Airborne contact	Lichen planus	Reiter's syndrome
Atopic dermatitis	Mastocytosis	Scabies
Candidiasis	Nummular eczema	Seborrheic dermatitis
Contact dermatitis	Pemphigus foliaceus	Staphylococcal scalded skin syndrome
Dermatophytosis	Phytophotodermatitis	Stasis dermatitis
Icthyosis	Pityriasis rubra pilaris	Subacute cutaneous lupus erythematosus

Exfoliative dermatitis may be the initial presentation of an underlying preexisting dermatosis, or it may be the result of an exacerbation of a preexisting disease. Some commonly known dermatoses associated with erythroderma are atopic dermatitis, psoriasis, scabies, and seborrheic dermatitis. These and other associated dermatoses are listed in Table 55–1.

As the use of drugs has increased over the years, the list of drugs implicated in causing erythroderma has grown. Table 55–2 enumerates drugs known to be associated with inducing erythroderma and highlights the fact that any drug that a patient is taking should be considered as a possible offender.

Various malignancies are associated with erythroderma, but the one most recognized is cutaneous T-cell lymphoma (CTCL) (8 to 19%). Other, less frequently associated malignancies are Hodgkin's lymphoma (1%), non-Hodgkin's lymphoma (1%), leukemia (1%), myelodysplasia (1%), and various solid tumors (1%).[1–5]

Rarely, other diseases that do not fall into the categories previously discussed, such as human immunodeficiency virus (HIV) infections, congenital immunodeficiency syndromes, graft-versus-host disease (GVHD), and postoperative erythroderma, may be implicated as the underlying cause of erythroderma.

Finally, there is a subset of patients presenting with exfoliative dermatitis in whom no underlying cause can be found. The diagnosis of idiopathic erythroderma should be reserved only for patients in whom a diligent search for etiology over 10 to 12 months proves to be unfruitful.

TABLE 55–2

Drugs Associated With Erythroderma

Allopurinol	Dapsone	Phenothiazines
Aminoglycosides	Dimercaprol	Phenylbutazone
Amiodarone	Gold	Phenytoin
Arsenic	Hydroxychloroquine	Quinacrine
Aztreonam	Iodine	Quinidine
Barbiturates	Isoniazid	Ranitidine
Calcium channel blockers	Isotretinoin	Rifampin
Captopril	Lithium	Streptomycin
Carbamazepine	Mephenytoin	Sulfadiazine
[illegible]phalosporins	Mercurials	Sulfonamides
[illegible]roquine	Mercury	Sulfonylureas
[illegible]romazine	Mexiletine	Terbutaline
[illegible]pramide	Minocycline	Thiacetazone
	Neomycin	Thiazides
	Paracetamol	Trimethoprim
	Penicillins	Vancomycin

TREATMENT

Therapy for erythrodermas is targeted toward symptomatic relief and, if known, the causative dermatoses. Symptomatic relief (Table 55–3) is best provided by bedrest; tepid soaks or baths, which may include antipruritic agents (e.g., colloidal oatmeal [Aveeno]), liberal use of emollients, and systemic antihistamines. Low-potency or midpotency topical steroids (e.g., triamcinolone, fluocinolone) can be helpful but should be used with caution, as there can be significant systemic absorption of the steroid through denuded or erythrodermic skin. Significant fluid loss may occur owing to the shedding of scale and can lead to prerenal azotemia and high-output cardiac failure in patients with borderline renal and cardiac status, respectively. Hypothermia can occur in patients with widespread erythroderma owing to the body's compensatory increase in basal metabolic rate and heat production that leads to increased heat transport to the skin and overall total thermal loss. Therefore, patients may benefit from being in a warm, humid room with extra blankets and covers as needed. Because drugs may be the offending agents, any oral medication that a patient is taking that is unnecessary should be discontinued. Systemic antibiotics should be considered only if signs of a clinically significant secondary infection of the skin are present and not responsive to topical agents.

Once the acute phase of exfoliative dermatitis has passed and the erythroderma has improved, the underly-

TABLE 55-3

Symptomatic Therapy of Erythroderma

Soak in tepid bath without soap for 10–15 minutes twice daily; pat body dry with soft towels; colloidal oatmeal (Aveeno) may be added to water
Apply medium-strength topical steroid ointment (triamcinalone 0.1% or fluocinolone 0.05%) to entire body after each bath
Use antihistamines such as hydroxyzine 25–50 mg tid or qid or benadryl 50 mg tid or qid to sedate and control itch
Rest in bed with blankets in a warm, humid environment
Eat a high-protein diet
Discontinue unnecessary or potentially causative drugs

Abbreviations: tid, three times daily; qid, four times daily.

ing etiology may become more obvious. If CTCL is diagnosed, therapies to consider depend on the CTCL stage and include psoralen plus ultraviolet A radiation (PUVA), topical nitrogen mustard, electron beam radiation, extracorporeal photopheresis, and systemic chemotherapy.[1, 5] If chronic idiopathic erythroderma is diagnosed, the use of PUVA, systemic steroids, or other immunosuppressive drugs may be empirically used if emollients and topical steroids are ineffective for at least 3 to 4 weeks or if the erythroderma progressively worsens despite more conservative therapy.

PITFALLS AND PROBLEMS

As with treatment, the course and prognosis of exfoliative dermatitis in any given patient depend on the underlying etiology. A potential pitfall is not being diligent enough in the search for the underlying etiology. If the erythroderma is due to drug reactions, it may or may not resolve within 2 to 6 weeks after discontinuation of the offending medication. If it is due to preexisting dermatoses, the symptomatic phase of erythroderma often lasts 3 to 12 weeks. Erythroderma due to malignancies and miscellaneous causes such as HIV infection and GVHD runs a course commensurate with the prognosis of these underlying diseases.

Another potential pitfall is not treating the acute manifestation of erythroderma aggressively. The mortality rate for exfoliative dermatitis has not been well delineated. Various retrospective studies report deaths of 18 to 64% of their patients owing to causes related to exfoliative dermatitis. A major reason for morbidity and mortality is sepsis due to infection through the denuded skin. The threshold for admitting a patient with erythroderma for intensive skin care and systemic antibiotics should be low if any signs or symptoms of systemic infection or vascular instability are present.

REFERRAL/CONSULTATION GUIDELINES

The primary physician should begin symptomatic therapy as soon as possible. Any patient sick enough to be admitted to the hospital may benefit from dermatologic consultation to delineate the cause of the erythroderma and to assist with intensive skin care programs. Individuals with erythroderma who are managed in the outpatient setting should also have consultation if the eruption persists for more than 3 weeks of symptomatic treatment despite removal of the suspected offending drug or if the clinician is unfamiliar with dealing with erythroderma and its complications. Consultation may also be useful to initiate the often complex therapy necessary to treat the disorder responsible for erythroderma.

REFERENCES

1. Wilson DC, Jester JD, King LE: Erythroderma and exfoliative dermatitis. Clin Dermatol 1993; 11:67–72.
2. Botella-Estrada R, Sanmartin O, Oliver V, et al: Erythroderma: A clinicopathological study of 56 cases. Arch Dermatol 1994; 130:1503–1507.
3. King LE: Erythroderma: Who, where, when, why, and how. Arch Dermatol 1994; 130;1545–1547.
4. Wong KS, Wong SN, Tham SN, Giam YC: Generalised exfoliative dermatitis—A clinical study of 108 patients. Ann Acad Med Singapore 1988; 17(4):520–523.
5. Thestrup-Pedersen K, Halkier-Sorensen L, Sogaard H, et al: The red man syndrome: Exfoliative dermatitis of unknown etiology: A description and follow-up of 38 patients. J Am Acad Dermatol 1988; 18:1307–1312.

CHAPTER 56

Lyme Borreliosis

John W. Melski

CLINICAL APPEARANCE

Definition

Lyme borreliosis (LB) is a multistage, multisystem infection by a spirochete in the genus *Borrelia* (*B. burgdorferi* in North America and Europe; *B. garinii* and *B. afzelii* in Europe and Asia). LB is acquired primarily from an infected nymphal tick in the genus *Ixodes* that has been attached to skin for at least 24 hours. This chapter describes the diagnosis and treatment of early LB associated with one or more expanding, red, skin lesions called *erythema migrans* (EM; previously called *erythema "chronicum" migrans*).[1–3]

Typical Lesions and Symptoms

Primary EM

Primary EM (see Fig. 56–1 on Color Plate 21) is a solitary lesion that occurs at the site of inoculation of *Borrelia*. The punctum, a minute crust at the point of insertion, is almost always gone by the time EM forms, but there can be a persistent papule or postinflammatory pigmentation or scale. The most consistent morphology of primary EM is a solid red circle or oval that expands over days. The size depends on the time to presentation. The Centers for Disease Control and Prevention uses 5 cm for case definition, but *Borrelia* have been recovered from lesions as small as 3 cm, and lesions larger than 20 cm are not rare. The long axis is usually parallel to a line of maximal skin tension.

Inflammatory variants are presumably due to hypersensitivity to one or more tick antigens or, possibly, coinfections. In the absence of such reactions, erythema and discomfort (usually itch) are mild to moderate and elevation and induration are minimal to absent. As primary EM expands (see Fig. 56–2 on Color Plate 22), concentric rings of different shades of erythema can form, with the centralmost being dull or "dusky." Central erythema can fade, resulting in a complete annulus of erythema. An incomplete annulus (arciform lesion) is not seen unless the entire lesion is fading.

Although annular EM has been emphasized, solid erythema is more common when lesions are less than 15 cm. The border of EM is often less well demarcated than that of either urticaria or classic erysipelas. The central transitions of redness are even less distinct. When primary EM occurs below the knee, there can be faint pigmentation, edema, or mild purpura, as seen with any inflammatory lesion. Faint pigmentation and an expanding collarette of scale are possible postinflammatory sequelae of primary EM.

Constitutional symptoms are often absent with primary EM. When present, they are usually less severe than with secondary EM. As with secondary EM, only a third of patients will recall a recent tick bite.

Secondary EM

Secondary EM consists of multiple lesions at sites of hematogenous dissemination. A larger primary lesion may still be present when secondary EM appears (see Fig. 56–3 on Color Plate 22), but usually the primary has faded or is no longer obvious. Patients are often unaware of their secondary lesions. The morphology of secondary EM (see Fig. 56–4 on Color Plate 22) is similar to that of primary EM, but local symptoms are less severe and sequelae of a tick bite are absent. The number of secondary lesions can vary from 2 to more than 80. Lesions appear in "crops" that have similar size, color, and orientation. When the face, hands, or feet are involved, there is mild swelling and erythema that is poorly marginated. Discrete lesions of palms and soles are uncommon and faint when present.

Constitutional symptoms are usually present and often severe with secondary EM. Symptoms include fatigue, fever, headache, stiff neck, joint pains, muscle pains, and loss of appetite. Although described as flulike, respiratory symptoms are uncommon. Organ system involvement includes oligoarticular arthritis, meningitis or subtle encephalitis, cranial neuritis (especially facial nerve palsy), motor or sensory radiculoneuritis (especially in Europe), atrioventricular block, myopericarditis or pancarditis, and ocular involvement including panophthalmitis. Many other manifestations have been described.

Atypical Presentations and Alternative Forms

Otherwise typical EM can be difficult to recognize owing to the normal topology of the face, perineum, hands, or feet. Other confounding factors are thick hair, large lesions wrapped around the trunk or an extremity, and local comorbidity such as stasis dermatitis.

Primary EM

Inflammatory variants of primary EM are probably due to hypersensitivity to tick antigens or, possibly, coinfections. Variants include persistence of central erythema resulting in a bull's-eye pattern, central vesiculation and necrosus, lymphangitic streaks, and postinflammatory sequelae including transient focal alopecia.

Secondary EM

Multiple small secondary lesions can be mistaken for urticaria. Occasionally, secondary lesions are so elongated that they resemble erythematous bands rather than ovals. When secondary lesions collide, the erythema is suppressed in the region of overlap, resulting in polycyclic patterns and unusual shapes that may not be recognized.

DESCRIPTION OF DISEASE

Demographics

As with all tick-borne diseases, the incidence of LB is highly focal and depends on habitats suitable for (1) *Ixodes* ticks, (2) mice and other rodent and small animal reservoirs of *Borrelia* for uninfected larval ticks ("seed" ticks), and (3) deer or other large mammal hosts suitable for matings of adult ticks. Risk is from exposure to endemic areas, usually between late spring and mid fall. Risk is reduced by avoiding brush where ticks are questing, wearing protective clothing, using insect repellents, and inspecting for ticks after each day of exposure. Embedded ticks should be removed by grasping close to the site of attachment with forceps and without squeezing the body. Application of an antibiotic ointment may be helpful. The site should be inspected daily for 1 month if there is a possibility that the tick was *Ixodes* and attachment was for longer than 24 hours. If tick analysis is available, the tick can be saved in a sealed jar along with a piece of moist tissue paper.

Natural History

LB has three stages. Primary or "early localized" LB occurs days to weeks after the tick bite. Secondary or "early disseminated" LB occurs weeks to months later. Late or "tertiary" LB occurs after more than 1 year. As with syphilis, progression without treatment is difficult to predict. EM eventually fades, with reports of occasional recurrences.

Skin lesions in later stages are (1) Borrelial lymphocytoma: a solitary, persistent, inflammatory nodule often near the earlobe, nipple, or axillary fold; and (2) acrodermatitis chronica atrophicans: an insidious, parchment-like atrophy with sensory changes and juxta-articular fibrotic nodules, often in an extremity that was inflamed in an earlier stage. These lesions occur mainly in Europe. The relationship of LB to morphea, lichen sclerosus, or Jessner's benign lymphocytic infiltrate remains controversial.

Laboratory and Pathology

Serology is unreliable in primary EM but usually positive in secondary EM, especially if a sensitive immunoglobulin M (IgM) assay is used.[4] Treatment with antibiotics can blunt the antibody response. Skin culture for *Borrelia* is not widely available, but it can be positive in up to 75% of primary EM and 100% of secondary

EM. Why some primary lesions are culture-negative is unclear. Possible reasons include misdiagnosis, fastidious strains, self-limited disease, and small numbers of organisms. Culture is rarely needed with secondary EM, since the clinical features are usually diagnostic. Polymerase chain reaction is an evolving tool, and sensitivity and specificity of available primers need to be better defined. In secondary EM, there can be mild anemia, elevations of sedimentation rate, neutrophils, and platelets, and occasionally, a cholestatic liver enzyme profile. An electrocardiogram to search for heart block is not routinely indicated, but this should be obtained if there is a history of lightheadedness or palpitations or if the pulse is irregular.

Biopsy is useful only to rule out other diseases (Table 56–1). The histology of EM is generally nonspecific, and primary EM is often confounded by tick bite reactions. Unlike the more tightly coiled and rigid spirochete of syphilis, the spirochete of LB is loosely coiled and irregular in tissue, similar to elastic and other fibers.

TABLE 56–1

Differential Diagnosis of Erythema Migrans Based on Examination

Solid Erythema
Delayed hypersensitivity (e.g., arthropod, contact, injection)
Cellulitis
Fixed drug eruption
Large urticaria
Wells' syndrome
Localized mucinosis
Atypical infiltrates, lymphocytic and other
Annular Erythema
Erythema annulare
Granuloma annulare (macular form)
Involuting lesions (e.g., arthropod bites, urticaria, psoriasis, eczema)
Inflammatory morphea
Subacute cutaneous lupus
Annular granulomatous reactions (e.g., sarcoid, leprosy)
Purpura annularis telangiectodes
Benign lymphocytic infiltrates

Pathogenesis

There are many unresolved questions concerning the pathogenesis of the erythema itself and the relationship of disease sequelae to the immune response and to tissue tropism and intracellular sequestration of spirochetes.

TREATMENT

Therapeutic Expectations

The response of early LB to treatment is usually satisfying for both physician and patient. A transient increase in constitutional symptoms (Jarisch-Herxheimer reaction) occurs in about 20% of patients. Bright erythema is always gone after a week of treatment, and systemic symptoms and signs are usually markedly improved. Local postinflammatory changes in the skin usually resolve within a month, but faint dull erythema may persist longer. Recurrent EM is rare, but relapses of LB in other organ systems can occur, especially with secondary EM. Relapses usually respond to retreatment. Adverse outcomes of pregnancy are rare even in endemic areas.

Moderate fatigue, unresponsive to antibiotics, can persist for several months or longer in patients with prominent constitutional symptoms. Some patients are subsequently diagnosed as having chronic fatigue syndrome or fibromyalgia.[5] These possibly identical disorders are poorly understood and may improve with nonantibiotic therapies or simply with time.

First-Line Therapy

Safe, effective, and inexpensive antibiotics have long been available. Optimal use of these agents remains uncertain, despite numerous studies of more expensive antibiotics. For localized disease in adults, oral doxycycline (100 mg bid) or amoxicillin (500 mg tid) for 10 days to 3 weeks is recommended. The author favors 3 weeks, since the incremental risks of adverse reactions and the costs are small. Prophylactic antibiotic treatment after tick bites is controversial, but most favor watchful waiting. This author favors 10 days of antibiotics if there is proven exposure (*Borrelia* demonstrated in a tick embedded for more than 24 hours) or possible exposure and unreliable follow-up.

For disseminated LB without neurologic signs and without heart block, the treatments previously discussed can be extended to 4 to 6 weeks. Also, doxycycline can be increased to 100 mg tid or amoxicillin to 1000 mg tid, especially for large patients. Adding probenecid to amoxicillin is not recommended owing to added toxicity (contraindicated in pregnancy), lack of empirical justification, and possible decreased transport of amoxicillin into cerebrospinal fluid.

Age Considerations

Amoxicillin (20 mg/kg/day divided tid) is the drug of choice for children. The dose can be doubled for children under 8 years of age with disseminated disease but without serious complications (see later in this chapter).

Alternative Therapeutic Options

When both doxycycline and amoxicillin are inappropriate, cefuroxime axetil (500 mg bid in adults, 40 mg/kg/day divided bid in children) can be used, although the cost will be more than tenfold higher. Oral azithromycin (500 mg on day 1 and 250 mg on days 2 to 5) seems to be effective for localized LB but has a higher relapse rate for disseminated LB than 20 days of amoxicillin (500 mg tid). Two 5-day courses given 5 days apart may be effective, but this needs further study. First-generation cephalosporins, penicillin, erythromycin, and sulfa antibiotics are poor choices.

PITFALLS AND PROBLEMS

The diagnosis of EM requires skilled examination, especially for primary lesions when constitutional symptoms are absent and where serology is unreliable. However, the pathognomonic nature of EM has been greatly overstated. There are non-LB skin lesions that mimic EM (see Table 56–1), and a detailed history of the present illness should always be considered. A complete review of systems, complete skin examination, and pertinent systems examination are also indicated for patients with constitutional symptoms or secondary EM.

Lesions that enlarge within hours or take months to enlarge are uncharacteristic of EM. Prominent scale, overlying erythema, arciform patterns, and nodularity also reasonably exclude the diagnosis. Failure to respond to treatment should prompt consideration of other possibilities including coinfection such as ehrlichiosis. Lesions of more than 1 month's duration without positive serology are probably not EM, and biopsy may be indicated. The vast majority of cases of LB occur after exposure to an *Ixodes* habitat between late spring and mid fall. Exceptions should be reviewed critically.

REFERRAL AND CONSULTATION GUIDELINES

Consultation is appropriate if there are serious complications such as complete heart block or neurologic signs with cerebrospinal fluid pleocytosis. Intravenous antibiotics for 2 to 4 weeks may be needed. Choices include ceftriaxone (2 g/day for adults, 50 to 100 mg/kg/day for children up to 40 kg), cefotaxime (2 g every 8 hours for adults, 100 to 200 mg/kg/day divided qid for children up to 50 kg), and penicillin G (3.3×10^6 units every 4 hours for adults, 250,000 units/kg/day divided qid for children up to 40 kg).

Consultation is also appropriate if the practitioner is not confident in the diagnosis after history and examination or if there is the possibility of coinfection or a pyoderma. Doxycycline will cover coinfection with *Ehrlichia,* also transmitted by *Ixodes* ticks. A mixture of amoxicillin and clavulanic acid should treat both LB and *Staphylococcus aureus*. Consultation should also be considered for infections acquired during pregnancy, failure to respond to treatment, and comorbidity such as renal or hepatic insufficiency or immunosuppression.

REFERENCES

1. Melski JW: Lyme borreliosis: Lessons in diagnosing and treating erythema migrans. Fitzpatrick's J Clin Dermatol 1994; May/June, pp 14–25.
2. Melski J, Reed KD, Mitchell PD, Barth GD: Primary and secondary erythema migrans in central Wisconsin. Arch Dermatol 1993; 129:709–716.
3. Steere AC: Current understanding of Lyme disease. Hosp Pract 1993; 28:37–44.
4. Mitchell PD, Reed KD, Aspeslet TL, et al: Comparison of four immunoserologic assays for the detection of antibodies to *Borrelia burgdorferi* in patients with culture-positive erythema migrans. J Clin Microbiol 1994; 32:1958–1962.
5. Steere AC, Taylor E, McHugh GL, Logigian EL: The overdiagnosis of Lyme disease. JAMA 1993; 269:1812–1816.

CHAPTER 57

Rocky Mountain Spotted Fever

Debra Karp Skopicki

CLINICAL APPEARANCE

Definition

Rocky Mountain spotted fever (RMSF) was first described in the United States during the late 19th century.[1] A potentially fatal member of the spotted fever group of rickettsial infections, RMSF is the most prevalent rickettsial disease in the United States.[1] It is heralded by the classic triad of fever, rash, and a history of recent tick exposure.

Typical Lesions and Symptoms

The incubation period for RMSF varies from 2 to 14 days, beginning with a prodrome that includes malaise, anorexia, and chills.[2] Abruptly, patients may next experience headache, fever, myalgias, conjunctival erythema, nausea, and photophobia. Skin lesions develop that are typically erythematous macules and papules, beginning on the wrists and ankles, and becoming hemorrhagic or purpuric while spreading centripetally to the trunk (Figs. 57–1 and 57–2). The palms and soles may also be affected.[3] As the disease disseminates, multiple organ systems become involved, including the gastrointestinal, reticuloendothelial, central nervous, and cardiovascular systems. Patients may develop abdominal pain, diarrhea, hepatosplenomegaly, meningismus, confusion, hypotension, myocarditis, noncardiogenic pulmonary edema, and gangrene of acral sites. The clinical differential diagnosis includes meningococcemia, measles, atypical measles, idiopathic thrombocytopenic purpura, encephalitis, drug reaction, infectious mononucleosis, enteroviral infection, ehrlichiosis, and other rickettsial diseases.

Laboratory abnormalities generally peak 4 to 9 days after the onset of the illness. Hematologic abnormalities include anemia and thrombocytopenia. Leukocytosis is commonly not seen, and in fact, a mild leukopenia may be observed. Severely ill patients also demonstrate laboratory evidence of disseminated intravascular coagulation with increased fibrin split products and prothrombin time as well as thrombocytopenia. Renal dysfunction may manifest with an elevated blood urea nitrogen, whereas gastrointestinal involvement can result in hypoalbuminemia, elevated alkaline phosphatase, serum glutamic-oxaloacetic transaminase, and bilirubin.[1] Patients who develop jaundice appear to have fulminant disease and a poorer prognosis. These patients may have a glucose-6-phosphate deficiency, resulting in hemolysis rather than a primary liver function abnormality.[3] Hyponatremia may be present, and although inappropriate secretion of antidiuretic hormone may be partly responsible, the etiology is likely multifactorial.[4] Cerebrospinal fluid is abnormal in up to 60% of patients as demonstrated by an elevated protein level and a mononuclear pleocytosis, although polymorphonuclear leukocytes may be present.[4]

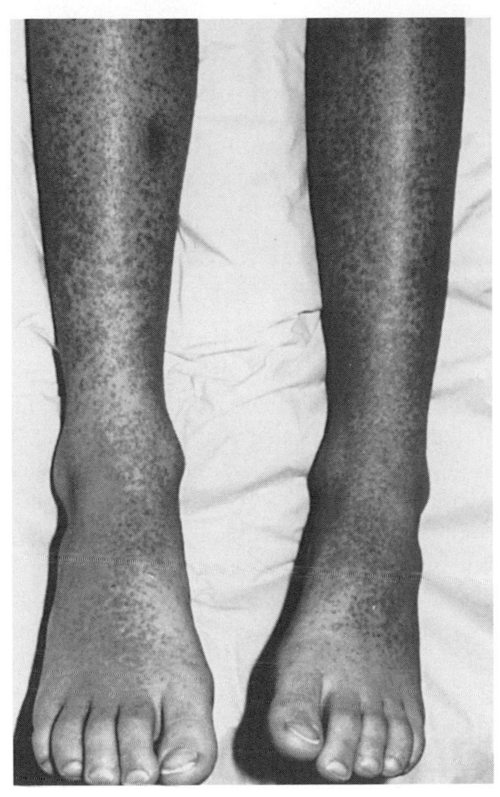

FIGURE 57–1
Erythematous and violaceous macules and papules are confluent on the lower extremities of a patient with Rocky Mountain spotted fever (RMSF).

Atypical Presentations or Alternative Forms

Patients under 15 years tend to have more typical disease. Those older than 15 years appear to develop the eruption later, have less frequent history of tick exposure, and have more severe systemic illness including pneumonia, stupor, cardiac arrhythmias, and death.[3]

The actual site of the tick bite may be clinically inapparent, for instance, if it occurs in an area covered by hair (Fig. 57–3). In addition, the cutaneous eruption does not develop in up to 15% of all confirmed cases of RMSF.[5] Even if the rash does appear, it may be more difficult to appreciate in African Americans. Moreover, features that are associated with late stages of the disease may, in fact, occur quite early.[3] These include abdominal pain, diarrhea, conjunctivitis, and lymphadenopathy.

RMSF may result in complications even in patients who receive treatment. Neurologic complications are the most frequently encountered and include encephalopathy, neuropathy, seizures, and permanent motor deficits.[4] In addition, renal or hepatic insufficiency, congestive heart failure, and permanent hearing or vision loss may be seen.

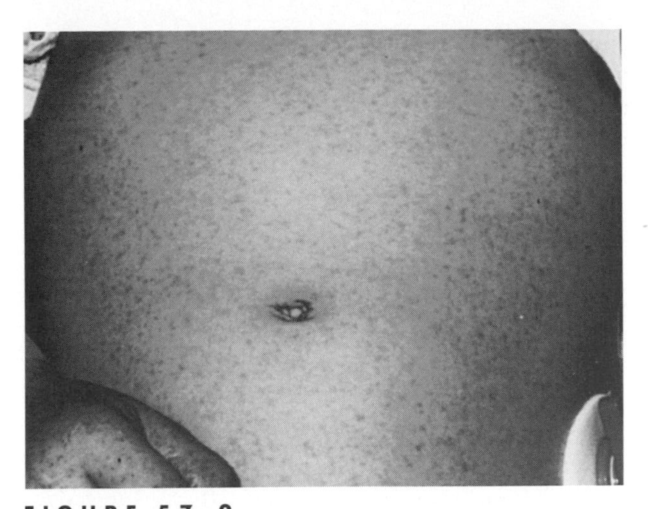

FIGURE 57–2
Petechial papules are located on the abdomen of a child with RMSF, having spread centripetally from the distal extremities.

DESCRIPTION OF DISEASE

RMSF is caused by *Rickettsia rickettsii*, a small, pleomorphic, obligate intracellular coccobacillus. It survives

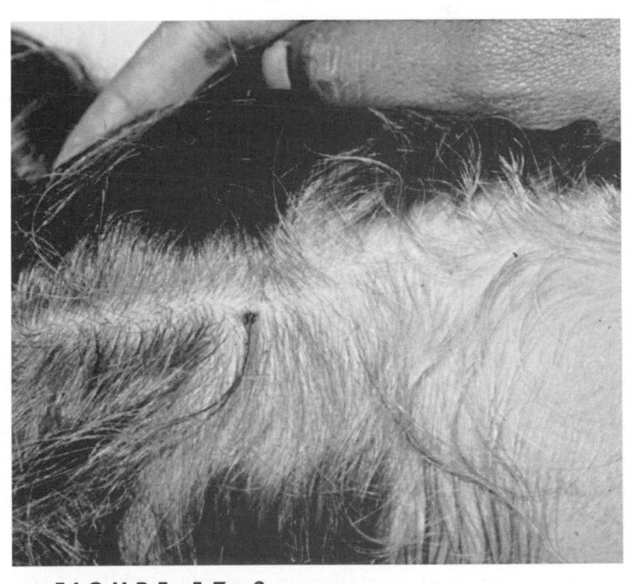

FIGURE 57–3
A tick bite site is hidden in the scalp of a child with RMSF.

only briefly outside a host and is transmitted by infected blood-sucking arthropods, the natural reservoir of many rickettsiae. Transmission occurs during their 6 to 10 hours of attachment.[1] In the Western United States, the wood tick *Dermacentor andersoni* and, in the East, the dog tick *Dermacentor variabilis* are the most common vectors.[1] Most infections occur in April through September. Although RMSF is distributed widely across the United States, the incidence is highest in the South Atlantic and South Central States, usually in rural or suburban areas; however, an outbreak of RMSF was documented in New York City.[2] Children ages 5 to 9 years old seem to be the cohort at highest risk for infection.[2]

Death from RMSF can occur as early as 3 to 6 days after the onset of the infection, so early diagnosis and initiation of therapy are imperative. Unfortunately, the mean time for documenting diagnostic titers by routinely available testing is approximately 10 days.[4] The Weil-Felix reaction, a nonspecific serologic test, measures agglutinins to selected antigens from *Proteus vulgaris* strains (OX-19, OX-2, and OX-K). In RMSF, antibodies to *Proteus* OX-19 or OX-2 but not to OX-K appear in the second or third week, disappearing a few weeks after the febrile period has passed.[2] The rickettsia-specific antigens can be incorporated into complement fixation, agglutination, passive hemagglutination, radioimmune precipitation, indirect fluorescent antibody, or enzyme-linked immunosorbent assay tests. Group-specific and even species-specific diagnostic testing is becoming more widely available. At the present time, the most efficient and rapid diagnostic technique is demonstration of the pathogen by direct immunofluorescence or immunoperoxidase staining of skin biopsy specimens.[5] Whenever possible, patients should receive a skin biopsy, which may result in a definitive diagnosis. However, treatment should be initiated empirically if the diagnosis is suspected on clinical grounds. Polymerase chain reaction to identify *R. rickettsii* in blood or tissue may eventually become the diagnostic test of choice.

The characteristic histopathologic feature of disseminated rickettsial infection is a vasculitis of arterioles, capillaries, and venules in the skin, brain, heart, and kidneys.[5] *Rickettsia* damage the endothelial cells, resulting in medial necrosis, endothelial hypertrophy, and proliferation, which along with platelet and fibrin thrombosis, causes vascular occlusion. The inflammatory response is generally lymphocytic or lymphohistiocytic, with macrophages and plasma cells arriving late.

TREATMENT

Therapeutic Expectations

Patients who do not receive treatment have a mortality of 15 to 20%, which decreases to 3 to 6% for those who are treated.[2]

First-Line Therapy

Daily inspection for ticks on people living in endemic areas is essential. If a tick is found, forceps, not bare fingers, should be used for its removal, since infectious fluid or feces from the tick may enter a break in the skin. Although antibiotics are not chemoprophylactic against RMSF, they may delay the onset of the disease.[2]

As soon as the diagnosis of RMSF is suspected, treatment with tetracycline or chloramphenicol should be initiated. Adults should be treated with oral tetracycline (500 mg four times daily). Hospitalization and intravenous treatment with tetracycline (2 g in four divided doses) or intravenous chloramphenicol (50 to 100 mg/kg in four divided doses) may be necessary in those with more severe illness. Antibiotic therapy should be continued for 5 to 7 days and for at least 48 hours after the resolution of fever and clinical improvement are observed.[1] Supportive therapy includes fluid replacement and, when necessary, the treatment of disseminated intravascular coagulation and shock.

Age Considerations

Children over 8 years of age can be treated with oral tetracycline (25 to 50 mg/kg/day in four divided doses). When tetracycline is contraindicated—for instance, in young children and pregnant women, when staining of the teeth and bones may occur—intravenous chloramphenicol (50 to 75 mg/kg/day to a total of 3 g in four divided doses, switching to 50 mg/day orally) can be given. The dose should be reduced to 25 mg/kg/day for infants less than 2 weeks of age.

PITFALLS AND PROBLEMS

Physicians must remain aware that patients may not present with the classic clinical features and history typically associated with RMSF. In fact, although patients tend to visit their physician in the first 2 days after the onset of their illness, only 3% have the classic triad of fever, rash, and history of tick exposure at the time.[3] Patients without a definite history of tick exposure tend to be older and have a longer interval between the onset of the illness and the cutaneous eruption.[3] Importantly, fatalities more commonly occur when a history of tick bite is not elicited and a recognizable eruption does not develop.

Delayed diagnosis and late treatment usually result because of atypical presenting symptoms or late appearance of a rash. Systemic complaints occurring early in the illness such as abdominal pain and diarrhea may result in a diagnosis of acute viral gastrointestinal disease rather than RMSF. In fact, the most frequent initial misdiagnosis is nonspecific viral illness or fever of unknown origin.[3]

Ultimately, clinicians must remember to consider the diagnosis of RMSF early and to realize that RMSF may present in nonendemic areas, during seasons not considered classic, and with no rash or history of tick exposure.

REFERRAL AND CONSULTATION GUIDELINES

Clearly, any patient with a cutaneous eruption that is difficult to diagnose, particularly if accompanied by fever or other constitutional symptoms, should be referred to a dermatologist early. The potentially life-threatening consequences of a delay in the appropriate diagnosis and therapy of RMSF underscore the need for early treatment referral.

Physicians working in endemic areas should remain especially vigilant, not only for the cases of RMSF that display the classic triad of fever, rash, and history of tick exposure but also for the cases in which the eruption is absent or a history of tick exposure is not elicited. Empirical therapy should be started, and referral to a dermatologist should be initiated.

REFERENCES

1. Spach DH, Liles WC, Campbell GL, et al: Tick-borne diseases in the United States. N Engl J Med 1993; 329:936–947.
2. Weber DJ, Walker DH: Rocky Mountain spotted fever. Infect Dis Clin North Am 1991; 5:19–35.
3. Helmick CG, Bernard KW, D'Angelo LJ: Rocky Mountain spotted fever: Clinical, laboratory, and epidemiological features of 262 cases. J Infect Dis 1984; 150:480–488.
4. Kirk JL, Fine DP, Sexton DJ, et al: Rocky Mountain spotted fever. A clinical review based on 48 confirmed cases, 1943–1986. Medicine 1990; 69:35–45.
5. Dumler JS, Walker DH: Diagnostic tests for Rocky Mountain spotted fever and other rickettsial diseases. Dermatol Clin 1994; 12:25–36.

CHAPTER 58

Toxic Epidermal Necrolysis and Stevens-Johnson Syndrome

Robert S. Stern

CLINICAL APPEARANCE

Stevens-Johnson syndrome (SJS) and toxic epidermal necrolysis (TEN) are related mucocutaneous blistering reactions most often due to drugs. They are characterized by the development of erythematous macules and epidermal necrolysis. In SJS, cutaneous manifestations include erythematous or purpuric macules, some of which blister, atypical flat target lesions, or larger areas of erythema that may go on to blister. Epidermal necrosis is evident in many lesions of SJS (see Figs. 58–1 on Color Plate 22 and 58–2 on Color Plate 23). True target lesions (see Fig. 58–3 on Color Plate 23) are unusual in cases of SJS and TEN. Instead, these lesions are typical of past infectious erythema multiforme, a less serious condition (see Chapter 19: Erythema Multiforme). TEN represents the most severe manifestations of this blistering reaction. Initially, TEN may be indistinguishable from SJS. In some cases, the initial skin presentation of TEN is widespread erythema. To be classified as TEN, the area of skin detachment should exceed 30% of body surface area. Mucous membrane involvement almost always occurs in both SJS and TEN, with oral involvement most frequent. Fever is an almost universal symptom of these diseases.

The greatest challenge to the clinician is separating out patients who present with limited disease to determine whether they have erythema multiforme (EM), a usually self-limited disease most often related to infections, especially herpes simplex virus infection, or SJS, a more serious condition, which in some cases, may evolve to TEN. SJS and TEN are most often related to the use of drugs.

Patients with SJS and TEN often initially present with fever and symptoms of mucosal inflammation including sore throat, dysphagia, sore mouth, and photophobia. The initial cutaneous lesions tend to be concentrated more on the trunk than on the extremities, whereas the opposite is often the case with postviral EM. Fever, mucosal symptoms, and general malaise are almost always present in persons with SJS and TEN and may begin before cutaneous or mucosal lesions are evident. Skin lesions may be painful or may sting. Itching is relatively uncommon. In most cases, the eruption evolves rapidly, with the full extent of involvement typically occurring within a few days after the first skin lesions appear.

DESCRIPTION OF DISEASE

Demographics

SJS and TEN occur in individuals of all ages and sexes. Since exposure to drugs is the primary cause of the reaction, the incidence is higher among older persons who are more likely to be using the drugs that cause this reaction. Patients with human immunodeficiency virus (HIV) infection, especially those with acquired immunodeficiency syndrome (AIDS), as well as individuals with other immunologic abnormalities, including systemic lupus erythematosus and bone marrow recipients, are at higher risk of developing this reaction, even after the greater number of medications these patients use is considered. Overall, the incidence in the general population without immunologic abnormalities of SJS and TEN is about 1 to 3 per million person-years. The risk associated with sulfonamides in HIV-positive individuals may approach 1 per 1000 such persons exposed to this drug.

Natural History of Disease

The first signs of SJS and TEN are nonspecific. Malaise and signs of mucosal inflammation such as sore throat or photophobia are frequent. The initial cutaneous lesion often begins as erythematous macules, which may be stinging or painful, but are unlikely to itch. These are most marked on the trunk (see Fig. 58–4 on Color Plate 23). Flat, atypical target lesions and purpuric macules are also seen. Blisters may be seen in association with the lesions. As the skin lesions increase in number and size, they may coalesce to give widespread erythema. As epidermal necrosis develops, blistering occurs.

TEN may begin with a clinical picture identical to that of SJS or as a severe morbilliform eruption or with bright red macules. The hallmark of TEN is widespread necrosis of the epidermis (see Fig. 58–5 on Color Plate 23). As a result, the epidermis is easily separated from the underlying dermis with the slightest trauma. This is called the *Nikolsky sign.*

Pathologic examination is helpful in ruling out other blistering diseases and separating out SJS and TEN from EM. In SJS and TEN, one typically sees full-thickness epidermal necrosis. Early on, there is relatively little inflammatory infiltrate in the skin. In EM, more dermal inflammation and less epidermal necrosis are observed.

Etiology/Pathogenesis

Most cases of SJS and TEN are drug-induced. A recent case-controlled study established the relative risk of frequently prescribed drugs in association with this condition. Drugs most often associated with these conditions are listed in Table 58–1. The positive association with short-term corticosteroid use (less than 2 months) as well as a higher risk in persons with immunologic disorders is especially notable.

TABLE 58-1

Drugs Most Strongly Associated With Stevens-Johnson Syndrome and Toxic Epidermal Necrolysis

Sulfonamides	Carbamazepine (≤2 months)
Trimethoprim-sulfamethoxazole	Phenytoin (≤2 months)
Aminopenicillins	Valproic acid (≤2 months)
Quinolones	Oxicam NSAIDs (≤2 months)
Cephalosporins	Allopurinol (≤2 months)
Tetracyclines	Corticosteroids (≤2 months)
Phenobarbital (≤2 months)	

Abbreviation: NSAIDs, nonsteroidal anti-inflammatory drugs.

The exact pathogenesis of these disorders is unknown. Their usual onset is 1 to 2 weeks after beginning treatment with the responsible drug, and the presence of CD8 cells and killer T cells in blister fluid suggest to some that these disorders are immunologic reactions. Reexposure to a causative drug is likely to lead to a more extensive and serious reaction within days (or even hours) of the reexposure, a finding also consistent with an immunologically mediated mechanism.

The morbidity and mortality associated with SJS and TEN are a result of the necrosis of the skin and mucous membranes. Secondary infections, fluid and electrolyte balance problems, pain, and negative catabolic states cause acute complications. Therefore, sequelae can be predicted from which sites are involved and the extent of involvement. Prognostic factors associated with lower survival include greater extent of involvement and underlying illnesses such as diabetes or immunosuppression. Among survivors, the most frequent sequelae are ocular. Eye involvement can lead to corneal scarring and blindness. Sometimes, oral or genital involvement will be so severe as to lead to scarring and synechiae formation. Cutaneous scarring is also seen.

TREATMENT

General

The key to treatment is the prompt withdrawal of possible causative agents. Any drug started within 2 months should be considered as a possible cause. Those agents most often associated with this reaction (see Table 58–1) and started within 2 weeks should of course be especially suspect.

Unfortunately, many drugs will persist in a patient for hours or days, even after their ingestion is discontinued. Therefore, one should be sure to consider as possible causes drugs that were stopped before the first symptoms of the reaction appeared, especially if they have long half-lives.

One problem in the treatment of SJS and TEN is the fact that these are rapidly progressive diseases, with the full extent of necrolysis often occurring within 12 to 48 hours of the first cutaneous symptom. Therefore, any early intervention that might halt extension of the process is difficult to institute during this brief critical time window. Further, no treatment has proved effective in controlling the evolution of the eruption. In addition, it is not possible to predict the ultimate extent of necrolysis from a patient's initial presentation. The key to therapy is support of the affected individual, especially one with extensive areas of skin necrosis. Treatment should parallel that for a second-degree burn of the same extent. Therefore, experience from the treatment of patients with thermal burns is essential in anticipating and attempting to avoid the problems associated with these diseases. For individuals with extensive necrolysis, treatment in burn units is indicated. For individuals with less extensive necrolysis, a setting that would be appropriate for a similar extent of a second-degree thermal burn is appropriate.

The principal problems of SJS and TEN are fluid loss, secondary infection, impaired thermal regulation, increased susceptibility to infection as a result of immune suppression and loss of the normal skin barrier, and increased metabolic needs. Therefore, fluid and electrolyte replacement as well as hyperalimentation should be instituted if necrolysis is extensive. Signs of skin infection should be carefully monitored. Central lines should be avoided when possible, as these may increase the risk of infection. The prophylactic use of antibiotics should be avoided, but infection should be rapidly and aggressively treated. The increased metabolism of these individuals requires careful metabolic monitoring and appropriate therapy to compensate for these stresses. An individual expert in the treatment of burns is best able to manage these diseases. In addition, because of the high frequency of ocular involvement and the sometimes devastating nature of its complications, ophthalmic consultation is desirable in any case where a patient has clinical evidence of ocular involvement.

Alternative Therapeutic Options

There is general agreement about the desirability of applying the principles of management of burn treatment to patients with SJS and TEN. There is general disagreement about the appropriateness and utility of systemic corticosteroids or other immunosuppressive therapies in these patients. Although some individuals strongly advocate high-dose (1 to 2 mg/kg/day) prednisone and some even advocate pulse therapy with very high doses of corticosteroids beginning at the first recognition of these diseases, studies suggesting that this is beneficial are lacking. Clearly, systemic corticosteroid therapy increases the risk of infection, the primary source of mortality in these cases. Corticosteroid therapy also complicates fluid and electrolyte balance and delays healing. Another argument against the use of systemic steroids is that the evolution of the disease process is generally so rapid that by the time the patient is diagnosed and care is instituted, the potential beneficial effect of corticosteroids cannot be realized, as the disease has progressed too far. For these reasons, in most cases, the risks of corticosteroids are likely to outweigh their potential benefit. Use of other immunosuppressive agents has been advocated on the basis of case reports, but credible evidence for these agents' safety and efficacy in the treatment of these disorders is lacking.

PITFALLS AND PROBLEMS

The key to optimal therapy of SJS and TEN is early diagnosis, so that drugs can be withdrawn and measures can be instituted to decrease the risks of infection, electrolyte imbalance, and scarring that accompany epidermal necrosis and mucosal inflammation. All recently instituted drugs that are not essential to the patient should be withdrawn, and the relative risks and benefits of continuing any recently introduced drug must be viewed from the perspective that this medication might be worsening the disease.

REFERRAL/CONSULTATION GUIDELINES

Patients with ocular involvement should be seen by an ophthalmologist. Patients with extensive necrolysis (more than a few percent of body area) should be monitored for fluid or electrolyte metabolic and infection risk. For cases with substantial epidermal loss, care by experts including those experienced in the treatment of thermal burns should be instituted. Patients with TEN and necrolysis in excess of 30% of body area should be considered as candidates for care in burn units.

BIBLIOGRAPHY

Assier H, Bastuji-Garin S, Revuz J, Roujeau JC: Erythema multiforme with mucous membrane involvement and Stevens-Johnson syndrome are clinically different disorders with distinct causes. Arch Dermatol 1995; 131:539–543.

Cote B, Wechsler J, Bastuji-Garin, et al: Clinicopathologic correlation in erythema multiforme and Stevens-Johnson syndrome. Arch Dermatol 1995; 131:1268–1272.

Roujeau JC, Kelly JP, Naldi L, et al: Medication use and the risk of Stevens-Johnson syndrome or toxic epidermal necrolysis. N Engl J Med 1995; 333:1600–1607.

Roujeau JC, Stern RS: Severe adverse cutaneous reactions to drugs. N Engl J Med 1994; 331:1272–1285.

CHAPTER 59

Toxic Spider Bites

Philip C. Anderson

CLINICAL APPEARANCE

Almost every U.S. spider is venomous, but only a few can puncture human skin and commonly cause important disease. Wolf spiders *(Lycosa),* garden spiders (argiope), orb weavers, and *Chiracanthium* surely can hurt us and cause tiny necrosis in skin with sterile, venom-induced, ascending lymphangitis. Tarantulas (a *Lycosa* variant), kept as pets, usually bite with the impact of wasps. None is of concern. The bite of the black widow spider causes no skin lesion but can produce a moderate neurologic overstimulation in children, a disorder that is readily managed with diazepam (Valium) and calcium gluconate. Even in rural areas, such bites have become very rare since the horse barn and the outhouse have disappeared into history. Only the brown recluse spider *(Loxosceles reclusa)* concerns us (see Fig. 59–1*A* on Color Plate 24).

After an envenomating bite by a North American brown recluse spider, individuals who are not immune will endure a sudden sequence of painful and frightening changes at the site, principally rapid necrosis of the skin (see Fig. 59–1*B* on Color Plate 24). Occasionally, a few unfortunate people may experience a rapid acute hemolysis of up to two thirds of their red blood cell mass. However, many recluse spider bites are entirely trivial because the spiders often put little or no venom in their bite. The usual necrotic cutaneous injury is an acute episode lasting 10 to 15 days, concluding with uncomplicated, if slow, healing and no important scarring.

DESCRIPTION AND ETIOLOGY

How does the spider bite? Almost invariably, the spiders are caught against the skin while the destined patient is wrapped in bedclothes at night or is dressing in the morning, and so, most bites are on the covered torso, almost never on exposed skin. Reliably, most people feel pain in 2 to 3 hours and fall ill about noontime, or 4 to 6 hours after the bite. The lesion is an acute infarct of skin caused by rapid blood coagulation within the vessels. The lesion is a sinking macule, pale dead gray in color, slightly eroded in the center, and at the margins is a halo of very tender inflammation and hemorrhage. The entire lesion usually is about the size of the palm of the hand, and the necrotic core is about 1 to 2 cm across. The bite of *Loxosceles* will be a single bite, not multiple. By the time patients reach the physician, they may be mildly ill, in pain, usually intensely anxious, with low fever, malaise, nausea, and sometimes, they have a bright red, generalized toxic erythema that resembles an exanthem. The erythema may contain many petechia, and a few patients may show purpura or even ecchymoses. Those who have hemolysis will be sicker, will have free hemoglobin in their urine, and may even report passing black urine.

Bites by *Loxosceles* are almost always mild. Many people residing in the habitat of the *Loxosceles* repeatedly have no response when bitten, and perhaps, they are protected by antibodies to the venom. On the other hand, the author has seen proved recluse spider bites that involve broad necrosis of skin (60 cm across) and push deeply into muscle. Some patients have only a small necrosis of skin but have severe generalized toxic skin reactions with alarming facial edema, swelling of hands and feet, and impressive malaise for 4 or 5 days. Severe hemolysis may require admission to the hospital or even the intensive care unit.

Entomologists have determined the range of the

brown recluse spider, which is across the more southern portion of the verdant Appalachian forest or, more simply, a zone roughly south of I-70, west of the Blue Ridge mountains but east of the arid plains of Kansas or Colorado. Outside of this well-defined area, no one should report loxoscelism in the medical literature without having promptly recovered some *Loxosceles* spiders, taken in the immediate vicinity, and verified by an experienced entomologist. The relevant medical literature has been thoroughly distorted by reports of necrosis of skin that the authors call recluse bites, without any evidence of *Loxosceles* at all. Such reports are not useful, lacking any reliability. Readers should ignore clinical reports that lack particular physical verification of the presence of the *Loxosceles* spider. The spider is a tree-bark arachnid, prefers river country and wet forests, but has adapted as a house spider to life (partly) in the walls of cardboard boxes. The spider makes every effort to avoid people. No one has any reasonable estimate of the prevalence of loxoscelism. No validated deaths from loxoscelism have been acceptably reported in the medical literature, but it is credible that a very few may have occurred.

The spider is characteristic. If it is safe, try to have the patient bring in the spider. Always solicit a trained entomologist to work with you. Experienced entomologists can identify *Loxosceles* even from fragments of a crushed spider.

PATHOLOGY

As stated, cutaneous loxoscelism is a sterile infarction, and biopsy will give no decisive evidence for the diagnosis. Some dozen different diseases can produce sterile focal infarcts in skin. Biopsy is useful in diagnosing early acute necrotizing fasciitis.

TREATMENT

For the usual case of cutaneous loxoscelism, no persuasive medical evidence demonstrates any benefit for any systemic treatment on the patient's outcome. A tetanus booster may be due. Routine wound care is needed, as is relief of pain, splinting and rest, padding, and a long explanation to the patient, with good telephone support later, to control fear and anxiety. For the rare large or complicated bite, consider an early consultation on diagnosis. Antibiotics, nitroglycerin, heparin, dapsone, and steroids are not required; the patients will recover exactly as well without these drugs, and all of these drugs have complications of their own.

The case of a child or of the rare adult with severe hemolysis is an emergency, needing expert attention. Therapy is aimed at homeostasis. Peritoneal dialysis may be needed if anuria occurs. Often, there is great worry among physicians, but the illness is self-limited. A team of pediatrician, intensivist, nephrologist, hematologist, entomologist, and dermatologist is valuable. Treatment with antibiotics or steroids does not appear to be any more beneficial than simple conservative care.

Early débridement of cutaneous loxoscelism with skin grafting was tried too often in the period 1960 to 1980 and proved to be expensive, disabling, painful, and not beneficial. These infarctions have delayed healing, but reliably they do heal. By waiting 5 to 10 days, we often see reduction of the apparent necrotic injury down to one fifth of the initial size. Haste is counterindicated. Consider surgery for very large lesions only after at least 4 to 6 weeks of good wound care.

PITFALLS AND PROBLEMS

The most important pitfall for the physician is to fail to diagnose necrotizing fasciitis. Cutaneous loxoscelism is almost never multiple lesions. Tender lymphadenopathy is not an early response to venom, and ascending lymphangitis is not seen. Rapid progression after 12 hours is common with necrotizing fasciitis, but not typical with cutaneous loxoscelism. The author has seen leukocytosis over 25,000 with proven loxoscelism, but usually such high white blood cell counts are an indication of streptococcal fasciitis. Enormous leukocytosis with bands is typical of fasciitis. General toxicity is much greater with fasciitis. When the question about fasciitis is appropriate, take two or more disk biopsies from the core and halo. Do a smear. Have all of these immediately stained with hematoxylin and eosin and with bacterial stains. The diagnosis can usually be resolved quickly. Cultures are not suitable for early diagnosis.

A second pitfall is to overlook the hemolysis. All patients seen with bites larger than 2 cm at the necrotic core are advised to have urinalysis and perhaps, a follow-up examination 2 days later. Patients can watch for dark urine. All children should be followed carefully. In our series of six proven cases, the severe hemolysis has been Coombs'-negative, often severe, and associated with problems of disseminated intravascular coagulation. All our patients with severe hemolysis have shown complete recoveries as regards hematologic and renal problems, without residual.

REFERRAL/CONSULTATION GUIDELINES

Large bites produce such concern as to be worth referral promptly. Early consultation to resolve the pitfalls is advisable.

CHAPTER 60

Vasculitis

Nicholas A. Soter

CLINICAL APPEARANCE

Definition

The term *necrotizing vasculitis* describes clinical disorders in which there is segmental inflammation and necrosis of blood vessels. Clinical syndromes are based on the gross appearance and histologic alterations of the lesions, the caliber of the affected blood vessels, the involvement of specific organs, and laboratory abnormalities (Table 60–1). The form of necrotizing vasculitis that most frequently affects the skin involves venules and has been called *cutaneous necrotizing venulitis* and *leukocytoclastic vasculitis.* The cutaneous vascular lesions may be a feature of an underlying chronic disorder, may develop after defined precipitating events, or may occur as a variety of idiopathic syndromes (Table 60–2). Systemic necrotizing vasculitis, which is accompanied by skin lesions but does not correspond to any diagnostic category, is termed *systemic polyangiitis.*

TABLE 60–1

Necrotizing Vasculitides

Polyarteritis nodosa
Classical polyarteritis nodosa
Allergic granulomatosis and angiitis (Churg-Strauss syndrome)
Systemic polyangiitis
Mucocutaneous lymph node syndrome (Kawasaki disease)
Hypersensitivity angiitis
Coexistent chronic disorders
Recent precipitating events
Idiopathic disorders
Wegener's granulomatosis and variants
Giant cell arteritis

Typical Lesions and Symptoms

The signature lesion of cutaneous necrotizing venulitis is an erythematous papule that does not blanch when the skin is pressed; it is known as *palpable purpura* (see Fig. 60–1 on Color Plate 24). A variety of other lesions may be present, including pustules, vesicles, ulcers, necrosis, and livedo reticularis. The vascular eruption most frequently develops on the lower extremities or over dependent areas. The lesions appear in episodes that may recur over weeks to years. Palpable purpura persists from 1 to 4 weeks; hyperpigmentation or atrophic scars may develop. Lesional symptoms include pruritus or burning and, less commonly, pain.

An episode of cutaneous vascular lesions may be associated with fever, malaise, arthralgias, or myalgias. Systemic involvement most commonly occurs in synovia, voluntary muscles, peripheral nerves, gastrointestinal tract, and kidneys.

Involvement of small arteries in the skin occurs in polyarteritis nodosa, which is recognized as nodular lesions along the course of an artery, and in giant cell arteritis, which may be present as erythema with or without necrosis. Both allergic granulomatosis/angiitis and Wegener's granulomatosis affect vessels of all sizes. These disorders are not considered in this chapter.

Atypical or Alternative Forms

Urticarial vasculitis is an edematous form of necrotizing venulitis that occurs in patients with serum sickness,

TABLE 60–2

Cutaneous Necrotizing Venulitis

Coexistent chronic disorders
Rheumatoid arthritis
Sjögren's syndrome
Systemic lupus erythematosus
Hypergammaglobulinemic purpura
Paraneoplastic vasculitis
Cryoglobulinemia
Ulcerative colitis
Cystic fibrosis
Antiphospholipid or antineutrophil cytoplasmic antibody syndromes
Precipitating events
Bacterial and viral infections
Therapeutic and diagnostic agents
Idiopathic disorders
Henoch-Schönlein syndrome
Recurrent urticaria/angioedema syndrome and variants
Erythema elevatum diutinum
Nodular vasculitis
Livedoid vasculitis
Acute hemorrhagic edema of childhood

connective tissue disorders, infections, an immunoglobulin M M component, and an idiopathic disorder. The skin lesions appear as wheals that may last up to 3 to 5 days. Other skin manifestations include foci of purpura in the wheals, angioedema, livedo reticularis, and bullae. The lesions are pruritic or may possess a burning or painful quality; transient contusions or hyperpigmentation may develop. The episodes of urticaria are recurrent, range in duration from months to years, and vary in frequency.

Erythema elevatum diutinum presents as indolent erythematous plaques disposed over the extensor surfaces of the extremities and the gluteal area that may be accompanied by arthralgias. Associated conditions include immunoglobulin A (IgA) monoclonal gammopathy, multiple myeloma, and myelodysplasia.

Nodular vasculitis occurs as painful red nodules over the lower extremities, especially the calves, without systemic manifestations. Erythema induratum represents a form of nodular vasculitis, which is associated with *Mycobacterium tuberculosis.*

Livedoid vasculitis appears as recurrent, painful ulcers of the lower extremities in association with livedo reticularis of a persistent nature; it results in sclerotic pale areas surrounded by telangiectases called *atrophie blanche.* Livedoid vasculitis is especially prominent in patients with systemic lupus erythematosus and central nervous system involvement.

Acute hemorrhagic edema develops in children and appears as painful, edematous areas with petechiae and ecchymoses on the head and distal extremities. Systemic features are usually absent.

DESCRIPTION OF DISEASE

Epidemiology

In children, cutaneous necrotizing venulitis is most commonly described as the Henoch-Schönlein syndrome. Acute hemorrhagic edema has been confused with Henoch-Schönlein syndrome.

In adults, cutaneous necrotizing venulitis presenting as palpable purpura is often associated with flares of the coexistent chronic disorder. The natural history of most idiopathic forms is unknown.

The prevalence and natural history of idiopathic urticarial vasculitis remain unknown. The development of Sjögren's syndrome and of systemic lupus erythematosus has been reported in one patient each. Deaths have resulted from pulmonary disease, sepsis, and myocardial infarction.

Histopathology

In routinely prepared skin biopsy specimens, the histologic criteria required for the diagnosis of cutaneous necrotizing venulitis include necrosis of the endothelial cells with the deposition of fibrinoid material and dermal cellular infiltrates consisting of various numbers of neutrophils with nuclear debris, mononuclear cells, and extravasated erythrocytes. The dermal inflammatory infiltrates vary in intensity and are usually perivenular in location but at times are dispersed widely. The fibrinoid material consists predominantly of fibrin but also contains necrotic endothelial cells and deposited immunoreactants.

By direct immunofluorescence techniques, perivenular fibrin deposition has been identified routinely in lesional biopsy specimens. Immunoglobulin G is the most commonly deposited immunoglobulin. IgA alone is deposited around blood vessels in the skin, intestine, and kidney in the Henoch-Schönlein syndrome. C3 is the only complement protein that has been sought with any frequency.

Etiology/Pathogenesis

The most frequently postulated mechanism operative in the production of cutaneous necrotizing venulitis is the local deposition of circulating immune complexes or the formation of immune complexes in the skin. Certain types of immune complexes may activate the complement system with the generation of C4a, C3a, and C5a anaphylatoxins that degranulate mast cells; in addition, C5a may attract neutrophils that release lysosomal enzymes. The neutrophil superoxide generating system may produce oxygen-derived free radicals, which cause tissue injury. The generation of the chemoattractant leukotriene B4 from infiltrating neutrophils would further enhance the influx of neutrophils.

In patients with cutaneous necrotizing venulitis, circulating immune complexes have been demonstrated in serum directly as cryoproteins and indirectly by a variety of assays such as C1q binding. Their presence is inferred also by the presence of serum hypocomplementemia.

In lesional tissues, immune complexes were detected by direct immunofluorescence techniques and by ultrastructural observation. In humans, the antigen has been identified in only a few instances, in which bacterial or viral proteins have been detected by direct immunofluorescence techniques combined into complexes with immunoglobulins and complement proteins.

Areas that could potentially be important in the pathogenesis of cutaneous necrotizing venulitis include the participation of mast cells, lymphocytes, and monocyte-macrophages and the capacity of cutaneous dermal microvascular endothelial cells to produce adhesion molecules, cytokines, and inflammatory mediators.

Laboratory Evaluation

Laboratory studies that should be obtained in all patients with cutaneous necrotizing venulitis are listed in Table 60–3. An elevated erythrocyte sedimentation rate is the most consistent laboratory abnormality. The platelet count is usually normal. Other abnormalities reflect either a coexistent underlying disorder or the involvement of an additional organ system.

TABLE 60–3

Laboratory Studies for Cutaneous Necrotizing Venulitis

- Erythrocyte sedimentation rate
- Complete blood count with differential analysis
- Platelet count
- Urinalysis
- Blood chemistry profile
- Serum protein electrophoresis
- Hepatitis A, B, C antigens
- Cryoglobulins
- Total serum hemolytic complement
- Antinuclear antibody
- Rheumatoid factor
- Antiphospholipid and antineutrophil cytoplasmic antibodies
- Skin biopsy

TREATMENT

Therapeutic Expectations

When cutaneous necrotizing venulitis is associated with a precipitating event, withdrawal of the medication or treatment of the infection results in resolution of the cutaneous lesions. If a coexistent chronic disorder is present, treatment of the underlying disease may improve the skin. The treatment of the skin in cutaneous necrotizing venulitis can be divided into two phases (Table 60–4), each of which depends on an analysis of the degree of cutaneous disability as well as the toxicity and side effects of the therapeutic agents.

First-Line Therapy

Initially, an oral H_1 antihistamine, such as hydroxyzine hydrochloride 25 mg four times daily, in combination with a nonsteroidal anti-inflammatory agent, such as indomethacin 25 to 50 mg three times daily, should be administered. Depending on the therapeutic response, colchicine 0.6 mg three times daily or hydroxychloroquine sulfate 200 mg daily can be added to or substituted for these agents. If there is still no benefit, dapsone may be used. Cutaneous ulcers are generally managed by local measures.

TABLE 60–4

Treatment of Cutaneous Necrotizing Venulitis

- Phase one
  - H_1 antihistamines ($\pm$ H_2 antihistamines)
  - Nonsteroidal anti-inflammatory agents
  - Colchicine
  - Hydroxychloroquine sulfate
  - Dapsone
- Phase two
  - Systemic corticosteroids
  - Azathioprine
  - Cyclophosphamide
  - Intravenous gamma globulin
  - Plasmapheresis

Age Considerations

Cutaneous necrotizing venulitis is treated similarly in children and in adults.

Alternative Therapeutic Options

If there is no beneficial response with the use of first-line therapy, a major therapeutic decision occurs, since the use of the medications listed in phase two requires a careful analysis owing to their side effect profile. Although all of the therapeutic agents listed have been reported to be of benefit, controlled clinical trials are usually not available.

PITFALLS AND PROBLEMS

The episodic lesions characteristic of cutaneous necrotizing venulitis may be a manifestation of systemic hypersensitivity angiitis, may be associated with necrotizing angiitis of larger blood vessels, or may be restricted to the skin. When thrombocytopenia occurs in association with nonvasculitic cutaneous papules resulting from other causes, palpable purpura may result. A skin biopsy specimen should be obtained, since palpable purpura should be considered to be vasculitis until proved otherwise. The cutaneous manifestations of disseminated intravascular coagulation, also called *purpura fulminans,* appear as extensive areas of purpura with a slate-gray color and may or may not be palpable. Septic emboli occur as finite numbers of hemorrhagic pustules, papules, and vesicles over acral areas.

Cutaneous nodules may be a manifestation of erythema nodosum, panniculitis, superficial forms of thrombophlebitis, and fat necrosis associated with pancreatic disease.

REFERRAL AND CONSULTATION GUIDELINES

Cutaneous necrotizing venulitis associated with systemic disorders should be referred to the appropriate specialist depending on the sites of internal involvement. If cutaneous necrotizing venulitis restricted to the skin does not respond to agents such as an H_1 antihistamine, indomethacin, or colchicine, consultation with a dermatologist should be obtained. The atypical or alternative forms of cutaneous vasculitis also require consultation with a dermatologist.

BIBLIOGRAPHY

1. Bloch DA, Michel BA, Hunder GG, et al: The American College of Rheumatology 1990 criteria for the classification of vasculitis: Patients and methods. Arthritis Rheum 1990; 33:1068–1073.
2. Burden AD, Tillman DM, Foley P, et al: IgA class anticardiolipin antibodies in cutaneous leukocytoclastic vasculitis. J Am Acad Dermatol 1996; 35:411–415.
3. Sanchez NP, Van Hale HM, Su WPD: Clinical and histopathologic spectrum of necrotizing vasculitis: Report of findings in 101 cases. Arch Dermatol 1985; 121:220–224.
4. Sánchez-Guerrero J, Gutiérrez-Ureña S, Vidaller A, et al: Vasculitis as a parapaneoplastic syndrome: Report of 11 cases and review of the literature. J Rheumatol 1990; 17:1458–1462.
5. Weimer CE Jr, Sahn EE: Follicular accentuation of leukocytoclastic vasculitis in an HIV-positive man: Report of a case and review of the literature. J Am Acad Dermatol 1991; 24:898–902.

SECTION IV

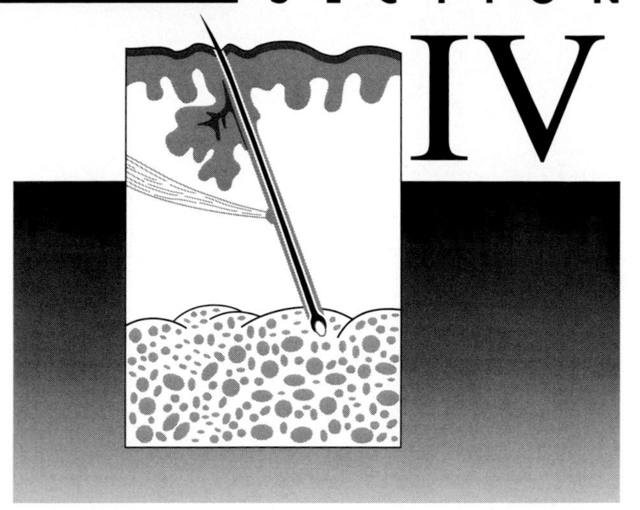

Procedures

CHAPTER 61

Biopsy (Punch, Shave, Saucerization, and Elliptical)

June K. Robinson

Biopsies are performed to establish a diagnosis, to remove a neoplasm and check its margins to ensure complete excision, and to assess the effectiveness of a therapeutic procedure on a previously diagnosed condition. The biopsy procedure results in a specimen, the histopathologic examination of which can aid the clinician. Because clinical examination is not always sufficient to make a definitive diagnosis,[1] support for a clinical diagnosis from histopathologic examination of tissue is frequently necessary. The manner in which the biopsy is performed depends on the anticipated depth of the disease process[2] and the potential consequences of placement of a scar from the biopsy procedure.

The area that is most representative of the disease process and is uncomplicated by changes unique to the anatomic region should be selected. For instance, when a drug eruption is suspected and areas of the trunk and extremities are involved, the biopsy should be taken from a fully developed lesion on the trunk rather than a similar lesion on the lower leg. In general, biopsies of the lower leg, even in young persons, heal very slowly and show stasis vascular changes that complicate the interpretation of the histologic presentation. Similarly, biopsy of the palm and sole should be avoided whenever possible. For a generalized eruption, the trunk, arms, and upper legs are the more favorable biopsy sites. The elbows and knees are subjected to pressure and friction in everyday life and should likewise be avoided.

Once having decided that a biopsy is necessary, the physician must choose among various modalities: punch biopsy, shave biopsy, saucerization biopsy, and elliptical excisional or incisional biopsy. A superficial disease process such as a seborrheic keratosis, solar keratosis, or a wart, in which the pathologic changes are largely limited to the epidermis, is easily biopsied by the shave technique with an acceptable cosmetic result. A deep-seated lesion such as a cyst or lipoma is best approached by an incisional technique with a scalpel, using sterile technique and a three-layer closure of muscle, fascia, and subcutaneous tissue.[3] Each of the principal biopsy techniques and its particular advantages and disadvantages are discussed (Table 61–1).

Whenever possible, the biopsy specimen should include subcutaneous fat because, in many dermatoses, characteristic histologic features are found in the lower dermis or subcutaneous fat. Punch biopsies that are 3 or 4 mm in diameter are the usual procedure for obtaining specimens for histopathologic examination. Since it may not be possible to obtain adequate amounts of subcutaneous tissue by punch biopsy, elliptical incisional biopsies often are advisable for the study of subcutaneous lesions or panniculitis.[4] In the case of pigmented lesions that are clinically suspected of being malignant and fungating or nodular processes, an incisional biopsy that extends beneath the deepest part of the lesion and includes as much of the lesion as possible should be obtained.

TABLE 61-1

Selected Examples of Diseases Correlated With Type of Biopsy Most Likely to Assist in Diagnosis

Disease	Punch	Shave	Excision by Saucerization	Excision or Incision With Ellipse
Pigmented lesion suggestive of malignancy[5, 8]	Yes as a sampling technique	No	Yes	Yes
Fungating or nodular process	No	No	Yes	Yes
Basal cell carcinoma	Yes	Yes	Yes	Yes
Keratoacanthoma, squamous cell carcinoma	No	No	Yes	Yes
Wart	No	Yes	No	No
Seborrheic or solar keratosis[6]	Yes if need to rule out malignancy	Yes	No	No
Inflammatory processes[7]	Yes	No	Yes	Yes
Panniculitis, scleroderma, morphea, atrophic diseases, erythema nodosum	No	No	No	Yes
Alopecia areata[5]	Yes transversely sectioned	No	No	No
Blistering disorders	Yes	No	No	No
Hypertrophic lichen planus	No	No	Yes	Yes
Oral lesions[11–14] Persistent ulcerations Leukoplakia Vesicular lesions Pigmented lesions	Yes	No	No	Nodular lesions Leukoplakia Pigmented lesions

From Robinson JK, LeBoit PE: Biopsy techniques. *In* Robinson JK, Arndt KA, LeBoit PE, Wintroub BU (eds): Atlas of Cutaneous Surgery. Philadelphia: WB Saunders, 1996, p 42.

TYPES OF BIOPSY

Punch Biopsy

Depending on the size of lesion involved and the instrument used, the punch biopsy may be either incisional, resulting in partial removal of the lesion together with a section of normal skin, or excisional, resulting in removal of the entire lesion. Punch biopsy is performed with a circular cutting instrument or punch, which is commonly available in sizes ranging from 1.5 to 8 mm. The 3- or 4-mm disposable punch, which is light in weight and sharp every time, is most frequently used.

The biopsy site is cleaned gently with alcohol, leaving scales and vesicles intact. If the demarcation of a lesion is subtle, such as is the case with urticaria, the boundaries of a lesion can be outlined with a pen prior to injecting anesthesia. The site is injected with local anesthesia by raising a skin wheal with 0.2 to 0.5 ml of anesthesia injected into the deep dermis. When the circular incision with the punch has been carried to the subcutaneous fat, the punch is removed. Shallow punch biopsies to the level of the dermis are easily misinterpreted, require more manipulation to extract, and do not give the patient the complete benefit of the procedure. At this stage, there may be considerable oozing of blood. Applying firm pressure around the perimeter of the defect allows adequate visualization of the base. The small cylinder of tissue is gently lifted with the tip of a needle or a forceps, and the base is transected at the level of the subcutaneous tissue with a small scissors, such as an iris scissors. When the punch is removed, an oval defect is left (Fig. 61–1).

Hemostasis can be obtained by placing a suture or applying direct pressure with a chemical agent such as aluminum chloride 25% in isopropyl alcohol 50%, for 5 to 10 minutes. Also a Gelfoam pledget may be placed into the base of the wound and pressure applied. If a suture is used to stop the bleeding, no chemical hemostatic agent is placed in the wound. If an artery is

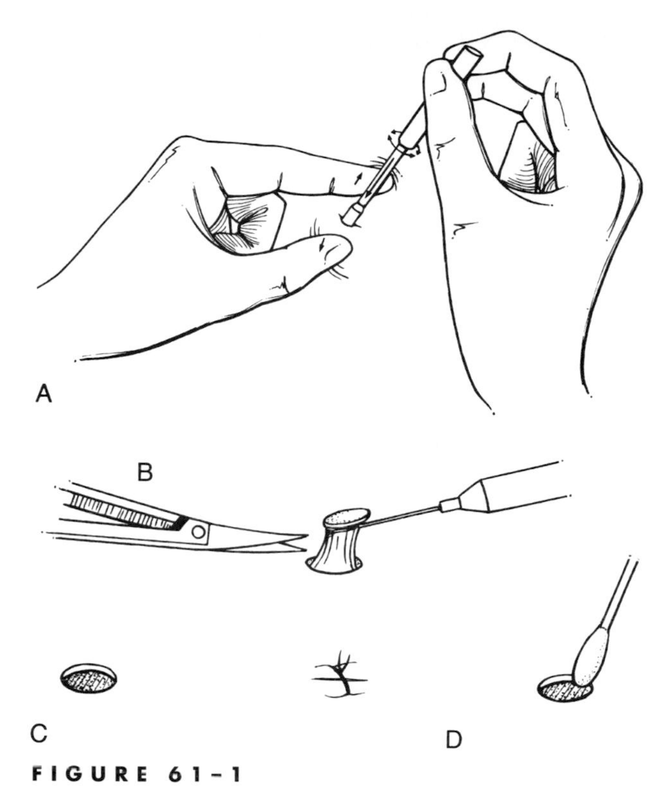

FIGURE 61-1
Punch biopsy. *A,* After the area to be biopsied is anesthetized, the skin around the area is infiltrated with anesthesia and drawn taut with the thumb and forefinger of the physician's free hand. *B,* The orifice of the punch is applied firmly to the skin surface with the handle held perpendicular to the skin. A gentle but firm downward pressure is exerted at the same time that the handle is rotated between the thumb and the forefinger. This motion will carry the punch through the subcutaneous fat.

Care is required in removing the specimen made with a punch. If a toothed forceps is used, there is a tendency to crush the tissue as it is being lifted from its bed. This produces an artifact that may interfere with the pathologist's ability to make an accurate diagnosis. This artifact may be avoided by a simple maneuver. Downward pressure on the skin around the cylinder will cause it to pop up. The cylinder can then be lifted with the tip of the needle that was used to administer the anesthesia.

C, The direction of tension should be along the line of elective incision. This force will cause the eventual defect to be oval rather than round.

D, It can be closed with a single suture, resulting in a closure as close to a linear one as possible, or a hemostatic agent is applied with a cotton swab and the area heals by second intention. (*A–D,* From Robinson JK, LeBoit PE: Biopsy techniques. *In* Robinson JK, Arndt KA, LeBoit PE, Wintroub BU [eds]: Atlas of Cutaneous Surgery. Philadelphia: WB Saunders, 1996, p 43.)

transected by the punch, the two ends will retract under the edges of the wound. Since it is difficult to gain enough exposure through a 3-mm circular defect to be able to place two clamps on the severed artery, the wound may have to be lengthened to expose the artery. When a lesion is located on the face over arteries that may be superficial enough to be injured by a punch biopsy, it is preferable to plan another type of biopsy, for example, temporal artery lateral to the eyebrow, the angular artery at nasolabial fold junction with the ala, and the supraorbital artery at the medial end of the brow.

One of the disadvantages of the punch biopsy is that the small size of the specimen may lead to difficulty in histopathologic interpretation. Sampling error can be minimized by care in deciding which portion of a lesion to biopsy. In inflammatory conditions, the 4-mm punch is generally preferable. Removal of a specimen smaller than 4 mm in diameter may allow histologic confirmation of a tumor but is often inadequate for diagnosis of inflammatory processes. The punch biopsy is usually inadequate to diagnose diseases of adipose tissue, for example, morphea, panniculitis, erythema nodosum. In these instances, an elliptical incisional biopsy is more likely to yield a sufficient quantity of tissue for diagnosis. Similarly in pigmented lesions suspected of being a melanoma, an elliptical biopsy that encompasses the entire lesion with border of 1 to 2 mm and is carried through the fat is preferable.[5] Smaller pigmented lesions may be encompassed by a 3- to 6-mm punch biopsy; however, if the lateral extent of the lesion cannot be obtained within this size then the elliptical excision should be performed.

A round cosmetic defect may result from using a large (5- or 6-mm) punch. This cosmetic result usually cannot compare with that of an elliptical excision. In some cases, the removal for cosmetic reasons of a 2- or 3-mm circular lesion by the punch technique with suture closure of the wound yields a result as good as that with elliptical excision. When closing defects created by the 4-mm punch and ones larger in size, dog ears commonly result and may be revised at the time of the procedure.

Shave Biopsy and Saucerization Biopsy

The difference between a shave biopsy and a saucerization biopsy is the depth achieved in excising the specimen. Shave biopsy removes the portion of the skin elevated above the plane of surrounding tissue either because of the exophytic nature of the process, the manner of injection of local anesthetic, or the manner of stabilizing the skin by pinching it between the thumb and the forefinger (Fig. 61–2). Saucerization biopsy excises below the surface of the surrounding skin (in a circular manner around the lesion) down into the level of the subcutaneous fat (Fig. 61–3). The decision to perform a saucerization or shave biopsy requires good

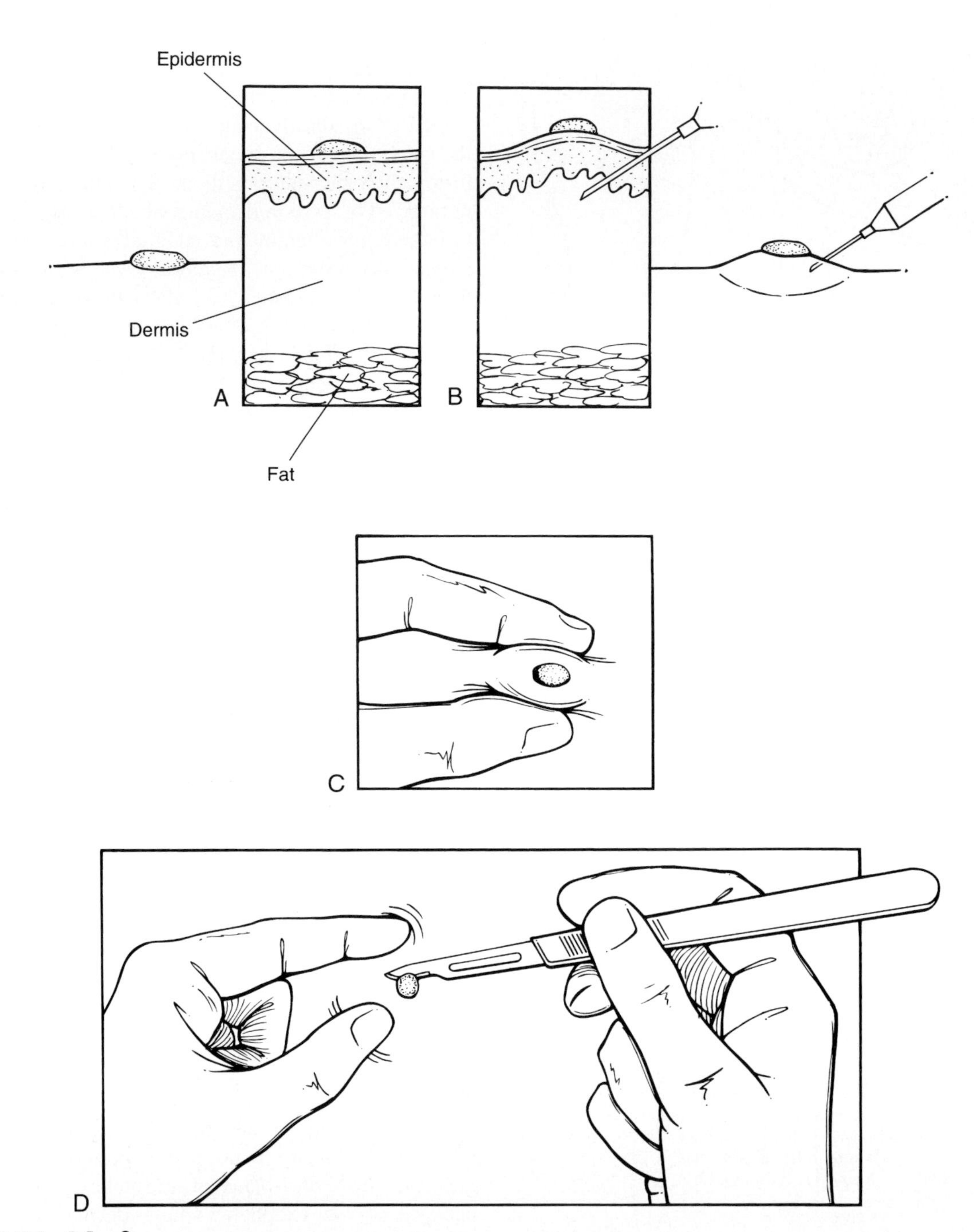

FIGURE 61-2
Shave biopsy. *A* and *B,* The epidermal process is elevated above the surrounding tissue by injecting local anesthesia or (*C*) by pinching the skin between the thumb and the forefinger. *D,* If the skin is elevated by the bleb of anesthesia and a biopsy at the papillary dermis is required, then the skin can be made taut and the blade moved under the lesion in a horizontal plane parallel to the skin surface. (*A–D,* From Robinson JK, LeBoit PE: Biopsy techniques. *In* Robinson JK, Arndt KA, LeBoit PE, Wintroub BU [eds]: Atlas of Cutaneous Surgery. Philadelphia: WB Saunders, 1996, p 45.)

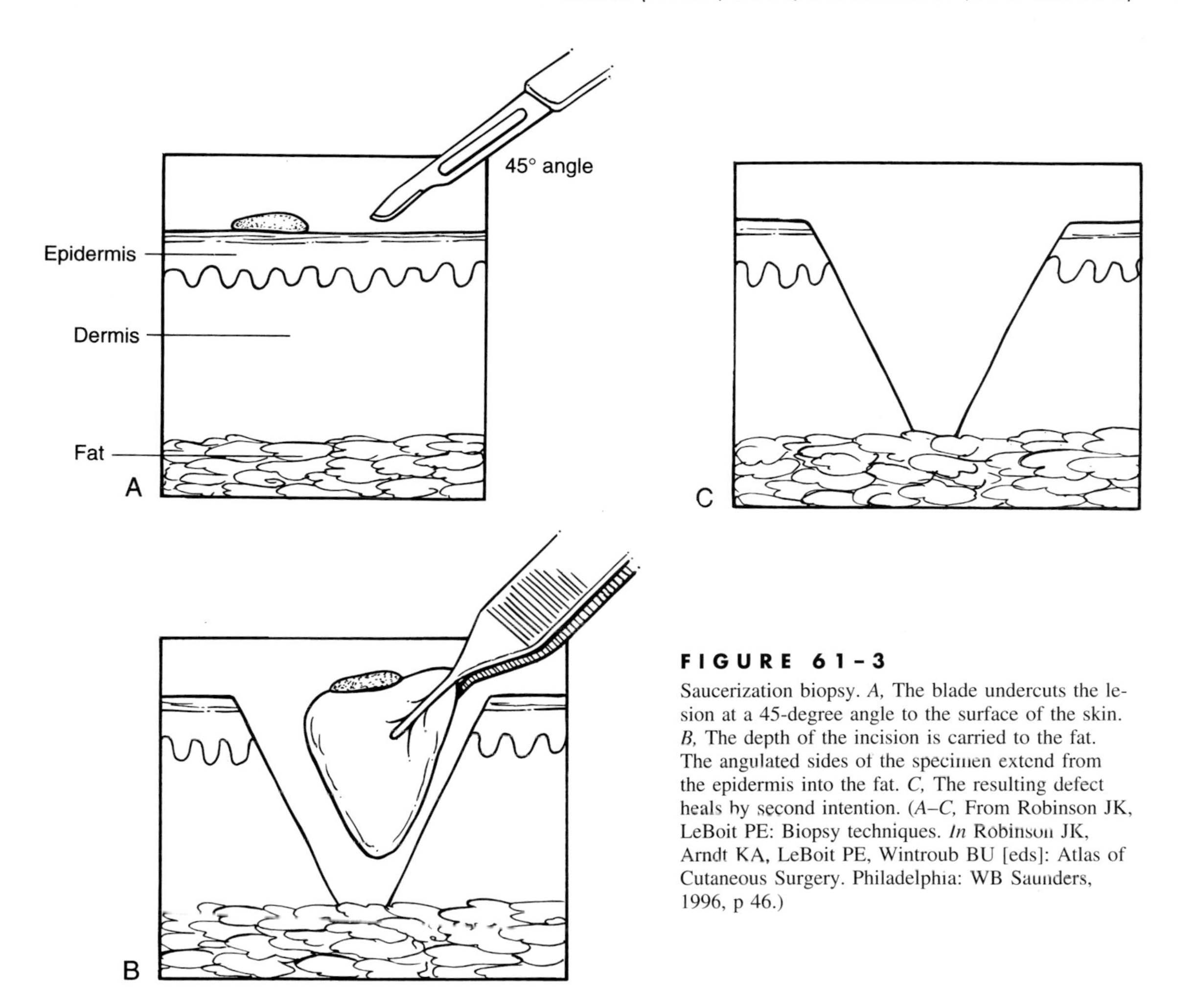

FIGURE 61-3

Saucerization biopsy. *A,* The blade undercuts the lesion at a 45-degree angle to the surface of the skin. *B,* The depth of the incision is carried to the fat. The angulated sides of the specimen extend from the epidermis into the fat. *C,* The resulting defect heals by second intention. (*A–C,* From Robinson JK, LeBoit PE: Biopsy techniques. *In* Robinson JK, Arndt KA, LeBoit PE, Wintroub BU [eds]: Atlas of Cutaneous Surgery. Philadelphia: WB Saunders, 1996, p 46.)

judgment and an accurate clinical impression of the preoperative diagnosis.

Shave biopsy is an appropriate technique for superficial exophytic conditions such as seborrheic keratoses, solar keratoses, and warts and for cosmetic removal of some melanocytic nevi.[6] The shave is made at a depth between the deep papillary dermis and the midreticular dermis. This procedure produces a cosmetically acceptable result. Because it leaves the lower portion of the dermis intact, it also gives maximal flexibility in selecting a postbiopsy treatment plan for basal cell carcinoma. This is important if the biopsied tumor will be subsequently treated by curettage and electrosurgery. The "hammock" of dermal connective tissue remains intact to scrape against. A dermal defect would allow the curet to slip into the subcutis where it would flounder around, thus interfering with defining the deep extension of the skin cancer with the curet.[5]

Shave biopsies are not suitable for inflammatory skin diseases in general,[7] neoplasms that clinically appear to infiltrate the dermis, or pigmented lesions where there is even a faint clinical suspicion of melanoma. For such lesions, fusiform incisional biopsy through the "heart" of the lesion to and including a portion of fat is recommended. Whenever possible, excisional biopsy of pigmented lesions that may be melanomas is recommended.[6] Accurate measurement of the deepest penetration of the melanoma cells in serial sections of a histopathologic specimen guides the assessment of prognosis. Shave biopsies that fail to encompass the entire breadth of a lesion compromise the evaluation of such key features as width, circumscription, and symmetry.[8]

Since a saucerization biopsy (see Fig. 61–3) is essentially a circular excision to the depth of fat, it can be performed for lesions that involve the dermis, for example, atypical nevi, melanoma, or squamous cell carcinoma. In choosing to perform this type of biopsy, the location and size of the defect must be considered to provide good second-intention wound healing, for example, lateral canthus of the eye. A hypopigmented, hyperpigmented, or hypertrophic scar may result.

The instruments used to perform both shave and saucerization biopsies are a scalpel and a toothed forceps. For shave biopsies, some experienced physicians prefer to use a hand-held razor blade.[9] Flexibility in contouring of curved surfaces of the body is obtained by using local anesthesia to elevate the lesion above the surrounding skin surface (see Fig. 61–2). With the operator's hand resting firmly in contact with a solid anatomic flat surface of the patient, the blade is lightly applied to the junction of normal-appearing skin and the slightly raised lesion. When saucerization is performed around a lesion suspected of being an atypical nevus, it is important not to transect the most peripheral cells. One way of ensuring this is to score the surface of the skin around the periphery of the lesions, allowing a 2-mm margin of normal-appearing skin, before beginning the procedure. In using a no. 15 blade, this initial cut is best made with the tip of the blade. The tip of the blade is always pointed slightly up to prevent going unnecessarily deep into the deeper dermis. When using a no. 10 blade to remove lesions larger than 1.0 cm in diameter, lead with the broad, flat cutting surface of the belly of the blade. The scalpel handle is held like a butter knife. This broader cutting surface lessens the opportunity of producing a jagged surface on the wound caused by ''sawing across'' the surface with two or three strokes of a no. 15 blade.

In performing shave biopsy, the operator's thumb and forefinger roll the skin, which has been infiltrated with anesthesia, in such a manner as to create a flat cutting surface for the scalpel blade and to provide a tamponade effect on the blood vessels in the surrounding skin. If a margin of tissue surrounding and below the lesion is desired, the shave should be done immediately after injecting the anesthesia while the tissue is maximally elevated by the fluid. If less depth is required, it is necessary to inject less anesthesia and wait a few minutes until the swelling subsides. A single, steady, sweeping motion of the blade over the junction of normal skin surface and the lesion and parallel to it will remove the elevated lesion. Sometimes, the last attachment to the skin is more easily severed with elevation of the specimen with a forceps. Bleeding can be stopped with application of a styptic such as aluminum chloride (35% in 50% isopropyl alcohol). If there is a slightly raised lip, this can be beveled down with the use of light electrodesiccation followed by the use of a 1-mm curet around the rim and light abrasion of this rim with a gauze pad.

The simplicity of shave biopsy favors multiple biopsies, and the ease of the procedure allows pathologic examination of tissue obtained under adverse conditions in children and hesitant adults. Although the technique or method is easily acquired and leads to a fine cosmetic result, it must be noted that nevi removed in this manner may return with central pigmentation.[10] This is especially common in patients under age 30 years who have nevi removed and who have dark hair and eyes and skin that is more deeply pigmented. If this happens and the pigmented area is biopsied again, it must be noted on the form that is submitted to the pathologist, as recurrent nevi can have features that a pathologist who is not aware of the prior removal of the nevus may misinterpret as melanoma.

Elliptical Incisional and Excisional Biopsy

None of the preceding biopsy techniques requires as much time, advance preparation of instruments and the surgical field, or skill as the elliptical biopsy. This type of biopsy also involves slightly more risk and discomfort to the patient. Nonetheless, use of the elliptical (fusiform) technique is absolutely essential when larger or deep specimens must be taken (see Table 61–1). Situations in which such a specimen is indicated are diseases with significant changes in the deep dermis extending to the fascia, for example, dermatomyositis, scleroderma, panniculitis, or mesenchymal neoplasms. In these examples, the specimen is removed from the most indurated portion of the skin. Another type of condition in which elliptical incisional specimens are necessary is when the specimen for microscopic examination must include a continuum from uninvolved normal skin through an indurated or inflammatory border into a necrotic central shallow ulcer, a thickened area of skin, or where the pathologic process may have skipped areas of normal skin between areas of active disease. Similarly, a specimen containing a continuum from normal to affected skin allows assessment of surgical margins and simplifies diagnosis of disease processes such as pyoderma gangrenosum, keratoacanthoma, and verrucous carcinoma. A final class of cases requiring this technique involves pigmented lesions that may be melanomas. If total excision for diagnosis is not possible, then the darkest area of the growth or the elevated portion are chosen for the site of incisional biopsy. It is essential that if the elevated portion of a melanocytic neoplasm is incised, the incision should be deep enough

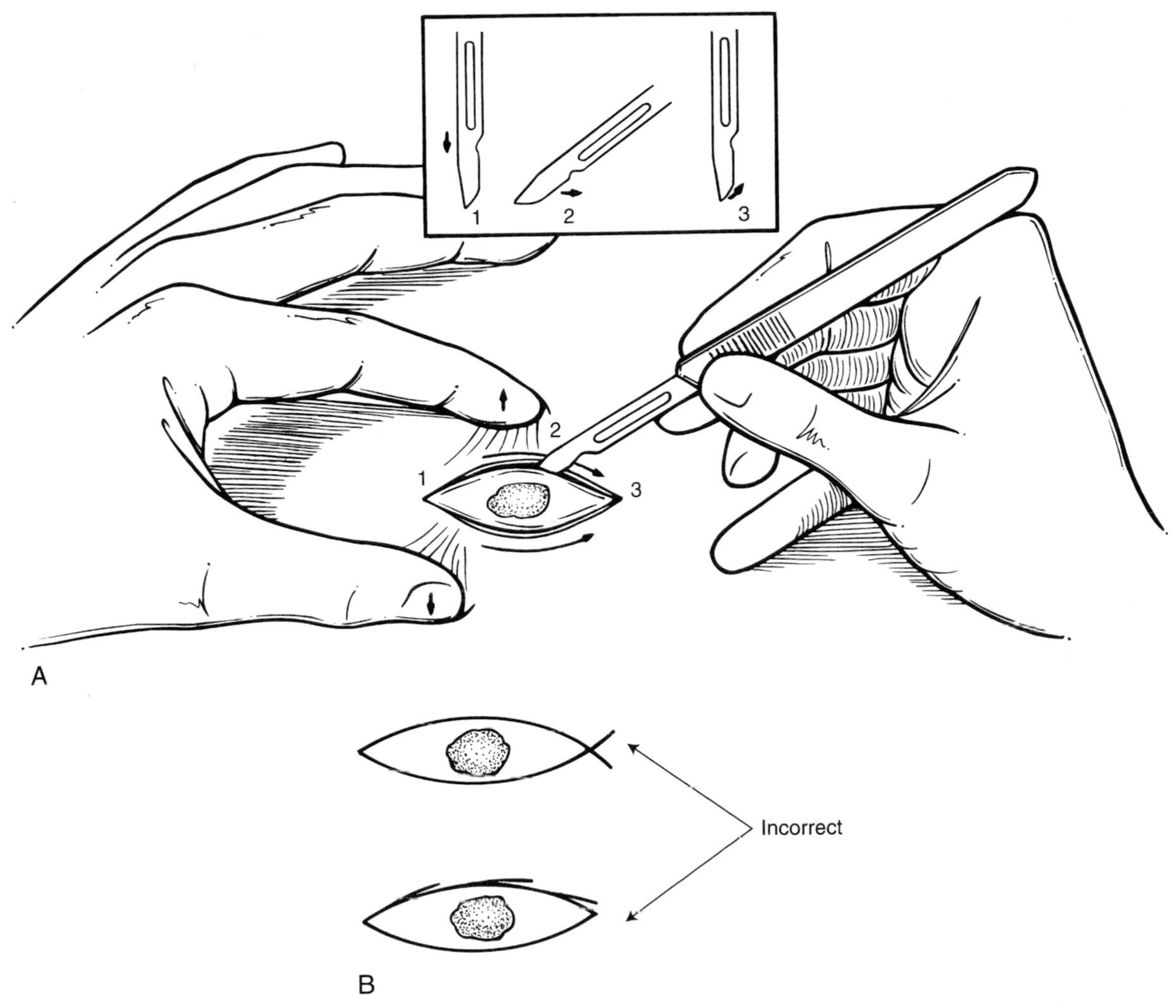

FIGURE 61–4

Elliptical excisional biopsy. *A,* The elliptical incision is planned with 30-degree angles at the apices and 3:1 length-to-width dimensions. The incision is started at the apex under traction. The tip of the blade is used at the apex (1). The blade rocks down to cut with the belly along the midportion of the incision (2) and then rocks up at the opposite apex to cut at the tip (3). *B,* A smooth, steady motion with the blade prevents unnecessary nicks at the apex or along the midportion of the incision. (*A* and *B,* From Robinson JK: Elliptical incisions and closures. *In* Robinson JK, Arndt KA, LeBoit PE, Wintroub BU [eds]: Atlas of Cutaneous Surgery. Philadelphia: WB Saunders, 1996, p 93.)

to encompass the deepest melanocyte in that area. The sections of a histopathologic specimen produced by such an excisional biopsy guide subsequent therapeutic surgical removal of the surrounding skin.

The optimal dimensions of the ellipse are a 3:1 ratio of length to width, thus producing angles of 30 degrees at the tips of the excision (Fig. 61–4). After marking the lines of elective incision to fall within natural creases of the skin by using the skin surface topography and relaxed skin tension lines, the skin is prepared with an antimicrobial solution such as chlorhexidine gluconate (Hibiclens), and local anesthesia is injected. The sterile tray of instruments contains a blade and blade handle, forceps, undermining scissors, two hemostats, a needle holder, a suture-cutting scissors, and the appropriate suture material.* In making the incision, the blade is held perpendicular to the skin surface—any deviation from the perpendicular will cause beveling of the edge that puts more stress on the suture line (see Fig. 61–4). The specimen is removed with the intention of maintaining an even base (Fig. 61–5). If the base is higher at the apices than at the middle, then additional tissue

*For additional information, see Robinson JK: Elliptical incisions and closures. *In* Robinson JK, Arndt KA, LeBoit PE, Wintroub BU (eds): Atlas of Cutaneous Surgery. Philadelphia: WB Saunders, 1996.

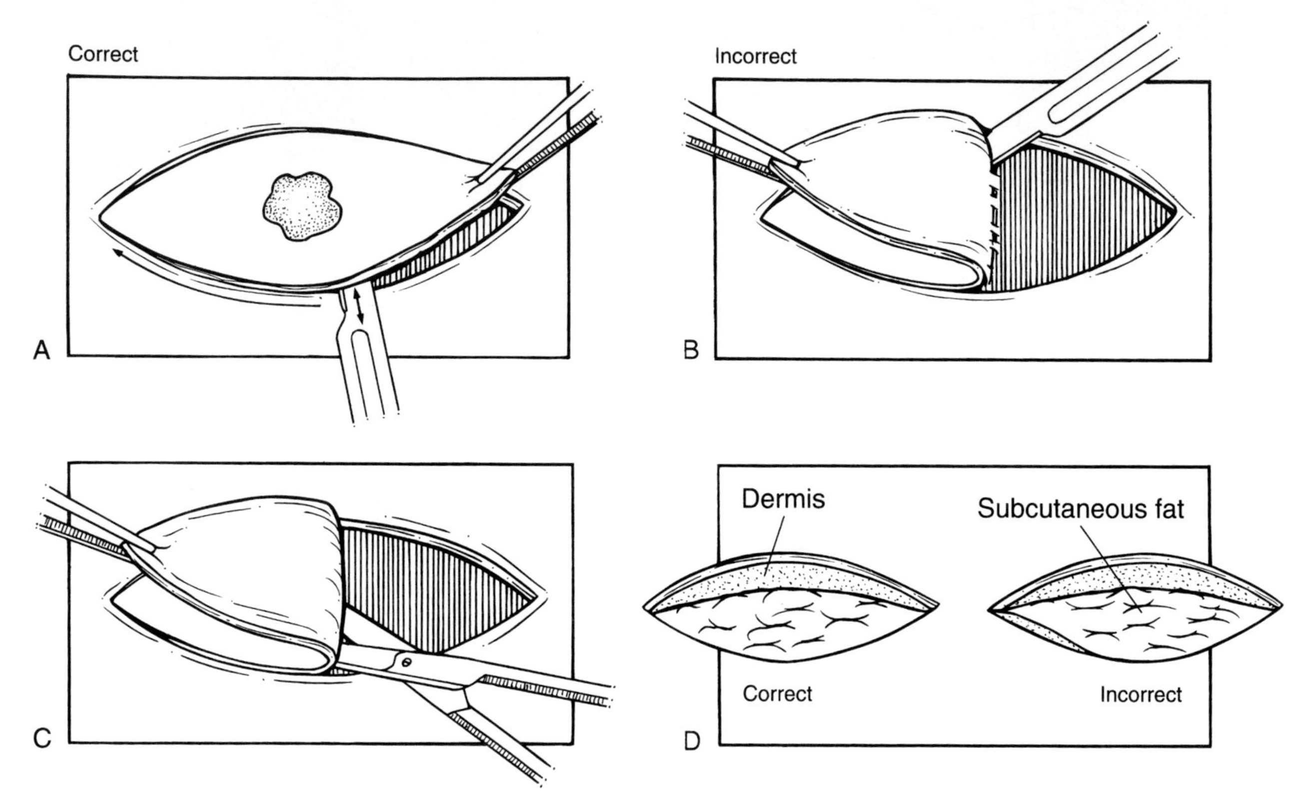

FIGURE 61-5

Removing the elliptical excision specimen. *A,* In undercutting the elliptical excision, an even plane throughout the base can be achieved by using the scalpel in a motion parallel to the surface of the skin. If tissue is pulled over the scalpel as the scalpel moves forward with a ''sawing'' stroke, then excessive depth in the center is avoided. *B,* Elevation of the tissue under tension leads to greater depth in the center of the wound. *C,* Some surgeons prefer to use the flat blades of the scissors resting against the wound base and to elevate the tissue to maintain the plane of removal. *D,* The final goal is even depth across the wound base. If excess fat or dermis is left at the apices of the wound, it elevates the apices and creates ''boating'' deformities. (*A–D,* From Robinson JK: Elliptical incisions and closures. *In* Robinson JK, Arndt KA, LeBoit PE, Wintroub BU [eds]: Atlas of Cutaneous Surgery. Philadelphia: WB Saunders, 1996, p. 94.)

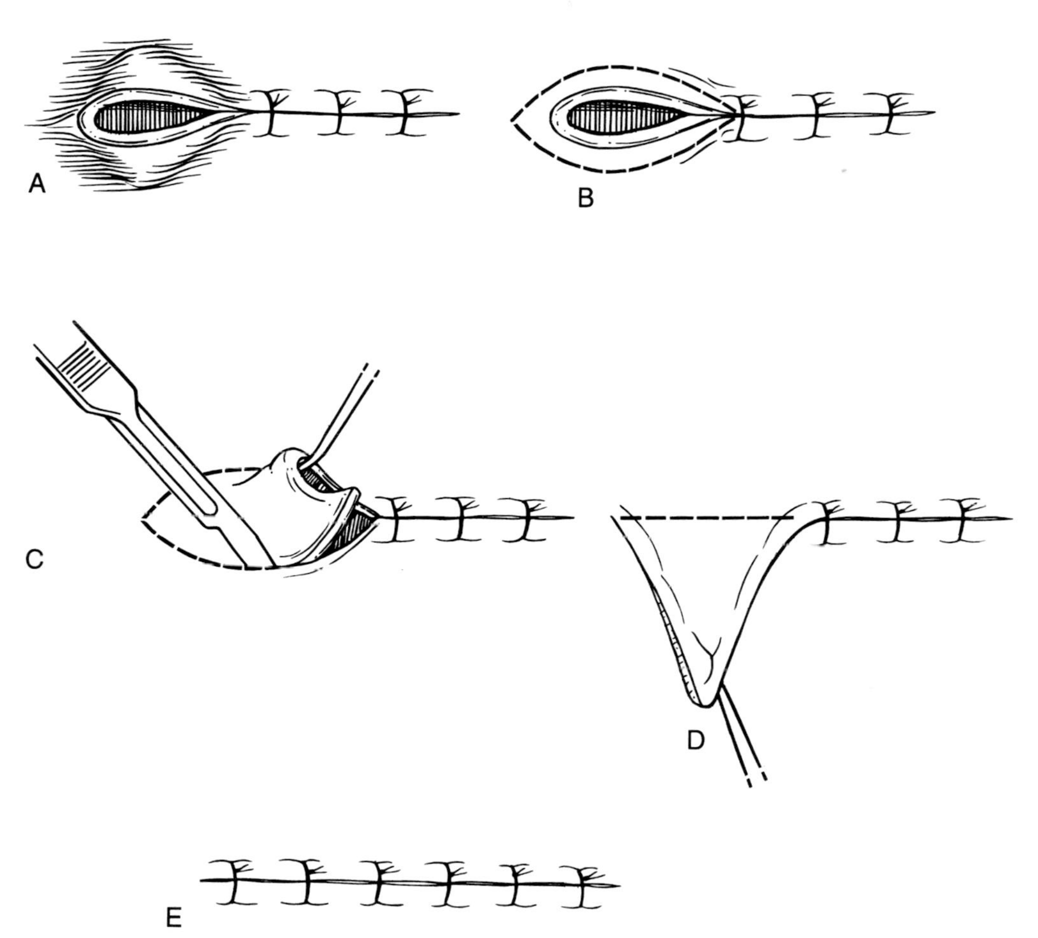

FIGURE 61-6

A–E, Dog-ear repair by extension of the line. The excess skin is tented up at the apex of the incision. Equal amounts of tissue on both sides of the wound are excised, thereby extending the original wound dimensions to 3:1. The final result is a longer, straight-line excision, which is useful for a long horizontal line such as on the trunk. (*A–E,* From Robinson JK: Elliptical incisions and closures. *In* Robinson JK, Arndt KA, LeBoit PE, Wintroub BU [eds]: Atlas of Cutaneous Surgery. Philadelphia: WB Saunders, 1996, p 101.)

is forced into the line of closure at the apices and pouches of redundant tissue form at the apices as standing cones. These standing cones are commonly referred to as *dog ears* and are revised. Selection of the particular method of revision used depends on the location of the incision and where it is better to place the additional incision made to revise the dog ear (Fig. 61–6). Wound closure is usually performed with buried subcutaneous sutures and interrupted cutaneous sutures.

All biopsy methods can result in hypertrophic scars, and most will leave a hypopigmented area.

REFERENCES

1. Lighthouse AG, Kopf AW, Garfinkel L: Diagnostic accuracy—A new approach to its evaluation. Arch Dermatol 1965; 91:497–502.
2. Pinkus H, Mehregan AH: A Guide to Dermatohistopathology. New York: Appleton-Century-Crofts, 1981.
3. Robinson JK: Surgical gems: Biopsy to and including muscle. J Dermatol Surg Oncol 1979; 5(8):595.
4. Crollick JS, Klein LE: Punch biopsy diagnostic technique [Letter]. J Dermatol Surg Oncol 1987; 13:839.
5. Bart RS, Kopf AW: Techniques of biopsy of cutaneous neoplasms. J Dermatol Surg Oncol 1979; 5:979–987.
6. Kopf AW, Popkin GL: Shave biopsies for cutaneous lesions. Arch Dermatol 1974; 110:637.
7. Ackerman AB: Shave biopsies: The good and the bad, the right and the wrong. Am J Dermatopathol 1983; 5:211–212.
8. Macy-Roberts E, Ackerman AB: A critique of techniques for biopsy of clinically suspected malignant melanomas. Am J Dermatopathol 1982; 4:391–398.
9. Shelley WB: The razor blade in dermatologic practice. Cutis 1975; 16:843–845.
10. Porter JM, Treasure J: Excision of benign pigmented skin tumors by deep shaving. Br J Plast Surg 1993; 46:255–257.
11. Jorizzo JL, Salisbury PL, Rogers RS, et al: Oral lesions in systemic lupus erythematosus. J Am Acad Dermatol 1992; 27:389–394.
12. Mashberg A: Erythroplasia vs leukoplakia in the diagnosis of early asymptomatic oral squamous carcinoma. N Engl J Med 1977; 297:109–110.
13. Chimenti S, Calvieri S, Ribuffo M: Malignant melanoma of the oral cavity. J Dermatol Surg Oncol 1981; 7:220–224.
14. Frim SP: Biopsy of lesions in the mouth. J Dermatol Surg Oncol 1981; 7:985–987.

CHAPTER 62

Destructive Methods

June K. Robinson

CRYOSURGERY

Cryosurgery is commonly performed to treat benign and premalignant disorders of the skin by using freezing temperatures to destroy tissue delivered by cotton swab, spray, or probe. The cotton swab affords less depth of freezing owing to the less efficient heat sink; however, it is usually adequate for the treatment of benign processes such as warts, molluscum, and sebaceous hyperplasia. If performed by dipping cotton swabs into liquid nitrogen in a cup, a new swab is used with each dip into the reservoir of the liquid nitrogen. The cryospray method involves the application of an intermittent spray directed toward the center of the lesion for a specified time period (Fig. 62–1 and Table 62–1). Cryosurgery is usually performed without local anesthesia; however, if the treated area is particularly large or cryosurgery is being combined with other methods of treatment, then local anesthesia is necessary. In treating particularly large (greater than 4 cm in diameter) seborrheic keratoses, local anesthesia may be injected and light curettage performed to remove the bulky portions of the lesion prior to freezing the base with cryosurgery. The treated area is characteristically red and slightly swollen initially. Then, it becomes crusted. The crust separates in about 10 days. Patients experience mild pain during freezing and thawing. If the treated location is on the scalp, forehead, or temple, transient headache may develop. When treating benign or premalignant lesions of the digit, care should be exercised if the lesion overlies the course of the nerve, as freezing the nerve may result in sensory loss, which usually resolves over a period of 6 to 12 months.

The cryoprobe technique, which is more commonly used for malignant lesions such as superficial or nodular basal cell carcinoma, involves selection of a probe size and type suitable for the lesion diameter. After the cryoprobe is precooled to prevent cryoadhesion, it is applied to the lesion with pressure for a specified time period. The treated lesion is characterized by circumscribed necrosis with early blister formation in some

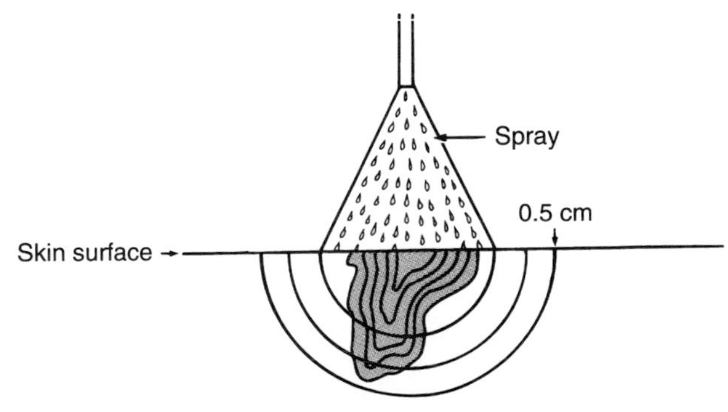

FIGURE 62–1

Cryosurgery with spray technique. The lateral spread of freeze extends 0.5 cm beyond the clinically apparent border of the premalignant lesion; however, if the process is clinically believed to be deeper than 0.5 cm, which could be true for a dermatofibroma, then the lateral spread of freeze should be greater than 0.5 cm. (Modified from Graham GF: Cryosurgery. *In* Robinson JK, Arndt KA, LeBoit PE, Wintroub BU [eds]: Atlas of Cutaneous Surgery. Philadelphia: WB Saunders, 1996, p 55.)

TABLE 62-1

Cryosurgery: Treatment Chart for Selected Lesions

Type of Lesion	Probe Tip or Swab	Time (seconds)	Target (mm)	Technique	Result
Warts	Swab	F = 5–10 T = 10–15	2	1 cycle	Excellent to good
Actinic keratosis	Swab B	F = 5–10 T = 10–15	2	1 cycle	Excellent to good
Seborrheic keratosis	Swab B	F = 10–20 T = 20–30	2.5	1 cycle	Good to fair
Dermatofibroma	Probe	F = 30–60 T = 60–90	3–4	1 cycle	Good to fair
Basal cell carcinoma	$<$1 cm = B $>$1 cm = A	F = 60–120 T = 60–180	3–4	2–3 cycles	Good to fair

F, freezing time using a probe or swab with a tip of approximately 0.03 inch; T, thawing time using a probe or swab with a tip of approximately 0.03 inch; B, medium-diameter tip for probe, approximately 0.0312 inch; A, large-diameter tip for probe, approximately 0.040 inch.

instances and with sloughing within 10 to 14 days. Although melanocytes are killed and the treated area remains depigmented, other tissues such as fibrous stroma, large arteries, nerves, and cartilage resist the cold injury and do not slough. At the time of tissue slough, there may be some bleeding.

The commonly used cryogens are carbon dioxide (solid, −78.5° C), nitrous oxide (liquid, −89.5° C), and liquid nitrogen (−195.8° C), the most efficient heat sink. To maximize tissue destruction, the following considerations are important: fast freeze to lethal temperature of −50° C, thaw slowly and completely, provide a short thaw interval between cycles, and repeat the freeze-thaw cycle for malignant lesions. For benign lesions such as warts, the commonly used technique is direct application of liquid nitrogen by a cotton swab to the surface of the lesion for about 5 to 10 seconds. A slight amount of pressure applied to the surface with the swab may slow the rate of warm blood entering the treated area and enhance the depth of freeze by the cotton swab method. The premalignant lesion actinic keratosis, with thick surface keratin, rapidly turns white, thus outlining the borders of the process against the surrounding normal skin. When this outlining is observed, the area of treatment may be extended until a 1- to 2-mm rim of normal tissue is frozen. Freeze times of 5 to 10 seconds with a thaw time of 10 to 15 seconds for common actinic keratosis are sufficient, but hypertrophic actinic keratosis may require 30 to 40 seconds of freezing. If the cryospray method is used, better control is obtained by intermittent spray rather than by continuous spray. Of the three basic spray patterns—solid central, spiral circular, and paintbrush—a solid central spray may be used on lesions smaller than 0.5 cm. A circular intermittent pattern can be used for slightly larger, 1- to 2-cm lesions, and a paintbrush pattern is used for lesions greater than 2 cm.

Cryosurgery is contraindicated in patients with cryoglobulinemia. In patients with deeply pigmented skin, cryosurgery may result in permanent depigmentation. Hyperpigmentation can also result after cryosurgery, especially on the lower leg.

ELECTROSURGERY

In electrosurgery, tissue is either cut or destroyed by heat generated by an electrosurgical apparatus. The actual extent of tissue destruction goes beyond the visible charred area produced at the time of surgery. Tissue destruction may also be achieved by combining electrosurgery with curettage of the area. Electrosurgical equipment in contact with blood should be either disposable or sterilized for each patient in the same way as all other surgical equipment contaminated by contact with blood is sterilized.

The two methods of generating heat are electrocautery and high-frequency electrosurgery. In electrocautery, metal is heated by electrical current and directly applied to tissue that is either desiccated, coagulated, or necrosed. When the current flows through the high-resistance wire of the tip of the unit, the temperature increases and the wire initially glows red and then turns white. The limited penetration of this heat injury to the dermis makes this an ideal method to treat superficial processes such as flat warts and seborrheic keratosis. The glowing needle tip lightly touches the surface of the lesion, which bubbles and then carbonizes. A crust develops and is shed in 7 to 10 days. It is possible to remove lesions that are entirely intraepidermal without scarring by this method. Electrocautery can also be used to produce coagulation in patients with pacemakers that would suffer interference from high-frequency electrosurgery units. For larger surfaces or deeper areas having greater bleeding, it is exceedingly time-consuming to stop bleeding with electrocautery.

With high-frequency electrosurgical apparatus, high-frequency current is conducted from the treatment electrode to the tissue. The tip of the electrode does not produce heat or become hot as it conducts oscillating electrical energy in a highly concentrated fashion to the tissue. The tissue offers a high degree of resistance to the electrical current, and the vibrating energy causes mechanical disruption of the cells and heat. The tissue

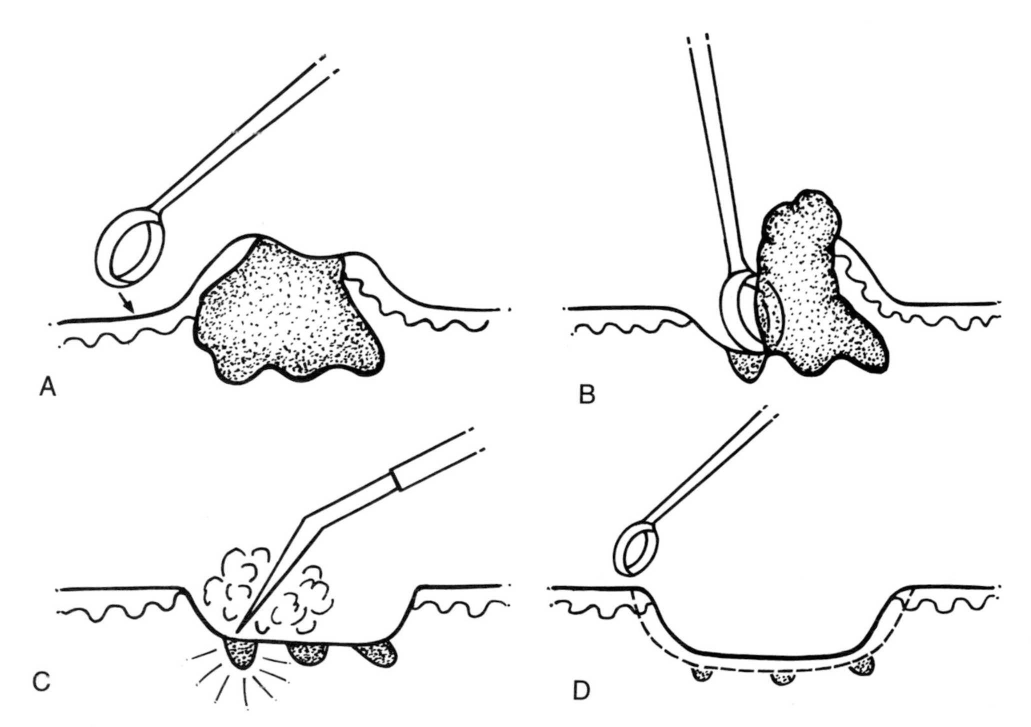

FIGURE 62-2

Curettage and electrodesiccation. *A,* Curette in position to remove a superficial basal cell carcinoma. *B,* Curette scooping out the gelatinous material. Islands of tumor remain at the base of the wound in three areas. *C,* Electrodesiccation with the needle tip in contact with the tissue. Smoke is created. Tissue damage extends into the dermis along the epidermis. *D,* A smaller curette is used to explore the margins and base of the lesion for pockets of tumor and charred material down to a firm base. (*A–D,* From Robinson JK: Electrosurgery. *In* Robinson JK, Arndt KA, LeBoit PE, Wintroub BU [eds]: Atlas of Cutaneous Surgery. Philadelphia: WB Saunders, 1996, p 64.)

is "boiled," with a loss of cellular architecture extending some distance beyond the field. Rapid clotting of blood is achieved, but electrocautery cannot stop forceful bleeding. Hemorrhage must be controlled by direct pressure, application of a hemostat, or suction. When bleeding is momentarily stopped by these means, final sealing of capillaries or vessels can be accomplished by short application of electrocoagulation current. The current is delivered to the hemostat or to a forceps that grasps the tissue. Electrocoagulation current delivered in this manner causes less adjacent tissue damage by limiting current flow to the small area between the tips of the forceps or hemostat.

Electrofulguration (sparking) dehydrates and produces superficial destruction of tissue with the needle not directly in contact with the tissue but with the current transmitted by an electrical arc or spark. Minimal heat is produced in the tissue. Electrodesiccation (drying) is the same as fulguration, but the needle is held directly in contact with the tissue. If the current is great enough, then coagulation by heat and destruction of tissue also occur. In removing epidermal processes (seborrheic keratosis, warts), electrofulguration may follow shave removal, follow or precede curettage, or be used alone with removal of coagulum by rubbing a piece of gauze across the treatment site. The briefest possible application of current while keeping the electrode in slow motion is used to lighten the lesion, and it will shrink in size. At the end of such treatment, hair follicles remain intact.

The majority of early small nodular and superficial basal cell carcinomas can be treated with curettage followed by electrocautery or electrodesiccation. After the area is anesthetized, a medium-sized curet is used to scoop out the gelatinous carcinoma (Fig. 62–2). Then the bleeding base is treated with either electrocautery or electrodesiccation and 1- to 2-mm perimeter of surrounding tissue is destroyed around the base. Then a small curet is used to explore the margins and the base of the lesion in at least three directions. The commonly used method employs two or three cycles of curettage followed by electrodesiccation. Healing occurs over 10 to 14 days and, in some locations, may be hypertrophic and is usually either hypopigmented or hyperpigmented.

When used in the cutting current mode for electrosection, the waveform differs from other uses, cells are exploded about the electrode, and there is little coagulation or carbonization of tissue. Facility in use of the cutting current is acquired by practicing the depth of the cut and the speed with which the electrode is moved. It can be used to debulk protuberant masses such as neurofibroma or condyloma.

Electrosurgery results in depigmented areas and certain locations, especially the upper lip and deltoid and presternal areas, may develop hypertrophic scars.

INTRALESIONAL CORTICOSTEROID INJECTIONS

Keloidal scars, inflamed cystic acne, treatment-resistant plaques of psoriasis, and limited circumscribed areas of alopecia areata are treated by intralesional corticosteroid injections. The dilution of the injectable material and its placement are dependent on the process being treated. There is a risk of localized cutaneous atrophy at the site of injection, and if the total systemic dose is large enough, there is the possibility of adrenal suppression. Keloidal scars generally require the greatest strength of intralesional triamcinolone. A previously untreated keloid can be injected initially with 10 mg/ml for a total of 2 to 3 ml. If there is no response in 6 weeks, then it can be injected with 20 mg/ml for a total of 2 ml. Rarely will higher dosages achieve a different result. Injections are given at 6-week intervals over a period of 6–8 months. The depth of injection is in the dermis at the bottom of the scar. As keloidal tissue is very firm, it is hard to inject and may require a great deal of force on the syringe. Three-ringed Luer-Lok syringes may be necessary. The keloid can be treated with a light spray of liquid nitrogen to induce edema prior to injection, thus making injection a bit less demanding of force. Cryosurgery alone is an effective treatment for keloids. Care should be exercised to ensure that the solution does not spill out beyond the borders of the keloid into the normal skin. If this happens, the result will be atrophy and hypopigmentation of the surrounding skin.

Alopecia areata is generally injected with either 2.5 or 5 mg/ml at the level of the deep dermis. Similarly, cystic acne lesions are treated with 5 mg/ml, but the depth of injection for an inflamed area may exceed the deep dermis, as the placement of the needle tip is just below the base of the lesion. Psoriatic plaques are injected with either 2.5 or 5 mg/ml, and the placement is relatively superficial in the dermis.

REMOVAL OF CYSTS AND INCISION AND DRAINAGE

If a cyst is hot, tender, and pointing or draining, then the appropriate systemic antibiotic is started and the area is drained; however, definitive removal is delayed until the inflammation has subsided, which may be 4 to 6 weeks. A previously ruptured, drained, or repeated inflamed cyst may have a great deal of scar tissue attaching its base to the surrounding tissue. The elliptical excision is planned to allow access to and mobilization of the scar tissue. This means that the incision line for a cyst that has been manipulated will be longer than one for a cyst that has not been ruptured.

An epidermal cyst that has not been ruptured will have a central punctum, and the cyst moves freely under the skin. A narrow ellipse that encompasses the punctum but does not extend to the lateral edges of the cyst can be used as a "handle" to elevate the cyst and undermine, using the firm cyst wall as the plane of dissection. If the intact cyst is delivered through the small aperture, the wound is closed. If the cyst ruptures during the procedure, then the wound is first irrigated to remove remnants of the cyst, and then the wound edges are closed.

INDEX

Note: Page numbers in *italics* refer to illustrations; page numbers followed by t refer to tables.